# NEUROANATOMY
## AND
# NEUROPATHOLOGY

*A Clinical Guide
for Neuropsychologists*

# NEUROANATOMY

## AND

# NEUROPATHOLOGY

## A Clinical Guide
## for Neuropsychologists

**Ralph M. Reitan**
Neuropsychology Laboratory
Tucson, Arizona

*Professor of Psychology*
*University of Arizona*
*Tucson, Arizona*

**Deborah Wolfson**
Neuropsychology Laboratory
Tucson, Arizona

Neuropsychology Press
Tucson, Arizona

Neuropsychology Press, 1338 East Edison Street, Tucson, Arizona 85719

Made in the United States of America

Library of Congress Catalog Card Number: 85-61660
ISBN 0-934515-03-4

# PREFACE

The unique aspect of neuropsychology that distinguishes it from other areas within psychology or psychology generally involves the emphasis on the neurological bases of behavior. Without this emphasis neuropsychology would be essentially similar to many other areas of psychology. It is imperative, then, that the neuropsychologist be familiar with the nervous system as well as psychology in order to deal effectively with their interrelationships.

Neuropsychology has been divided into experimental and clinical categories, but this distinction is far from perfect. The field of neuropsychology has emphasized animal brain- behavior relationships, but an increasing number of investigations in which variables are manipulated experimentally are now being performed with human beings. Clinical neuropsychology has traditionally focused on the application of knowledge of brain behavior relationships in human beings, especially concerning clinical problems, but the growth of clinical neuropsychology has been directly based upon carefully controlled experimental studies. In fact, clinical neuropsychology overlaps with many other areas of psychology (including animal and human branches) because it is concerned with behavior (psychology) and achieves its more unique characterization only through its emphasis on relating behavior to brain structure and function. Thus, neuropsychology includes such diverse content as endocrine function with relation to learning in rats, neuronal cell counts and behavioral changes in aging (both among animals and human beings), the clinical significance of cerebral damage in behavioral adjustment, and cerebral functioning with relation to learning disabilities. Although the content of experimental and clinical procedures may vary widely in neuropsychology, the unifying factor is represented by the continuing interest and concern in relating the brain to behavior.

This volume will concentrate on the structure and pathology of the brain, rather than the spinal cord, the peripheral nervous system or the relationships of nervous system functioning to other organs or systems of the body. The significance of other organs and systems for normal brain function is recognized and we refer to their importance throughout the text, particularly in the section on toxic and metabolic problems. Equally significant for behavior are the input mechanisms (the brain cannot be influenced unless it is reached by afferent impulses) and output mechanisms (the brain cannot respond unless it can control efferent impulses to effector organs). Despite their obvious importance, we do not attempt to provide a formal review of sensory (input) or motor (output) systems with relation to the brain. We shall only point out that an understanding of the biological bases of behavior, in its broader respects, requires knowledge and appreciation of reciprocal and integrative functions of the entire body and particularly of the peripheral and central divisions of the nervous system. We encourage the interested student to pursue such knowledge in the great number of sources already available, including, for example, the still impressive statements made by Walter B. Cannon in his volume, *The Wisdom of the Body* (1939).

As the reader is probably aware, there are several excellent texts available describing the neuroanatomy and neuropathology of the human nervous system; in fact, we have tried to select the best and included them in our reference list for the serious student to pursue. Why, then, another textbook on this subject? Hopefully, for several reasons. Most importantly, to provide the serious student and clinician with a reference book that is not only accurate and concise, but one that is *specifically* relevant to the field of neuropsychology. We have included over 100 medical illustrations, drawn especially for this text, to help the reader gain a better understanding of the concepts that we have described. Whenever possible, the neuroanatomy and neuropathology of a structure has been related to behavior, not left isolated and far-removed from the patient.

This book was written to complement *The Halstead-Reitan Neuropsychological Test Battery:*

*Theory and Clinical Interpretation* (Reitan & Wolfson, 1985). Together they present a comprehensive treatment of all of the facets of clinical neuropsychology. We have specifically attempted to avoid repetition; where overlap does occur it is intentionally done to emphasize a particular idea or present it from a different viewpoint. In order for the interpretation of test results to be relevant and significant for the individual patient, the neuropsychologist must have an understanding of the underlying biological condition of the brain that was responsible for producing the test results. We have tried to provide a vehicle toward that goal.

Many people were helpful in the production of this book. We would especially like to thank:

Jacquelyn Tarpy, for helping in all aspects of production and offering many useful suggestions.

Anthony M. Pazos, for doing over one hundred original and meticulously accurate medical illustrations.

Alan Hajek and David Roseman, for their technical expertise and patience.

Georgia Headley and Sharon Russell, for typing and proofreading the manuscript.

                        Ralph M. Reitan
                        Deborah Wolfson

Tucson, Arizona
August 1985

# CONTENTS

## SECTION IV

### NEUROLOGICAL DISEASES AND DISORDERS

# Section I

# Introduction

# INTRODUCTION

## AN OVERVIEW OF BEHAVIORAL FUNCTIONS OF THE CEREBRAL CORTEX

### Historical Contributions and Concepts of Brain-Behavior Relationships

The motor and sensory-perceptual functions of the cerebral cortex are very important, as illustrated by the fact that they predominate, together with similar functions subserved by other nuclei and pathways, the content of the neurological examination (DeMyer, 1980; Talbert, 1982). Higher-level functions (including intelligence and cognition) have also long been attributed to the cerebral cortex, although subcortical centers also appear to play some role in these functions. For the reader interested in more detailed information, historical reviews of theoretical developments and contributions to this body of knowledge have been published (Boring, 1929; Riese, 1959; Hécaen & Albert, 1978; Halstead, 1947).

These contributions, described by Halstead according to their theoretical outcome, can be divided into three categories: (1) holistic theory; (2) aggregation theory; and (3) regional localization theory. Halstead cited the work of Flourens (1843), based principally on extirpation of cerebral cortical areas in dogs, to support the theory that intellectual behavior is not differentially affected by extirpation of one area or another and appears to be a unitary function of the entire cerebral cortex. Flourens' position, which conflicted with Gall's teaching of phrenology, created a considerable amount of controversy when it was first proposed.

Despite intervening reports which had distinct implications for localization of function (e.g., Broca, 1861), positions supporting a **holistic theory** continued to be reported. Goltz (1881) found no evidence of localization of intelligence in his extirpation studies, but did note that removal of larger areas of cerebral cortex produced greater defects. He performed experiments in which quadrants of the brain were removed and compared, and he noted that, regardless of the area involved, impairment increased as the number of quadrants removed increased. The method of evaluation used by Goltz and other researchers at this time was primarily one of impressionistic observations. Based on his studies, Goltz concluded that cerebral impairment was essentially represented as a generalized dullness or defect in attention.

Ferrier (1886), who performed similar experiments with both dogs and monkeys, reached similar conclusions. Although he felt that the frontal lobes were of particular importance in integration of sensory and motor functions and therefore might be fundamental for higher intellectual functions, Ferrier did not believe that intelligence was localized. Conversely, he felt that the integrational process, necessary for intelligent behavior, was generally distributed.

Another researcher, Loeb, concluded that ablations of the cerebral cortex in dogs had little specific effect (1902). He noted that operations on only a single cerebral hemisphere caused little impairment and that extensive destruction of cerebral cortex in both hemispheres was necessary to produce clear evidence of deficit. He argued particularly against the hypothesis that the frontal lobes had any special function, even in cases with bilateral frontal resection. In fact, Loeb was so convinced of this position that he wrote that there was perhaps no operation as harmless for a dog as removal of its frontal lobes.

Probably the greatest influence toward a holistic (non-localization) view of cerebral cortical functions was made by Lashley (1929), who followed a very systematic procedure in extirpation of cerebral cortex in rats. Using maze-learning tests of varying difficulty, he made quantitative measurements of the performances of animals in these standardized learning situations and related the behavioral results to histological study and mapping of the brain lesion in each rat. His results supported a principal of *equipotentiality* (a lesion in any area of the cerebral cortex will produce equivalent deficits) and *mass action* (the resulting degree of deficit is a function of the amount of cerebral cortex destroyed). Lashley's findings went considerably further, especially in demonstrating the incremental impairment caused by a particular lesion with relation to the difficulty of the maze-learning problem, but the principles of equipotentiality and mass action were of major theoretical significance.

The **aggregation theory**, as described by Halstead, recognizes the existence of localized sensory areas within the cerebral cortex functionally joined by a large number of intracortical connections. The aggregate functioning of these sensory areas produces an integrated comprehension of sensory stimuli from the external environment and results in intelligent behavior.

This view of the neurological basis of intelligence was proposed particularly by Munk (1890). Von Monakow (1905) concurred with this theoretical conceptualization, but he criticized Munk for failing to adequately recognize the motor components of intelligence. Thus, von Monakow, instead of supporting primarily a sensory theory of intelligence, emphasized: (1) the importance of both sensory and motor fields which occupied localized areas in the cerebral cortex; and (2) the overall integration of these centers to represent intellectual behavior.

It should be noted that the aggregation theory of intelligence is not entirely incompatible with the holistic theory insofar as more extensive involvement of the localized sensory and motor centers would be expected to produce an increasing degree of intellectual impairment. However, in the aggregation theory the focus was on the sensory and motor centers and, in fact, served as the basis for additional theoretical formulations. For example, von Monakow's theoretical differentiation between transitory symptoms following an acute cerebral lesion and the residual or permanent effects of the lesion were represented by his term *"diaschisis,"* which refers to a loss of functional continuity between the various sensory and motor centers of the cerebral cortex. According to von Monakow, acute or transitory symptomatology was presumably a manifestation of temporary impairment of the functional continuity between centers; the permanent effects of the lesion represented a final disconnection between centers.

The existence of localized centers in the cerebral cortex was generalized to include not only sensory and motor areas but also many other abilities. Kleist, for example, subdivided the cerebral cortex into subdivisions which subserved many skills, such as reading, writing, and other functions almost reminiscent of phrenology (1934).

Positions of relatively extreme localization were also adopted by Henschen (1920-1922) and Nielsen (1946). The theories of extreme localization of specific abilities in various areas of the cerebral cortex have gradually eroded in their significance. The clinical tests that were used to identify these abilities were often relatively crude, and the abilities themselves (such as reading) in all probability are not unitary functions but require multiple psychological capabilities for adequate performance. Brain lesions in human subjects were rarely so exactly or specifically localized to permit a valid basis for initial proposal of the specific brain-behavior relationships or verification and validation in any significant number of individual subjects. Thus, the tendency toward mapping of specific abilities, skills, and functions in accordance with discrete cerebral cortical areas has largely been discontinued, especially with relation to higher-level behavioral and psychological functions.

The **regional-localization theory**, which postulates that areas within the cerebral cortex are differentially committed to separate psychological functions, is compatible with current findings of specialization of right and left cerebral functions. As early as 1836 Dax recognized that the left cerebral hemisphere was particularly involved with language and related symbolic communication (Benton, 1964). In 1861 Broca examined a patient with a long-standing limitation of ability in verbal communication who appeared to be normally intelligent and was able to communicate by use of signs. Broca had also been able to ascertain that the patient's peripheral mechanisms necessary for speech were intact. After the patient died, Broca examined the man's brain and found a large patho-logical area in the left cerebral hemisphere that extended from the frontal lobe to the posterior part of the parietal area and also included adjacent cortex of the temporal lobe. Broca, who believed that the frontal lobe was involved in speech as well as other motor functions, minimized the significance of the remainder of the lesion. He concluded that the posterior-inferior part of the left frontal lobe (which has come to be known as *Broca's area*) was the critical area in expressive speech and language. A great amount of additional evidence has been accrued to indicate the significance of this area in expressive language functions, although the remaining area of the lesion in Broca's patient has also long been recognized as being a significant part of the language area (Penfield & Roberts, 1959).

Broca's report of his findings with this patient (1861) as well as several others had a great influence on theories of cerebral cortical function with relation to behavior. Only a few years later Fritsch and Hitzig (1870) discovered the motor areas of the brain and their potential for eliciting movements, particularly on the opposite side of the body, with electrical stimulation. Hitzig pursued additional investigations and concluded that, in addition to motor and sensory areas, abstract thought was a function of the frontal areas of the brain even though intelligence or stored ideas and information was probably represented in all parts of the brain.

Up to this time the methods for evaluating the behavioral consequences of cerebral damage had been largely impressionistic. The experimenter merely observed and compared the behavior of the subject following the cerebral lesion (or, in experimental animals, before and after the cerebral lesion was imposed). Despite the carefully structured and standardized experimental testing procedures which have developed within the framework of psychology, impressionistic methods of evaluating behavior continue to be more common among neurologists and other physicians.

Franz (1907) was an experimental psychologist who adopted standardized testing procedures for evaluating cats and monkeys before and after the imposition of cerebral lesions. Using the type of puzzle boxes developed by Lloyd Morgan and Thorndike which permitted evaluation of acquisition and retention of "escape" skills, Franz concluded that the frontal lobes were particularly important in behavior. If the animal had been trained to a criterion of success before a brain lesion was imposed, destruction of the frontal lobes resulted in a loss of the habit; the animal retained the escape ability when lesions were placed in other portions of the brain. Unilateral lesions showed much less effect than bilateral lesions. Franz found that his animals with frontal lesions could relearn the task in about the same amount of time as initially required. In addition, he noted that frontal lesions impaired recently learned tasks but affected long-standing skills only minimally. He emphasized the importance of standardized experimental tasks, concluding that the deficits of the animals would not be noticeable using "simple observational methods." Franz also cited the need for "accurate physiological and psychological methods" in the study of brain-behavior relationships in man.

At this point it may be noted that two factors principally contributed to the difficulty of generating a full range of cross-validated knowledge of brain-behavior relationships: (1) the use of observational and impressionistic methods for evaluating the effects of brain lesions; and (2) a tendency, particularly by some investigators, to reach conclusions and establish theoretical positions based on relatively uncritical amalgamation of evidence derived both from lower animals and human beings. The obvious deficits, such as motor and primary sensory functions, would be noted but the more subtle aspects of brain functions (such as reasoning, judgment, abstraction, and ability to analyze complex situations) would be much more difficult to discern in lower animals. In addition, use of language for communicational purposes, a very important aspect of brain functions in human beings, is much more limited in lower animals. Thus, the repertoire and richness of behavior, as related to brain functions, is so much greater among human beings than lower animals that a theory of brain-behavior relationships faces extreme difficulties in accounting for observable facts of behavior across their entire range of manifestations.

### The Emergence of Contributions by Psychologists

Although Franz (Franz & Gordon, 1933) continued to influence psychology, the contributions of Lashley had a much broader interdisciplinary impact. Psychologists began to become very actively involved in the study of human brain-behavior relationships. The investigations of Jacobsen and his colleagues in extirpation of cerebral tissue in primates, followed by formal studies of learning and other psychological functions, was of great influence (Jacobsen, 1936; Jacobsen & Elder, 1936; Jacobsen & Nissen, 1937). Jacobsen, Wolfe, and Jackson (1935) reported that learning, particularly when in the context of delayed responses, was significantly impaired with frontal lesions. The frontal lobes are structurally large, especially in man, and at this time the pre-frontal areas were essentially without known significance. Thus, this large area of cerebral cortex was referred to as the *frontal association area* and naturally attracted the attention and curiosity of experimental investigators.

As indicated above, in many instances prior research had also suggested that the frontal association areas were of special significance regarding intelligence and cognition. Halstead (1939; 1940; 1945), Halstead and Settlage (1943), and Hebb (1939a; 1941) undertook extensive studies to evaluate the effects of frontal lesions in human beings, although to achieve specificity in their conclusions they compared such patients with persons who had cerebral lesions in other locations (Halstead, 1947; Hebb, 1939b). These studies by psychologists, which were based on monkeys and human beings, tended to emphasize the importance of the frontal association areas in higher intellectual functions (except for certain findings reported by Hebb). These investigators also introduced much greater scientific rigor into their experimental procedures than had been used previously, essentially establishing the scientific basis of animal and human neuropsychology. In this sense, the work of psychologists deviated from the traditional investigation of brain-behavior relationships pursued within the medical and neurological tradition. The psychologists who were contributors in the field at this time had all been trained in the area of physiological and comparative psychology. Jacobsen, Nissen and Hebb were still working principally with animals, although Hebb did some evaluations of human beings and published his findings. Halstead did his doctoral dissertation on the effects of cerebellar lesions in pigeons, but had a strong interest in human brain-behavior relationships; immediately after completing his doctorate he began investigative work at the University of Chicago in conjunction with two neurological surgeons, Percival Bailey and Paul Bucy.

Interest in the effects of brain lesions and the development of diagnostic testing procedures for brain damage was also expressed by the emerging field of clinical psychology, but its orientation was toward "brain damage" as a clinical entity rather than an attempt to relate critical aspects of lesions to specified behavioral outcome. The term *neuropsychology* was rarely used at this time. Psychologists interested in brain-behavior relationships, both in animals and in human beings, were classified as physiological and comparative psychologists and interest in the effects of brain lesions in clinical psychology was not sufficiently extensive to have merited a special designation.

Contributions made by physicians (especially neurologists but also psychiatrists and neurological surgeons) continued in the tradition of clinical examination and correlation with locations of underlying brain lesions. An excellent example of investigation in this tradition is the work of Gerstmann (1924; 1927) who, in his study of patients with brain lesions, felt that he had identified a syndrome of deficits (finger agnosia, agraphia, acalculia, and right-left confusion) which was caused by specific lesions of the left angular and supramarginal gyri. Gerstmann published results of patients who had these four deficits along with corresponding lesions in the parietal-temporal-occipital junctional area. This approach — correlating specific deficits with lesions in a particular location — has had a powerful influence in establishing conclusions regarding localization of functions in the cerebral cortex; unfortunately, the method is often inadequate in precise specification of the location of the lesion in human beings, in careful documentation of the exact nature of the behavioral deficit, and even in more general scientific criteria for the establishment of definitive conclusions. In this latter respect, for example, Gerstmann published cases in which the location of the lesion and the configuration of deficits corresponded; however, one must also ask the question regarding lack of correspondence. Even in the simplest set of contingency relationships between two variables, four cells are implied: (1) plus-plus; (2) plus-minus; (3) minus-plus; and (4) minus-minus.

It was not until 1964 that Heimburger, DeMyer, and Reitan investigated the presence and absence of Gerstmann's syndrome with relation to the presence and absence of lesions specifically involving the angular and supramarginal gyri. In a series of more than 400 cases, seven patients had lesions involving the area of the left cerebral hemisphere in question and none of them showed evidence of all four components of Gerstmann's syndrome. Thirty-two patients had all four components, but none had a lesion specifically involving the supramarginal and angular gyri. Gerstmann's syndrome was present more frequently in patients with left than right cerebral lesions, but the syndrome did not seem to have special value in localization within the left cerebral hemisphere.

The generalization to be drawn in terms of scientific procedure is that it is quite inadequate to establish a relationship between only two variables and ignore the instances in which correspondence between the two variables does not occur. This problem exemplifies the scientific dangers involved in drawing conclusions from individual cases. Even if a definite relationship is found, it is often difficult to be sure that the variables have a cause-and-effect relationship as contrasted with an incidental or statistical association. The way to overcome this problem is to determine the accuracy that can be achieved in predicting one variable from the other (i.e., predicting the location of the lesion on the basis of the behavioral manifestations or, conversely, predicting the behavioral manifestations with knowledge only of the lesion's location). If predictions in either direction are possible at a clinically acceptable accuracy level, one can conclude that the relationship is meaningful and sufficiently robust to withstand the possible effects of attenuating variables that are always present in individual human beings.

Despite methodological and scientific problems of the kind just described, investigations by physicians in the 1920s and 1930s continued with a gradual evolution toward identification of the frontal lobes as the seat of intellectual functions. Gelb and Goldstein (1925) were particularly influential in studying the behavioral effects of cerebral damage and attributing special significance to the frontal lobes. Differentiation between the investigations of psychologists and physicians was becoming more apparent as psychologists entered the field, particularly with the employment of specified and standardized psychological testing procedures. While Halstead's methodology was in the tradition of using standardized experiments (such as measurement of finger tapping speed, complex psychomotor performances, and abstraction and reasoning abilities), other investigators (e.g. Hebb, 1939a; 1939b; 1941) used standardized psychological tests, such as the Stanford-Binet Scale that had been developed for evaluation of normal individuals rather than persons with cerebral lesions.

Goldstein (1936) argued very strongly against use of formal psychological tests, preferring to observe the behavior of the subject and draw conclusions about brain functions based on observations of the subject's method of performing the task or solving the problem rather than upon qualitative scores. Goldstein insisted, for example, that a brain-damaged person and a person with a normal brain might achieve the same score on the Wechsler Scale but use different procedures to do so. Goldstein felt that ability to assume the abstract attitude was impaired in the case of the brain-damaged person, even though the problem might be solved by a very concrete approach. Thus, Goldstein had little use for quantitative scores (such as I.Q. values), believing that they did not contribute to an understanding of the qualitative nature of deficits shown particularly by persons with frontal lobe lesions. This is much the same position as espoused by Luria in his approach to brain-behavior relationships. Luria also believed that little information could be gained by attaching a number (quantitative score) to a performance of a brain-damaged individual and that it was necessary to observe the defective performance in order to appreciate the impairment shown by the individual subject. This procedural difference continues to be a major factor that differentiates the medical (neurological) field that has become known as *behavioral neurology* from the field of *clinical neuropsychology*, which is dominated principally by psychologists, even though both disciplines are devoted essentially to elucidating brain-behavior relationships.

A number of contributions identified the special importance of the frontal lobes with respect to intellectual performances. Ackerly (1935) described in detail a patient with bilateral anterior frontal atrophic lesions and wrote extensively about this man's emotional and mental deficits. Brickner (1936) published a book concerned with the intellectual functions of the frontal lobes, citing individual cases in great detail to substantiate his conclusion that the highest levels of intellectual functioning were subserved by the anterior frontal cortex. Jefferson (1937a; 1937b) described significant intellectual and behavioral deficits associated with both right and left frontal lobectomies in man.

It is not surprising, then, given this spirit of the time, that an operation to disconnect the prefrontal centers from emotional centers of the brain was conceived by Moniz (1936; 1937) to alleviate emotional interference with intellectual processes, as seen in many persons with mental illness. In 1935 Moniz and Lima introduced the operation referred to as *prefrontal lobotomy* (prefrontal leukotomy). This surgery was based on the hypotheses that (1) the hypothalamus

was intimately involved in emotional responses; (2) the dorsomedial nucleus of the thalamus received projections from the hypothalamus; and (3) surgical disconnection of the pathways from the dorsomedial nucleus to the pre-frontal cortex might serve to relieve emotional distress and dissociate emotional responsiveness of the brain from the higher integrative and intellectual functions of the individual. Prefrontal lobotomies were performed on thousands of individuals, particularly persons suffering from severe depression. Eventually the results of the collective wisdom of the scientific community emerged and the operation was essentially discontinued as a treatment for emotional illness. The procedure continued to be used for some years to alleviate the subjective appreciation of pain. Patients with intractable chronic pain who underwent pre-frontal lobotomy often found the pain to be more tolerable, although not necessarily reduced in intensity, after the surgery. Procaine injections into the pathway from the dorsomedial nucleus of the thalamus to the pre-frontal areas was also proposed as a procedure to alleviate pain. Rylander (1939) described the operation as a procedure for "ablation of the soul."

Halstead, Carmichael, and Bucy (1946) studied a series of patients before and after pre-frontal lobotomy and found variable neuropsychological test results. Halstead felt that the operation frequently caused changes in the individual subject, and that it was a procedure in which "knowns" were traded for "unknowns" (i.e., the patient's known condition of emotional disturbance before the operation was altered by the surgery and the patient changed in ways that could not be predicted).

Thus, there is no doubt that neurological "reasoning" based upon conclusions reached in the area of behavioral neurology have definite implications. Moniz was recognized with the Nobel Prize for his introduction of pre-frontal lobotomy as well as for more enduring contributions. The operation, although initially performed through frontal burr holes in the skull, reached such a routine position that is was often done as an office procedure by inserting a leukotome above the eyeball and through the thin bony plate of the orbital surface of the frontal lobe and into the frontal lobes before sectioning of the fibers. (Neurological surgeons generally disapproved of this "blind" procedure.)

The field of clinical neuropsychology, as mentioned above, was initially stimulated in its formulation by the research and writings of a number of physiological and comparative psychologists. Study of human beings in the psychological tradition was initiated by Ward Halstead, who organized the first full-time laboratory for study of human brain-behavior relationships at the University of Chicago. Halstead developed a number of standardized and formal testing procedures, based upon his personal observations of patients with cerebral lesions, that have formed the nucleus for the Halstead-Reitan Neuropsychological Test Battery. The basic research for these tests was done in a number of studies (Halstead, 1939; 1940; 1945; Halstead & Settlage, 1943) that culminated in his book *Brain and Intelligence*, published in 1947. Many other psychologists had become interested in testing and evaluating patients with cerebral damage, sometimes using instruments especially designed for this purpose (Hunt, 1940) and in other instances adapting instruments that had been developed for other purposes such as the Rorschach Test (Klopfer & Kelley, 1942; Beck, 1937) or the earlier versions of the Wechsler Scales (Aita, Armitage, Reitan, & Rabinovitz, 1947; Wechsler, 1955).

## Behavioral Neurology

The area of clinical neuropsychology has expanded very rapidly, focusing on (1) the generation of neuropsychological test results that have clinical significance for the individual subject; and (2) a basis of formal research procedures in which groups of comparable subjects are evaluated and compared using statistical methods. The area of behavioral neurology has also developed substantially, with conclusions being derived principally from careful, detailed evaluation of specific performances and deficits of individual subjects and correlated with the underlying condition of the brain. Behavioral neurology has concentrated on study of deficits that fall under the categories of aphasia, agnosia, and apraxia.

Outstanding contributors to behavioral neurology in recent years have included Luria, Geschwind, Hécaen, Heilman, Benson, and Albert. The tradition of studying specific, circumscribed deficits as they relate to lesions of the cerebral cortex is well represented by several excellent recent books, including those by Hécaen and Albert (1978), Benson (1979), and Heilman and Valenstein (1979). Each of these volumes deals principally with aphasia and related disorders.

Benson, for example, writes rather specifically about language and related disorders due to cerebral lesions, even relatively neglecting gestural disturbances (apraxias) that are frequently included with this subject matter. He reviews the history and background of aphasia, neurological diseases and disorders that may produce aphasia, the many types and categories of aphasic disorders, the neuroanatomical correlates of aphasic manifestations, and the range of additional neurological and psychiatric disorders that may be present in aphasic patients.

The consistency of content in the field of behavioral neurology is illustrated by the similarity of topics covered by Heilman and Valenstein (1979). These authors reviewed categories of aphasia and types of aphasic deficits, such as alexia, agraphia, acalculia, as well as associated deficits, including right-left confusion, apraxias, constructional deficits, agnosias, visual-spatial neglect, amnesic disorders and dementia, and frontal lobe deficits. Neither of these books includes reference to formal testing procedures in any detail, even for aphasia and related disorders; however, they do describe the impressionistic clinical methods customarily used by neurologists for eliciting and evaluating aphasic deficits.

Hécaen and Albert (1978) review the types and categories of aphasia, describe various apraxic deficits as well as specific visual and auditory losses, the visual and auditory agnosias, tactile and somesthetic deficits, disorders of memory and dementia, frontal lobe deficits, and the areas of cerebral plasticity and recovery of function. Some contributions in the area of behavioral neurology relate specific deficits caused by brain lesions to more general areas.

Rose (1984) reviews aphasia, apraxia, and agnosia as well as dementias, and, in an effort to focus on recent contributions, also considers topics such as prosody as an aphasic disorder, cognitive psychology and aphasia, the role of auditory verbal comprehension in aphasia, linguistic components of acalculia, and correlation of aphasic manifestations with findings on computed tomography of the brain.

It is apparent from these books that the principal content areas of behavioral neurology center around aphasia, agnosia, and apraxia. Although specific disorders of this kind are also included in the area of clinical neuropsychology, differences in both content and methodology are present. Behavioral neurology still emphasizes the "sign" approach in identifying the presence or absence of specific deficits (even though it is well recognized that the deficits may vary in severity). Behavioral neurologists depend upon their clinical observations rather than quantitative measurement and tend to base conclusions on the study of individual persons rather than use statistical comparisons of group results.

It is fair to say that clinical neuropsychology has been much more influenced by traditional scientific criteria stemming from experimental design, statistical evaluations, and the psychometric tradition of evaluation than has behavioral neurology. One may note in passing, however, that two of the three books on behavioral neurology noted above use the word neuropsychology in their titles and one is called *Clinical Neuropsychology*, despite the fact that there is little (if any) reference to the use of psychological tests. In fact, the authors or editors of these three books are all neurologists rather than psychologists. Nevertheless, their contributions stem from and represent studies of human brain-behavior relationships that long antedate the emergence of psychology, in any form, as a discipline and contain many valuable insights into brain-behavior relationships. As noted by Hécaen

and Albert (1978), behavioral neurology is fundamentally based upon clinical-anatomical correlation in which the nature, extent, and evolution of the brain lesion must be described, the associated signs and symptoms of behavioral disorder must be identified, and the significance of these disorders determined as well as their consistency and value in cerebral localization.

Neurologists overlap considerably with speech pathologists (Darley, Aronson, & Brown, 1975) in their description and evaluation of aphasic manifestations, but have concentrated more closely on correlation of the location of brain lesions with the specific manifestation of impaired language. However, the areas including aphasia, agnosia, and apraxia constitute the principal subject matter of behavioral neurology whereas speech pathologists include other areas of speech impairment and also have concentrated on remediation of speech disorders.

We will not review the area of aphasia in any detail at this point because it has recently been considered extensively by one of the authors (Reitan, 1984) and the interested reader is referred to that publication. Language functions have been thought of philosophically, psychologically, and neurologically as representing one of the outstanding differential characteristics of human as compared with lower animal behavior, even though primitive forms of language are clearly used by subhuman primates. We must also note, however, that approximately one-fifth of the cerebral cortex constitutes the primary language area (Penfield & Roberts, 1959) and even this area is pervaded by additional functions (such as abstraction and reasoning) with respect to non-language problems (Reitan, 1960). Thus, while language and verbal communicational skills may be attributed special significance in human behavior, the biology of the cerebral cortex, at least in terms of the amounts of tissue involved, has assigned language an extremely important but not predominant role.

A great number of language disturbances have been identified. Expressive deficits among aphasics are often obvious, but receptive deficits, which involve the sensory avenues through which language symbols are principally appreciated (such as vision and hearing), and tactile losses are also recognized as being important. **Aphasia** involves all of the means of verbal communications, including expressive speech, naming, spelling, writing, calculating, reading, and other aspects of both visual and auditory language comprehension. Neurologists and psychologists have identified many categories of aphasia (see any of the books referred to above or other excellent volumes, such as Albert, Goodglass, Helm, Rubens, and Alexander, 1981; Brown, 1972; or Sarno, 1981, for detailed information).

The *apraxias* represent impairment of the ability to carry out purposeful movements even though the individual has the basic motor skills that are necessary and is not so demented that understanding of the nature of the tasks is impossible. Hécaen and Albert (1978) have described a number of types of apraxic disorders. In *ideomotor apraxia* the subject has impaired ability to relate the idea involved to a simple type of motor performance, such as waving good-bye, giving a military salute, pretending to stir coffee with a spoon, etc.

*Ideational apraxia* is a term used to describe a disruption in the logical and harmonious progression or succession of movements necessary to carry out complex gestures even though the subject is able to perform the individual elements of the total act. *Constructional apraxia*, in which the ability to comprehend and deal with spatial relationships is impaired even though single movements are not affected, has been discussed at length by many authors. Constructional dyspraxia may be manifested in simple drawing procedures as well as in solution of three-dimensional tasks.

*Dressing apraxia* has also been described. It is demonstrated by problems in arranging clothing on one's own body, often by failure to place arms through sleeves, accomplish appropriate buttoning, etc. Dressing dyspraxia is often seen in persons with constructional dyspraxia and appears to represent a fundamental problem in dealing with visual-spatial and con-

structive performances. Hécaen and Albert state that constructional apraxia occurs about four times more frequently than dressing apraxia. However, such a conclusion obviously is limited by the methodology of behavioral neurology; because of variable sensitivity of the testing procedures, instances of mild dressing dyspraxia may be much more difficult to discern than occurrences of constructional dyspraxia. A number of other apraxias are frequently described. *Buccofacial apraxia* is illustrated by inability to stick out the tongue upon command although ability to use the tongue to lick the lips is intact. Obviously, a disorder of this kind may also be determined, at least in part, by impairment of auditory verbal comprehension or a failure to be able to associate the idea involved, as communicated by the person, with the act (*ideomotor apraxia*).

It is clear, however, that patients with cerebral lesions may suffer a breakdown in the ability to carry out functional acts, sometimes even ones that are quite simple in nature. It has been recognized that both afferent and efferent features may be involved in such deficits. Sometimes, for example, a patient may be grossly impaired in his ability to complete simple drawings (two-dimensional constructional apraxia) even though he recognizes very well that his drawing deviates from the sample being copied. In other cases a person may have a great problem in appreciating the visual-spatial characteristics of the figure to be copied, demonstrating a receptive difficulty. While apraxias customarily refer to losses in the ability to perform simple movements, agnosias refer to impairment in appreciating the significance of information receptively. Thus, there undoubtedly is interaction of receptive losses (agnosia) and expressive losses in the individual case.

**Agnosia** refers to instances in which the subject is not able to appreciate the significance of sensory information reaching the brain, despite intact sensory mechanisms. Many specific agnosias have been identified and they are often named for the sensory avenue involved. *Visual agnosia* includes color agnosia, spatial agnosia, and various other agnosias, including prosopagnosia (inability to recognize familiar faces). *Auditory agnosias* have been referred to as pure-word deafness, auditory agnosia for non-speech sounds, music agnosia, and auditory receptive amnesia. *Tactile agnosias* have included impairment of tactile form recognition and finger agnosia. In addition, some patients are impaired in their ability to identify and recognize body parts, and this deficit has been referred to as *autotopagnosia* or *body agnosia.*

In the traditional descriptions of agnosias and apraxias within the field of behavioral neurology relatively little direct reference is made to these types of deficits when language symbols are involved, apparently respecting the distinction of the area of aphasia. However, examination of aphasic patients makes it quite clear that agnosias (receptive losses) and apraxias (expressive losses) occur among aphasic patients in their attempts to deal with language and verbal communicational information. In fact, the evidence that aphasic patients do not show significantly greater general impairment of intellectual and cognitive functions than patients with comparable brain lesions but without aphasia (Reitan, 1960) strongly suggests that any specific intellectual component of aphasia has probably been overemphasized in many analyses of this condition. Reitan (1984) has pointed out that regardless of the content (verbal or non-verbal), sensory avenues must carry information to the brain where central processing of the information occurs. In order to complete the response circuit, motor effectors must be involved in some form of response. Thus, the basic and inescapable ingredients of a response circuit include (1) input; (2) central processing; and (3) output. This requirement exists regardless of the content of the information or response, including language and non-language data. As a result, we would suggest the advantage implicit in broadening the use of the terms agnosia and apraxia to emphasize their input (receptive) and output (expressive) nature. The central processing function which may be defective can be identified by the nature of the deficit (reading, writing, spelling, etc.).

It is sometimes difficult to determine whether the impairment is receptive or expressive in nature (an agnosia or an apraxia), and both receptive and expressive deficits are usually present in the same aphasic individual. Thus, terminology used to describe aphasic deficits in individual persons might be clarified by emphasizing the presence of agnosia or apraxia. Using such an approach, receptive aphasic losses would require identification by three words, including the sensory avenue involved, the content of the loss, and the term *agnosia* (or *dysgnosia*). An aphasic deficit characterized by a failure to be able to read printed or written material (alexia or dyslexia) could more descriptively be referred to as *visual word agnosia.* Aphasic impairment of verbal comprehension capability would be referred to as *auditory verbal dysgnosia.* Apraxic deficits in the language area would require only identification of the content. For example, a person who was impaired in naming common objects (dysnomia) would be referred to as having a *naming dyspraxia.* Such a system of terminology would also include non-verbal deficits, such as constructional dyspraxia, body dysgnosia, finger dysgnosia, etc.

Because of the significance of both language and non-language specific deficits in the area of behavioral neurology, a system of terminology that comprehensively included the entire range of deficits, without diminishing the identity of the specific deficit, would facilitate communication. Use of such a system of terminology also emphasizes the descriptive nature of terminology in this area and might tend to decrease the need for a great number of categories of aphasia which have been based on observation of individual manifestations of deficit even though they rarely serve as categories for grouping of individual patients. This conceptual framework for a better organized and integrated terminology generally referrable to deficits in the categories of aphasia, agnosia, and apraxia has recently been presented in detail and related to pathological responses elicited in using the Reitan-Indiana Aphasia Screening Test (Reitan, 1984).

# Section II

# Neuroanatomy and Neuropathology

# NEURONS AND NEUROGLIA

In general, the central nervous system tissue is composed of two types of cells: neurons and neuroglia. **Neurons** or nerve cells are specialized cells which conduct nerve impulses; therefore, they give the nervous tissue most of its functional characteristics. **Neuroglia** ("nerve glue"), often simply called glia, make up about half the total volume of the central nervous system. Besides providing structural support, they also have important metabolic functions, which will be described later.

The central nervous system consists of gray matter and white matter. The **gray matter** is found primarily in the core of the CNS, the corpus striatum (a large mass located near the base of each hemisphere) and the cortex, a sheet of gray matter that covers the cerebral hemispheres and the cerebellum. The gray matter contains the cell bodies of neurons, which contributes to its characteristic color. It also contains neuroglial cells and blood vessels. The **white matter** surrounds the central core of gray matter. The white matter is composed of the long processes (axons) of neurons, most of which are surrounded by myelin sheaths. Unlike the gray matter, it does not contain cell bodies. The white matter has a substantial amount of neuroglia, but fewer capillaries than the gray matter.

NEURONS. As noted above, neurons are cells which are able to conduct impulses. A CNS neuron is generally made up of three parts: the cell body, dendrites and axon. The *cell body* or soma is the part of the neuron which contains the nucleus and other various organelles, such as the nucleolus, mitochondria and Golgi bodies. The *dendrites* are processes which branch out from the cell and serve as the receptive areas for the neuron. The *axon* is the part of the cell that conducts the impulse away from the cell body. The axon is usually longer than the dendrite and in a human may extend for as long as a yard; giant pyramidal cells of the cerebral cortex may send axons to the caudal tip of the spinal cord (Carpenter & Sutin, 1983). The site where the axon originates

from the cell body is the *axon hilock* (*see* Fig. 2–4). Action potentials usually arise from the *initial segment* (the part of the cell body where it is joined by the axon) because of its high excitability. The point of contact between neurons or between a neuron and a muscle fiber is known as the *synapse* or junctional point. The detailed insert in Fig. 2–3 illustrates a synapse and the structures that will be described below.

The axon may have one ending or several branches; the complexity of the axon's design will determine the number of contacts it will have with other cells. Most long axons are surrounded by a *myelin sheath*. In the brain and spinal cord, oligodendroglia (described later) wrap part of their cytoplasm, jellyroll fashion, around an adjoining axon. (This same function is accomplished by the neurilemmal or Schwann cells in the peripheral nervous system.) The myelin sheath is composed of alternating concentric layers of lipids and proteins, which gives the axon a white, glistening appearance. It is the tracts of myelin sheaths which make up the bulk of the white matter. Most neurons destined to be myelinated have completed the process by the time of birth or shortly thereafter. Myelin allows an axon to conduct impulses quickly and efficiently.

At various points along the axon the myelin sheath is interrupted by areas of constriction called *nodes of Ranvier* and occur about every 1-2 mm (*see* Figs. 2–2 and 2–3). Nerve impulses are able to "jump" from node to node (*saltatory conduction*) and thereby achieve a high velocity.

Communication between cells can be effected through two mechanisms: chemical and electrical. Although detailed cellular physiology is beyond the scope of this volume, we will briefly review some of the basic concepts.

The final end of the dendrite is called the *bouton* (knob), or pre-synaptic membrane and the part of the cell receiving the impulse is covered by a post-synaptic membrane; the area separating the two membranes is the *synaptic cleft* (Fig. 2–3). Highly specialized structures, the *synaptic vesicles*, are found within the bouton. These vesicles contain a chemical transmitter substance which combines with specific molecular binding sites on the receptor and either excite or inhibit the post-synaptic neuron. This is accomplished by a series of chemical reactions which change the post-synaptic cell's membrane permeability and thus affects its concentrations of potassium and sodium.

The electrical transport of nerve impulses is also concerned with the permeability of the cell membrane. The membrane is highly permeable to potassium ions when the cell is in the resting state; when excited, the cell membrane becomes highly permeable to sodium ions. The reversal in permeability creates an *action potential* or nerve impulse, which is propagated along the membrane by local circuits of electrical current (Barr & Kiernan, 1983).

**Types of Cells.** Neurons can be classified either according to their function or according to the number of processes extending from the cell body. *See* Fig. 2–2 for illustrations of the types of neurons described below.

*Sensory* neurons relay information to the central nervous system from the periphery of the body. When these impulses are perceived, a type of sensation is appreciated. Sensory neurons are generally found in the olfactory membrane, the inner ear and the retina.

*Motor* or effector neurons carry impulses to the periphery to produce movement. In general, they are large cells with long myelinated axons. Most are multipolar neurons, with one axon and a number of branching dendrites.

**NEUROGLIA.** The neuroglia are the non-neural elements which form the interstitial tissue of the nervous system (Carpenter & Sutin, 1983). The central nervous system is composed almost entirely of neurons and neuroglia cells packed tightly together. Approximately half the total volume of the human brain is made up of neuroglial cells.

The functions of neuroglial cells has not been firmly established, although the role of oligodendrocytes in forming the myelin sheath has been accepted. It is also fairly well established that astrocytes are important in the repair of injuries in the brain.

**Astrocytes** or astroglia are the largest and most numerous type of glial cell. They are characterized by their star-like shape and their numerous processes extending from the cell body. Some of these processes attach to the surface of capillary blood vessels, forming the "foot plates" or "perivascular end feet" (*see* Fig. 2–4). These "sucker processes" cover about 80% of the external surface area of each capillary (Barr & Kiernan, 1983). Other end feet are found applied to the pia mater at the external surface of the central nervous system (superficial glial membrane) and around larger blood vessels.

A number of enzymes have been isolated from astrocytes, indicating that they may be involved in transport mechanisms between the blood and the brain. As noted before, they also provide support for the other cellular structures in the nervous system.

When there is injury to the brain or spinal cord through trauma or disease the astrocytes undergo hypertrophy. The number of their cytoplasmic processes increases and mature astrocytes may multiply by mitosis. A *glial scar* may form, filling in the gaps produced by diseased or injured tissue. Astrocytes also have some limited phagocytic properties.

An astrocytoma is a type of intrinsic primary neoplasm which arises from the astrocyte cells. It is described in detail in another chapter in this volume.

**Oligodendroglia.** As mentioned, the oligodendroglia produce and maintain the myelin sheaths around the axons in the central nervous system. In mammals the oligodendroglia react to injury by swelling and increased acid phosphatase activity.

Oligodendrogliomas make up a small fraction of the gliomas. In general, they involve the cortex and white matter and are slow-growing. Calcification of the tumor is often visible on skull x-ray.

**Microglia.** Microglia cells are most abundant in the gray matter. They appear to be inactive in the adult brain until a disease or injury occurs, at which time they proliferate rapidly and migrate toward the site of injury. Microglial tumors occur very rarely.

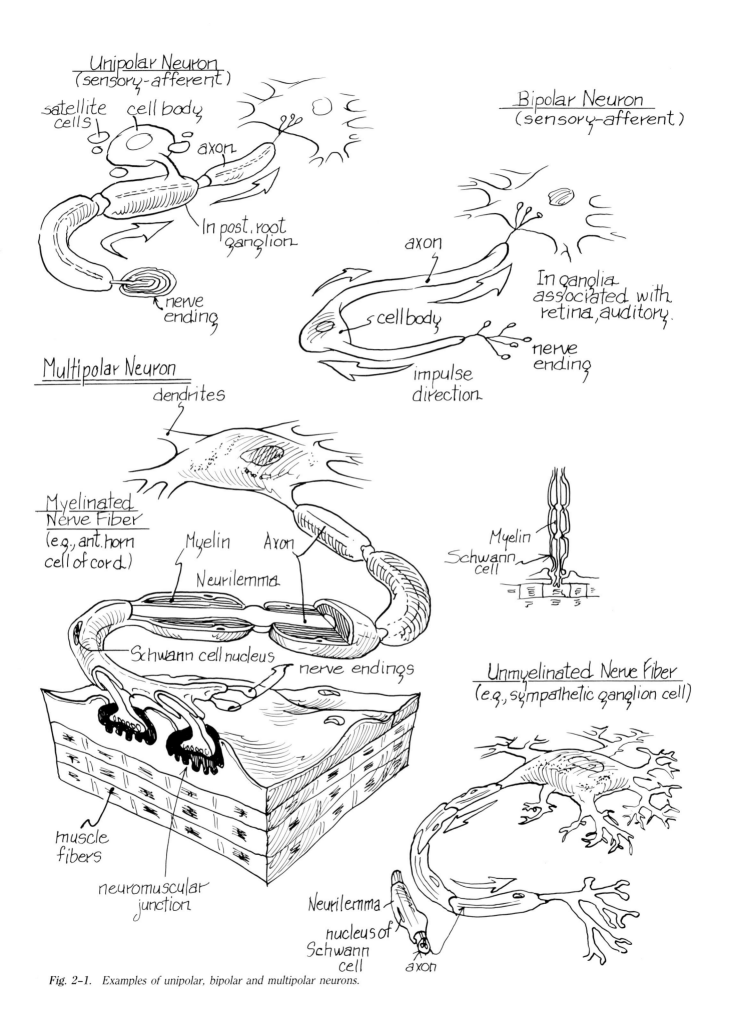

*Fig. 2–1. Examples of unipolar, bipolar and multipolar neurons.*

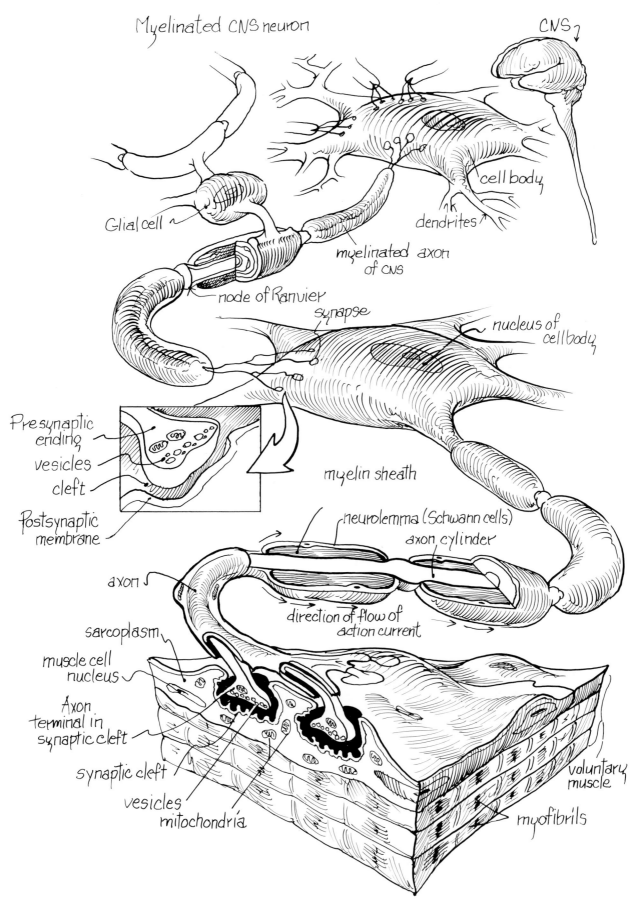

Myelinated CNS neuron

CNS

cell body

Glial cell

dendrites

myelinated axon
of CNS

node of Ranvier

synapse

nucleus of
cell body

Presynaptic
ending

vesicles

cleft

Postsynaptic
membrane

myelin sheath

neurolemma (Schwann cells)

axon cylinder

axon

direction of flow of
action current

sarcoplasm

muscle cell
nucleus

Axon
terminal in
synaptic cleft

synaptic cleft

vesicles

mitochondria

voluntary
muscle

myofibrils

**Fig. 2–2.** *Diagramatic representation of a myelinated neuron. Note relationship of glial cell to adjoining axon.*

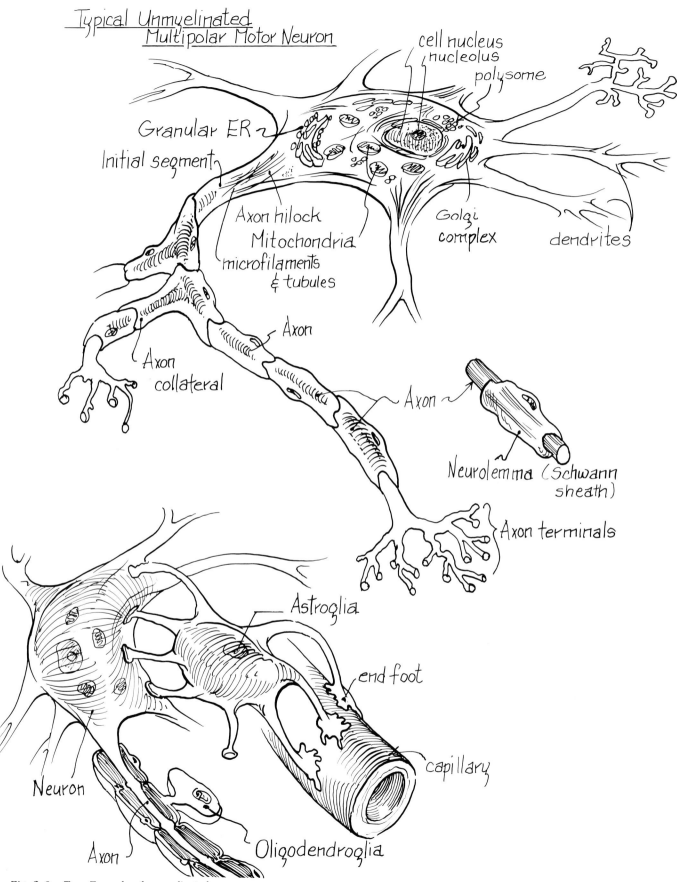

**Fig. 2-3.** Top: Example of unmyelinated neuron.

Bottom: Depiction of way in which astroglia gives structural support to surrounding structures (neuron and capillary). Up to 80% of the surface area of a capillary may be covered by astroglial end feet.

# CRANIAL NERVES

**I. OLFACTORY** (sensory). Cranial nerve I is actually a fiber tract of the brain. It arises from the olfactory bulb on the ventral portion of the frontal lobe and progresses posteriorly to end slightly lateral to the optic chiasm, where it penetrates the cerebrum. A lesion of the olfactory tract may cause *anosmia* (loss of sense of smell). A possible cause is a tumor at the base of the frontal lobe.

**II. OPTIC** (sensory). The optic nerves pass into the cranial cavity through the optic foramina and join to form the *optic chiasm*. Fibers from the nasal retina cross in the chiasm and join the uncrossed fibers from the temporal retina to form the optic tracts. (*See* the chapter entitled *The Visual Pathway* for a full discussion of the optic tract.)

**III. OCULOMOTOR** (motor). The oculomotor nerve supplies all of the orbital muscles except the lateral rectus and the superior oblique. Its functions include: (1) constriction of the pupil; (2) moving the eye upward, downward and medially; and (3) raising the upper eyelid. Lesions of the oculomotor nerve cause the eye to look downward and outward; the pupil does not constrict to light or accomodation.

**IV. TROCHLEAR** (motor). The trochlear muscle supplies the superior oblique eye muscle, which assists in turning the eye downward and outward. A lesion of nerve IV will cause the eye to look slightly upward.

**V. TRIGEMINAL** (sensory and motor). The *ophthalmic, maxillary* and *mandibular* nerves convey sensations of touch, pain and temperature from the eye, forehead, face, jaws, teeth, sinuses, nasopharynx and part of the dura mater. Lesions of the sensory components of the trigeminal nerve will produce anesthesia in the area of distribution. The motor component of the mandibular nerve supplies the muscles of mastication. Lesions of the motor part of the trigeminal nerve will cause paralysis of the jaws.

**VI. ABDUCENS** (motor). The abducens nerve supplies the lateral rectus muscle of the eyeball, which rotates the eye outwards. A lesion of the abducens nerve will turn the eye inward.

**VII. FACIAL** (motor and sensory). The sensory fibers of the facial nerve convey taste sensations from the anterior ⅔ of the tongue and soft palate. The motor fibers supply the muscles of the face and scalp; they control facial expression and aid in movements of mastication and speech. The secretory fibers innervate the sublingual salivary glands, the lacriminal glands and glands in the mucous membranes of the oral and nasal cavities. Lesions of the facial nerve may cause facial paralysis (Bell's palsy), decreased secretion of the gland of distribution and loss of taste sensation in the anterior ⅔ of the tongue.

**VIII. VESTIBULOCOCHLEAR** (sensory). The *vestibular* component of nerve VIII carries impulses concerned with balance, equilibration, position and coordination. A lesion of this nerve may cause vertigo and nystagmus. The *cochlear* component is the nerve of hearing. Lesions of this nerve may cause tinnitus and loss of hearing. Deafness will not occur unless there are bilateral lesions.

**IX. GLOSSOPHARYNGEAL** (motor and sensory). The motor component of nerve IX supplies the stylopharyngeus muscle in the neck. The sensory component conveys sensations from the pharynx, tonsil, tympanic cavity, auditory tube, mastoid cells and taste from the posterior ⅓ of the tongue. It also supplies the carotid body and sinus. Lesions of the glossopharyngeal nerve may cause (1) loss of gag reflex; (2) loss of taste in the posterior ⅓ of the tongue; (3) loss of constriction of the posterior pharyngeal wall when saying, "ah"; (4) tachycardia (from disturbances of the carotid sinus reflex; and (5) dysphagia.

**X. VAGUS** (motor and sensory). The motor fibers of the vagus nerve innervate the laryngeal muscles. Nerve X also provides parasympathetic supply to the heart and its vessels, the bronchi, trachea and alimentary canal. The sensory fibers convey impulses from the epiglottis. Lesions of the vagus nerve may cause (1) laryngeal paralysis; (2) aphonia (loss of voice); (3) dysphonia (impairment of voice); (4) dysphagia (difficulty swallowing); (5) loss of gag reflex; (6) coughing; (7) bradycardia; and (8) dilatation of the stomach.

**XI.  ACCESSORY** (motor). The accessory nerve supplies the sternocleidomastoid and trapezius muscles. Lesions of the accessory nerve will leave the patient unable to (1) rotate his head to the unaffected side; (2) shrug the affected shoulder; and (3) raise his chin.

**XII.  HYPOGLOSSAL** (motor). Nerve XII supplies the muscles of the tongue. A lesion of the hypoglossal nerve may cause contralateral hemiplegia and paralysis of the tongue.

# Cranial Nerves: Motor and Sensory Fibers

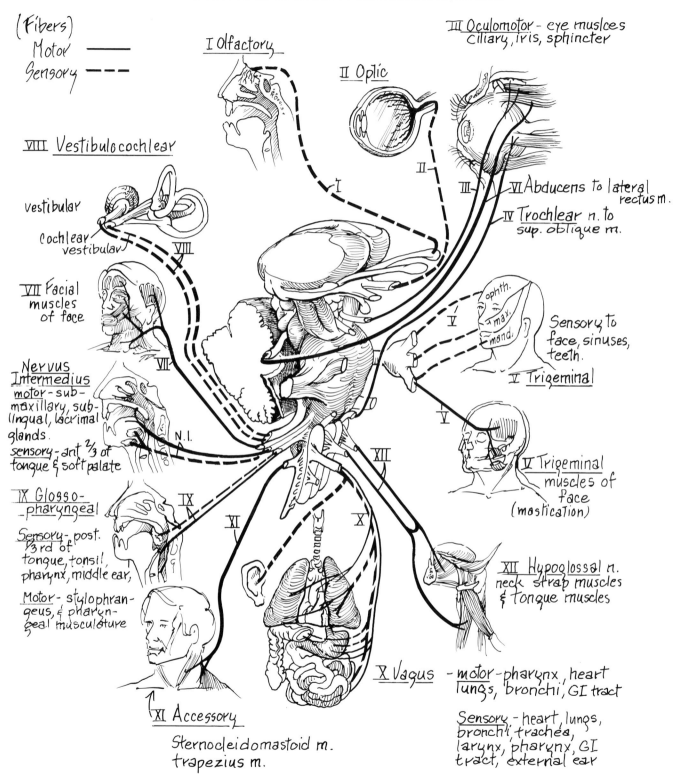

(Fibers)
Motor ———
Sensory - - - -

I Olfactory

II Optic

III Oculomotor - eye muslces
Ciliary, iris, sphincter

VIII Vestibulocochlear

vestibular

cochlear
vestibular

VIII

VII Facial
muscles
of face

VI Abducens to lateral
rectus m.

IV Trochlear n. to
sup. oblique m.

ophth.
max.
mand.

Sensory to
face, sinuses,
teeth.

V Trigeminal

Nervus
Intermedius
motor - sub-
maxillary, sub-
lingual, lacrimal
glands.
sensory - ant. 2/3 of
tongue & soft palate

N.I.

V Trigeminal
muscles of
face
(mastication)

XII

IX Glosso-
pharyngeal

IX

Sensory - post.
1/3 rd of
tongue, tonsil,
pharynx, middle ear,

Motor - stylophran-
geus, & pharyn-
geal musculature

XI

X

XII Hypoglossal n.
neck strap muscles
& tongue muscles

XI Accessory

Sternocleidomastoid m.
trapezius m.

X Vagus - motor - pharynx, heart
lungs, bronchi, GI tract

Sensory - heart, lungs,
bronchi, trachea,
larynx, pharynx, GI
tract, external ear

*Fig. 2–4.   The emergence of the cranial nerves from the brain.*

# ANATOMY OF THE CEREBRAL VASCULATURE

Since oxygen and glucose are necessary in a nearly steady supply for normal brain functioning, the blood flow to the brain is of great importance. An understanding of brain vascularization requires some knowledge of the vascular anatomy involved. Figs. 2–5 to 2–10 illustrate various aspects of the cerebral vasculature.

## THE ARTERIAL SYSTEM

Arteries arising from the aortic arch supply blood to the brain through the **carotid** and **vertebral-basilar artery systems**. On the right side the **brachiocephalic artery** arises from the aortic arch and divides into the **right common carotid artery** and the **right subclavian artery**. On the left, the **left common carotid artery** and the **left subclavian artery** usually arise directly from the aortic arch.

The subclavian arteries give rise to the **left and right vertebral arteries** which converge to form the **basilar artery**, giving rise to the **vertebral-basilar system**. This system supplies blood to parts of the temporal lobes, the occipital lobe, most of the thalamus, the rest of the brain stem (midbrain, pons, and medulla oblongata), the cerebellum, the upper part of the spinal cord and the inner ear via the internal auditory artery.

The common carotid arteries divide into the **external and internal carotid arteries**. The internal carotid arteries provide the basic blood supply to the eyes, basal ganglia, most of the hypothalamus, the frontal and parietal lobes, and the greater part of the temporal lobes. The bifurcation of the common carotid artery into the internal and external carotid artery is just below the angle of the jaw in about 50% of the population, somewhat above this level in 30%, and below this level in the remaining 20%.

Before terminating as the **superficial temporal** and **maxillary arteries**, the external carotid artery gives off a number of branches, several of which supply blood to the dura mater. The **middle meningeal artery**, which arises from the maxillary artery, is the most important in supplying blood to the meninges. If the internal carotid artery is occluded, the external carotid artery acts as a collateral source of blood supply to the brain.

The internal carotid artery has many branches, but those that are most important clinically are the **ophthalmic, posterior communicating, anterior choroidal, anterior cerebral, and middle cerebral arteries**. These arteries, usually in the order given above, arise from the internal carotid artery shortly after it penetrates the dura mater.

The **ophthalmic artery** enters the orbital cavity beside the optic nerve and divides into many branches to supply blood to the contents of the eye. The most important branch is the **central artery of the retina** which enters the globe at the optic disk and supplies the retina. (These are the arteries viewed through an ophthalmoscope.)

The **posterior communicating artery** arises from the internal carotid artery just above the sella turcica and travels posteriorly, mainly on a horizontal course, to join the posterior cerebral artery. Since the posterior cerebral artery is the terminal branch of the basilar artery, and a part of the vertebral-basilar artery system, the posterior communicating artery, when sufficiently large, may serve to equalize pressure between the carotid and vertebral-basilar systems. Normally, however, blood in the two systems does not mix. The size of the posterior communicating arteries is generally quite variable and may vary greatly on the two sides of an individual's brain. Many perforating branches arise from the posterior communicating artery, with the anterior branches serving the hypothalamus and ventral thalamic area, the anterior third of the optic tract, and the posterior limb of the internal capsule; the posterior branches supply the subthalamic nucleus.

The **anterior choroidal artery** usually arises from the internal carotid artery just above the posterior communicating artery. However, at times it arises directly from the posterior communicating artery or the middle

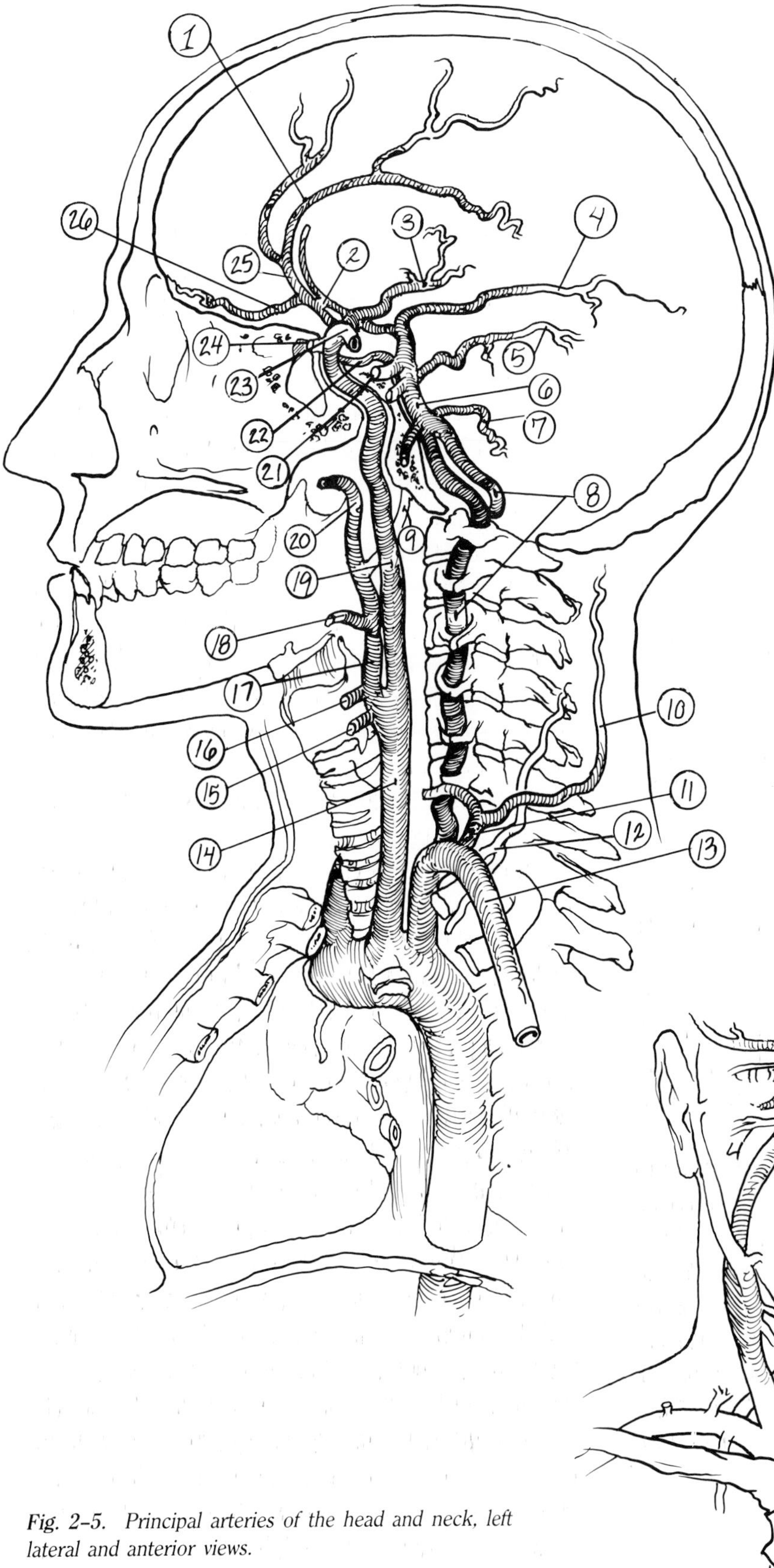

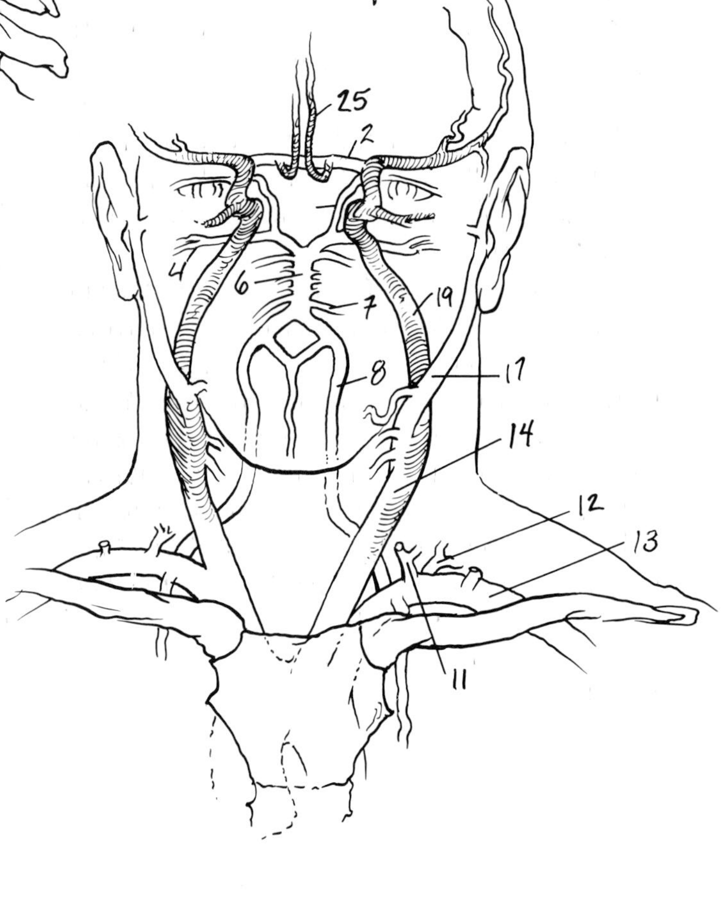

Fig. 2-5. Principal arteries of the head and neck, left lateral and anterior views.

## Arteries of the Brain

1. Pericallosal a.
2. Ant. Communicating a.
3. Right Middle Cerebral a.
4. Right Post. Cerebral a.
5. Right Sup. Cerebellar a.
6. Basilar a.
7. Inferior Cerebellar a.
8. Vertebral a.
9. Superficial Temporal a.
10. Deep Cervical a.
11. Thyrocervical trunk
12. Costocervical trunk
13. Left Subclavian a.
14. Left Common Carotid a.
15. Superior Thyroid a.
16. Lingual a.
17. External Carotid a.
18. Facial a.
19. Internal Carotid a.
20. Maxillary a.
21. Left Post. Cerebral a.
22. Post. Communicating a.
23. Left Middle Cerebral a.
24. Ophthalmic a.
25. Ant. Cerebral a.
26. Frontopolar a.

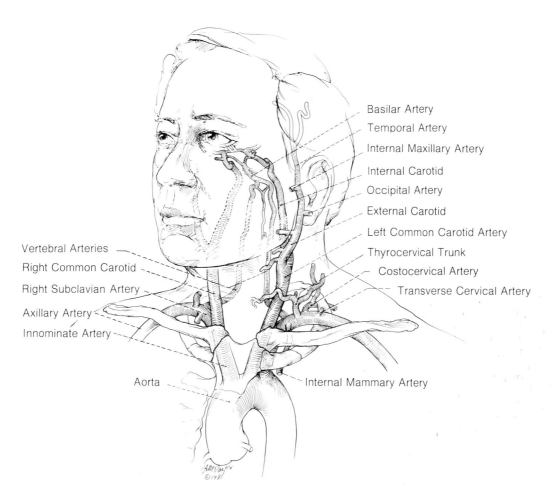

**Fig. 2-6.** *Pathways of internal, external carotid arteries and vertebral arteries. (© Edward B. Diethrich. Reproduced with permission.)*

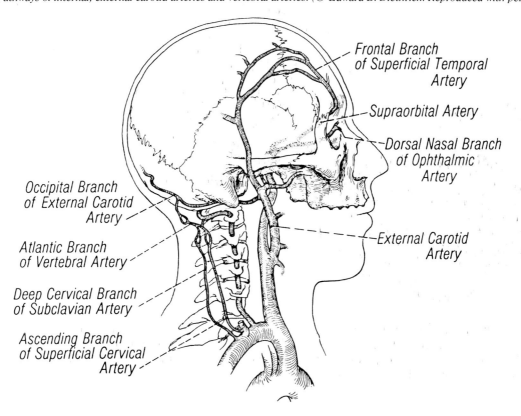

**Fig. 2-7.** *Extracranial cerebrovascular anatomy. Note the anastomotic connections between the external and internal carotid and between the occipital, cervical and vertebral arteries. (© Edward B. Diethrich. Reproduced with permission.)*

# Major Cerebral Arteries
## (medial & lateral views)

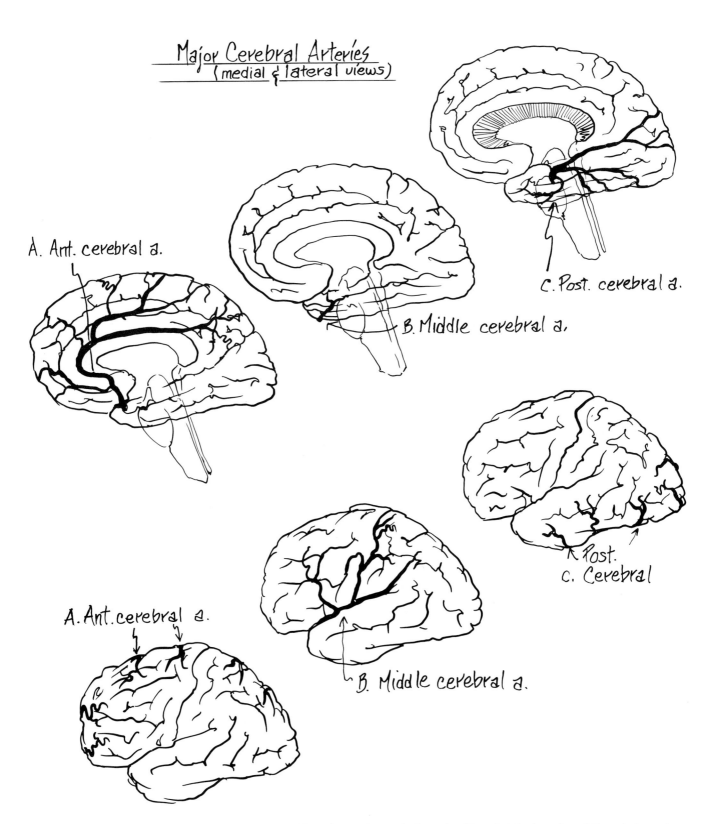

A. Ant. cerebral a.

B. Middle cerebral a.

C. Post. cerebral a.

R. Post. c. Cerebral

A. Ant. cerebral a.

B. Middle cerebral a.

**Fig. 2–8.** *Location and distribution of anterior, middle and posterior cerebral arteries. Note that the branches of the anterior and posterior cerebral arteries extend over the cerebral crest to the convexity of the hemisphere where they supply a region of 1-2 in (see arrows). The anterior cerebral artery supplies the medial surface of the brain up to the parieto-occipital sulcus. The posterior cerebral artery supplies the basal surface of the hemisphere and the cuneus.*

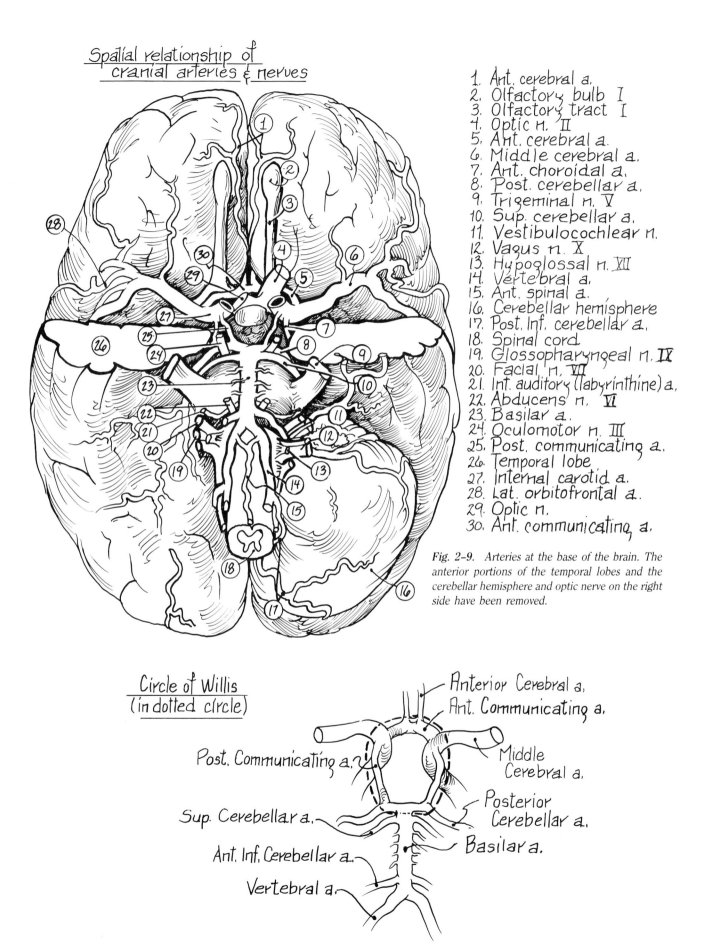

## Spatial relationship of cranial arteries & nerves

1. Ant. cerebral a.
2. Olfactory bulb I
3. Olfactory tract I
4. Optic n. II
5. Ant. cerebral a.
6. Middle cerebral a.
7. Ant. choroidal a.
8. Post. cerebellar a.
9. Trigeminal n. V
10. Sup. cerebellar a.
11. Vestibulocochlear n.
12. Vagus n. X
13. Hypoglossal n. XII
14. Vertebral a.
15. Ant. spinal a.
16. Cerebellar hemisphere
17. Post. Inf. cerebellar a.
18. Spinal cord
19. Glossopharyngeal n. IX
20. Facial n. VII
21. Int. auditory (labyrinthine) a.
22. Abducens n. VI
23. Basilar a.
24. Oculomotor n. III
25. Post. communicating a.
26. Temporal lobe
27. Internal carotid a.
28. Lat. orbitofrontal a.
29. Optic n.
30. Ant. communicating a.

*Fig. 2-9.* Arteries at the base of the brain. The anterior portions of the temporal lobes and the cerebellar hemisphere and optic nerve on the right side have been removed.

## Circle of Willis (in dotted circle)

Anterior Cerebral a.
Ant. Communicating a.
Post. Communicating a.?
Middle Cerebral a.
Sup. Cerebellar a.
Posterior Cerebellar a.
Basilar a.
Ant. Inf. Cerebellar a.
Vertebral a.

*Fig. 2-10.* Detailed diagram showing normal relationship of the arteries in the circle of Willis.

cerebral artery. It runs in a posterior direction passing beneath the optic tract and reaching the anterior part of the lateral geniculate body. At this point it divides into a number of branches and provides blood to the choroid plexus. In addition, it supplies blood to the posterior limb of the internal capsule, the globus pallidus, the optic tract and the lateral geniculate body. Many of the branches of the anterior choroidal artery which penetrate the brain are end-arteries and spread into a capillary network. The anterior choroidal artery on each side of the brain provides a degree of connecting blood flow of the internal carotid arteries. Together with the posterior choroidal arteries, the carotid system is linked with the vertebral-basilar system. Although occlusion of the anterior choroidal artery is quite infrequent, when it occurs it may cause homonymous hemianopia, hemiplegia, and hemihypalgesia.

The **anterior cerebral artery** arises from the internal carotid artery in the vicinity of the anterior part of the Sylvian fissure. It extends medially in a horizontal plane beneath the orbital surface of the frontal lobe, continues to the medial surface of the frontal lobe, circles around the anterior part of the corpus collosum, and extends posteriorly from that point. Numerous small branches of the anterior cerebral artery penetrate the brain as it runs along this general course, and small anastomoses between the two anterior cerebral arteries occur at various points. The **medial striate artery (Heubner's artery)** which supplies the orbital surface of the frontal lobe, is the first vessel of sufficient size to have a name. The next major artery given off by the anterior cerebral artery is the **frontopolar artery**, which supplies the anterior portion of the frontal lobe on its medial side. Next, the **callosomarginal artery** arises, supplying additional areas of the medial part of the frontal lobe and extending over the superior margin of the hemisphere on to the lateral surface in the area of the paracentral lobule. These arteries have many branches, forming an extensive network of surface vessels which penetrate the brain. In addition, the end branches of the callosomarginal artery anastomose with the terminal branches of the middle cerebral artery on the lateral surface of the cerebral hemisphere.

The **anterior communicating artery** provides a very important anastomosis between the carotid circulation on the two sides of the brain. This artery extends between the two anterior cerebral arteries just above the optic chiasm at the base of the brain and forms the anterior part of the circle of Willis.

The **middle cerebral artery** is the terminal extension of the internal carotid artery. After the internal carotid artery gives off the anterior cerebral artery, it becomes, by definition, the middle cerebral artery. In its initial portion this artery follows the Sylvian fissure, with the frontal lobe above and the temporal lobe below. The initial portion of the middle cerebral artery gives off many branches which supply the putamen, the head of the caudate nucleus, the globus pallidus, and the genu and posterior limbs of the internal capsule. The middle cerebral artery then divides into a number of branches called the **ascending frontal**, the **anterior and posterior temporal**, the **posterior parietal**, and the **angular arteries**. These arteries give off a large number of branches which essentially cover the lateral surface of the brain. The exact course of the branches varies greatly from one person to another, but the main branches can be identified either by angiography or visual observation.

The **anterior temporal artery** supplies the pole of the temporal lobe. The **ascending frontal arteries** cover the convexity of the frontal lobe and finally anastomose with the branches of the callosomarginal artery in the superior region of the hemisphere. The **posterior temporal artery** provides blood to the superior and lateral aspects of the temporal lobe. The **posterior parietal artery** extends in a posterior direction along the cerebral convexity and usually gives off a major branch called the **angular artery**. These arteries supply the lateral surface of the parietal lobe and superior portions of the temporal lobe.

The **middle cerebral artery** is the principal vessel among the arteries that provide blood directly to the cerebral cortex. This artery supplies the insula, the orbital frontal area, the inferior and middle gyri of the frontal lobe, parts of the precentral and postcentral gyri on either side of the central sulcus, the superior and inferior parietal lobules, additional portions of the parietal lobe, and the superior and middle temporal gyri of the temporal lobe. Approximately 80% of the blood received by the cerebral hemispheres is carried by the middle cerebral artery.

The vertebral-basilar arterial system of the brain consists essentially of the **subclavian arteries**, the **vertebral arteries**, the **basilar artery** (which leads to the circle of Willis) and the **posterior cerebral arteries**, which essentially represent the termination of the system. There are, of course, a number of additional arteries which arise from these vessels. The subclavian arteries give rise to the vertebral arteries and the vertebral arteries converge to form the basilar artery. This system supplies the posterior circulation of the brain. It is of vital significance, particularly because it supplies blood to the brain stem (including the ascending and descending tracts), the nuclei of most of the cranial nerves, and centers of vital significance in the maintenance and balance of bodily functions.

The **vertebral arteries** enter the skull through the foramen magnum and penetrate the dura mater shortly thereafter. They ascend along the ventral lateral aspects of the medulla oblongata and give off numerous small arteries that perforate the brain substance. The vertebral arteries join to form the basilar artery at approximately the junction of the pons and medulla. About 1 cm before this junction each vertebral artery gives off the **posterior inferior cerebellar artery**, the largest branches of the vertebral arteries. The posterior inferior cerebellar arteries supply blood to part of the medulla as well as the surface of the cerebellar hemispheres and possibly part of the dentate nuclei.

The **basilar artery** runs from the junction of the medulla and the pons along the ventral aspect of the pons and forms the two posterior cerebral arteries where the pons joins the midbrain.

In addition to the posterior inferior cerebellar arteries there are a number of significant branches of the vertebral-basilar system before it terminates in the posterior cerebral arteries.

The **anterior inferior cerebellar artery** supplies blood to the lateral portions of the tegmentum, the middle part of the brain stem, and parts of the cerebellum. It is extremely unusual for this particular artery to be selectively occluded, but if occlusion does occur the patient shows cerebellar signs, weakness of the facial muscles, impaired hearing, and loss of tactile sensitivity (touch, pain, and temperature) of the face on the same side as the lesion. In most cases the **auditory artery** represents a branch from the anterior inferior cerebellar artery, but sometimes stems directly from the basilar artery. This artery divides into the cochlear and vestibular branches. Particularly because of the sensitivity of vestibular function, the first evidence of disease in the vertebral-basilar system is often manifested by disturbances of equilibrium which, in turn, cause nausea, vomiting and vertigo. Sudden loss of hearing may be part of this set of symptoms, implying reduction of blood flow through the cochlear branch.

The **superior cerebellar artery**, and the **posterior and anterior inferior cerebellar arteries** are the three arteries that supply the cerebellum. The superior cerebellar artery also provides blood to the upper part of the brain stem and nuclei beneath the fourth ventricle. These three vessels have many anastomoses on the surface of the cerebellar hemispheres. Occlusion of the superior cerebellar artery is associated with manifestations of cerebellar dysfunction on the same side of the body as the lesion. Impairment of pain and temperature sensitivity may also be present, but this occurs on the contralateral side of the body.

The **mesencephalic artery** extends between the bifurcation of the basilar artery into the posterior cerebral arteries and the posterior communicating arteries of the circle of Willis. When this artery is occluded oculomotor (third cranial nerve) symptoms and a particular disturbance of vertical gaze may result.

The **posterior cerebral arteries** are terminal branches of the basilar artery, arising as continuations of the mesencephalic arteries. The posterior cerebral arteries anastomose with the posterior communicating arteries to complete the posterior portion of the circle

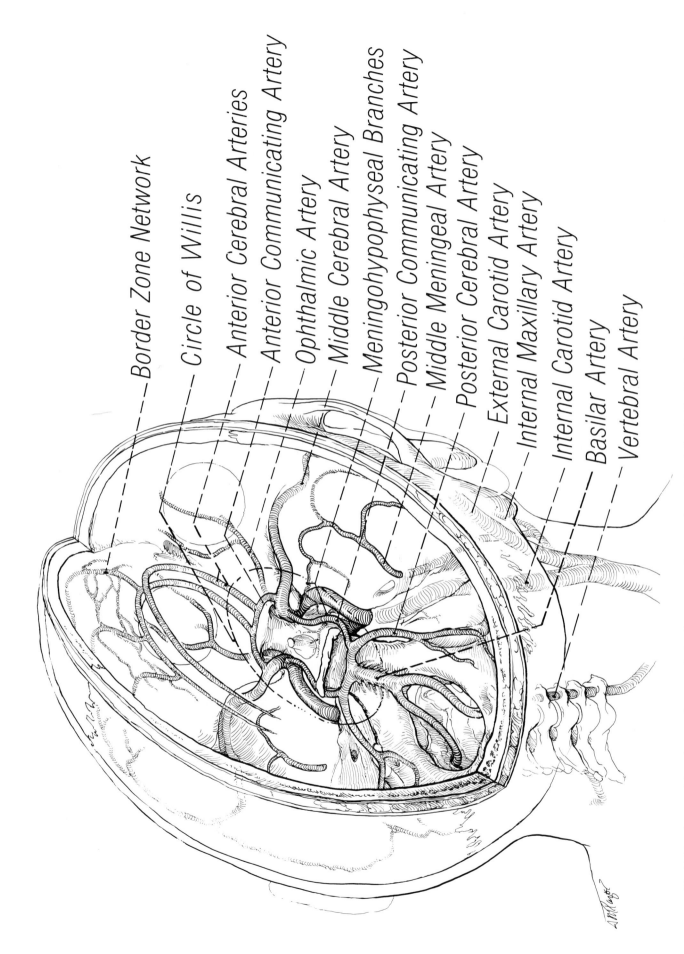

Border Zone Network

Circle of Willis

Anterior Cerebral Arteries

Anterior Communicating Artery

Ophthalmic Artery

Middle Cerebral Artery

Meningohypophyseal Branches

Posterior Communicating Artery

Middle Meningeal Artery

Posterior Cerebral Artery

External Carotid Artery

Internal Maxillary Artery

Internal Carotid Artery

Basilar Artery

Vertebral Artery

*Fig. 2–11.* Intracranial cerebrovascular anatomy showing anastomotic connections of the circle of Willis. Note that the principal blood supply to intracranial structures is via the carotid arteries. (© Edward B. Diethrich. Reproduced with permission.)

of Willis. They distribute blood principally to the medial, temporal and occipital parts of the cerebral hemispheres and terminate at the occipital pole. Small branches from the posterior cerebral arteries supply blood to the cerebral peduncle, the medial geniculate body, the superior and inferior colliculi, the pulvinar and other aspects of the posterior thalamus and the lateral geniculate body.

The **posterior choroidal arteries** also arise from the posterior cerebral arteries and terminate in the choroid plexus of the third ventricle. The inferior surface of the temporal and occipital lobes is supplied by the **anterior and posterior temporal arteries**, the **parieto-occipital arteries**, and the **calcarine arteries**. Ischemia or infarction of both occipital lobes may result in cortical blindness. In this condition pupillary responses to light are intact but vision is lost bilaterally. Some patients with this condition demonstrate *Anton's syndrome*, in which the patient believes that he is able to see, denies his blindness, and unhesitatingly offers descriptions of his environment that would require visual perception. Of course, occlusion of only a single posterior cerebral artery is likely to cause homonymous visual field losses on the contralateral side.

There are a number of extracranial anastomoses in the vascular system that supply blood to the brain. These anastomoses may be of definite assistance in reducing the neurological and neuropsychological deficits produced when lesions occur in these vessels. Intracranial anastomoses are also present. The anterior, middle, and posterior cerebral arteries have many branches over the surface of the cerebral cortex and form a diffuse network of arteries. The many arterial branches which enter and supply the gray and white matter of the cerebral hemispheres have few, if any anastomoses until they divide into their final capillary beds. Although the anastomoses among capillaries do not provide very effective collateral circulation, the interconnections among the three main arteries of each cerebral hemisphere permit blood to flow from one area to another with variable effectiveness in the individual case.

The **circle of Willis**, the principal point of interconnection of cerebral vessels, is located at the base of the brain (*See* Fig. 2–11). At this point, arteries form a polygon made up of both anterior cerebral arteries, both internal carotid arteries, both posterior cerebral arteries and both posterior communicating arteries, with the anterior portion of the polygon established by the single anterior communicating artery. The circle of Willis provides collateral circulation between the two sides of the brain and between the carotid and vertebral-basilar systems. Blood can flow in either direction in these vessels, depending upon pressure gradients determined by the areas of diminished blood supply.

## THE VENOUS SYSTEM

The cerebral venous system (*See* Figs. 2–12 and 2–13) receives far less attention than the arterial system, although lesions of the cerebral veins may impede drainage of blood from the brain and cause definite neurological disorders. It is likely that in most cases venous lesions (which consist principally of thromboses) are not specifically diagnosed.

As a brief overall statement of the cerebral venous system, it may be noted that blood leaves the brain by a large number of thin-walled veins divided into superficial and deep vessels. The **superficial veins** lie along the surface of the cerebral cortex and drain blood from the cortex and the adjacent white matter. The **deep veins** drain blood from the paraventricular white matter, basal ganglia and other deep centrally placed structures. The superficial and deep venous systems function separately with few collateral connections. However, both systems cross the subdural space to enter venous sinuses formed by two layers of dura mater. This system of sinuses empties into the **internal jugular veins** which course next to the carotid artery and the vagus nerve, joining the **subclavian veins** which lead to the **right and left brachiocephalic veins**. These, in turn, unite to form the **superior vena cava**, which empties into the right atrium of the heart.

The superficial venous system, which drains the cortex and underlying white matter, is divided into three groups: superior, middle, and inferior. The total superficial venous system consists of about 10 to 20

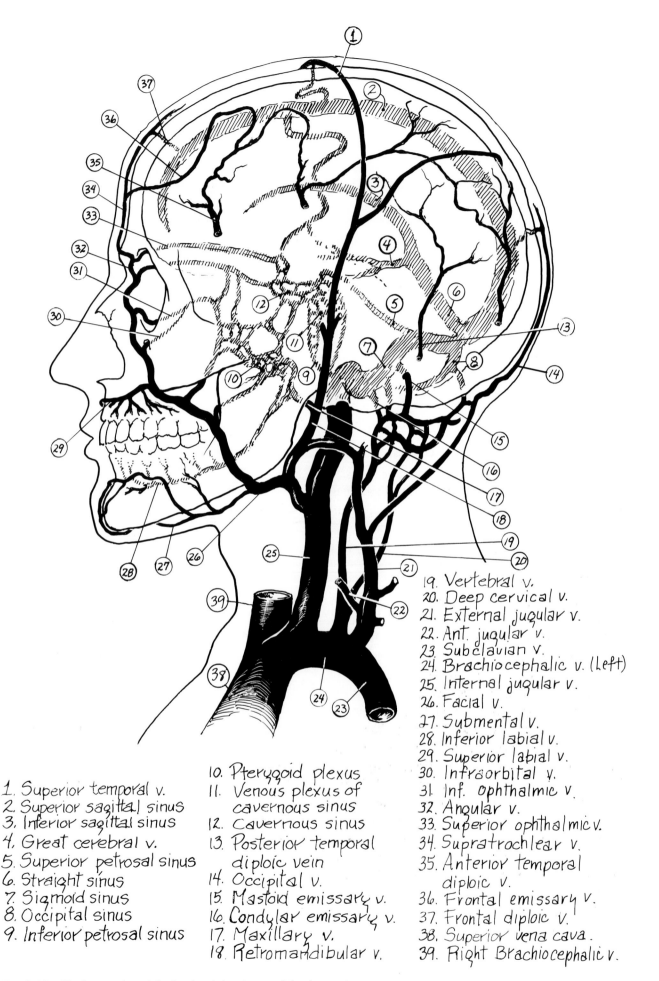

1. Superior temporal v.
2. Superior sagittal sinus
3. Inferior sagittal sinus
4. Great cerebral v.
5. Superior petrosal sinus
6. Straight sinus
7. Sigmoid sinus
8. Occipital sinus
9. Inferior petrosal sinus
10. Pterygoid plexus
11. Venous plexus of cavernous sinus
12. Cavernous sinus
13. Posterior temporal diploic vein
14. Occipital v.
15. Mastoid emissary v.
16. Condylar emissary v.
17. Maxillary v.
18. Retromandibular v.
19. Vertebral v.
20. Deep cervical v.
21. External jugular v.
22. Ant. jugular v.
23. Subclavian v.
24. Brachiocephalic v. (Left)
25. Internal jugular v.
26. Facial v.
27. Submental v.
28. Inferior labial v.
29. Superior labial v.
30. Infraorbital v.
31. Inf. ophthalmic v.
32. Angular v.
33. Superior ophthalmic v.
34. Supratrochlear v.
35. Anterior temporal diploic v.
36. Frontal emissary v.
37. Frontal diploic v.
38. Superior vena cava.
39. Right Brachiocephalic v.

Fig. 2-12. *The larger veins of the head and the sinuses of the dura mater.*

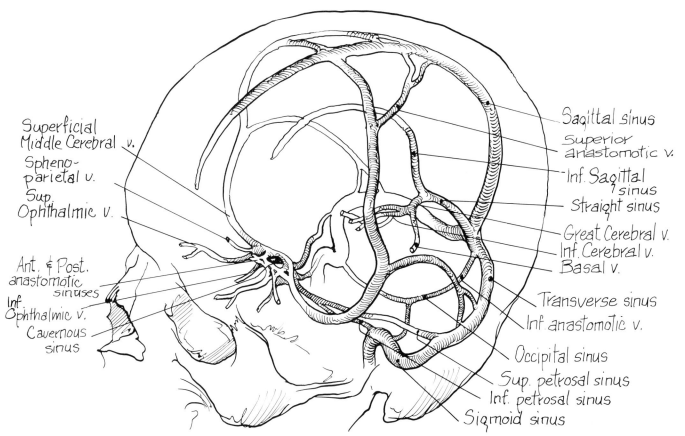

Superficial Middle Cerebral v.

Spheno-parietal v.

Sup. Ophthalmic v.

Ant. & Post. anastomotic sinuses

Inf. Ophthalmic v.

Cavernous sinus

Sagittal sinus

Superior anastomotic v.

Inf. Sagittal sinus

Straight sinus

Great Cerebral v.

Inf. Cerebral v.

Basal v.

Transverse sinus

Inf. anastomotic v.

Occipital sinus

Sup. petrosal sinus

Inf. petrosal sinus

Sigmoid sinus

*Fig. 2–13.* The venous drainage of the head.

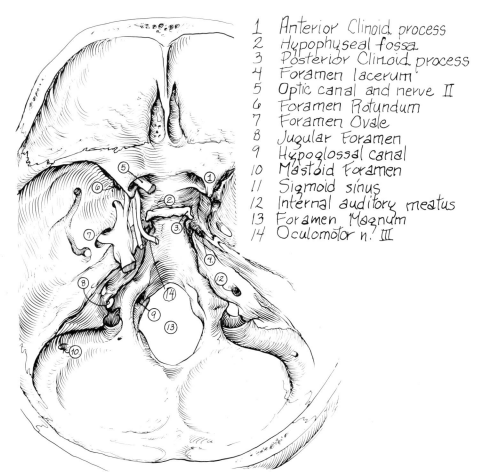

1  Anterior Clinoid process
2  Hypophyseal fossa
3  Posterior Clinoid process
4  Foramen lacerum
5  Optic canal and nerve II
6  Foramen Rotundum
7  Foramen Ovale
8  Jugular Foramen
9  Hypoglossal canal
10 Mastoid Foramen
11 Sigmoid sinus
12 Internal auditory meatus
13 Foramen Magnum
14 Oculomotor n. III

*Fig. 2–14.* Superior view of base of skull showing the principal foramina. The internal carotid artery enters the cranium through the foramen lacerum (4). The ophthalmic artery passes through the optic canal (5). The internal auditory artery passes through the internal auditory meatus (12). The vertebral arteries and the anterior and posterior spinal arteries traverse the foramen magnum (13).

veins which drain the entire surface of each hemisphere into the superior sagittal sinus. The deep venous system also consists of a considerable number of veins, with the principal ones being the **basal veins of Rosenthal** and the veins that make up the **galenic system** (particularly the great cerebral vein of Galen). As noted, these veins drain the deep structures of the brain.

The venous sinuses are formed by dural tissue and do not contain valves; therefore, unlike systemic veins, they do not collapse. The principal sinuses include (1) the **superior longitudinal (sagittal) sinus** (which lies in a midline position along the superior surface of the brain); (2) the **inferior longitudinal (sagittal) sinus** (which also lies in a midline position but deep within the brain structures); (3) the **straight sinus** (formed by the junction of the inferior longitudinal sinus and the great cerebral vein of Galen and lies deep within the brain structures); (4) the **sphenoparietal sinus** (which runs along the lesser wing of the sphenoid bone and terminates in the cavernous sinus); (5) the **cavernous sinuses** (paired structures on either side of the sella turcica which derive their name from the fact that the sinuses are divided into multiple cavities and have an extensive network of veins which provide many routes for drainage of blood from these sinuses); (6) the **transverse and sigmoid sinuses** (the transverse sinus begins at the internal occipital protuberance of the skull and runs anteriorly, curves downward to form the sigmoid sinus, and then drains into the internal jugular vein); (7) the **confluence of sinuses**, (a junction of the superior longitudinal, straight, and occipital sinuses with the transverse sinuses); (8) the **superior petrosal sinus** (connecting the cavernous with the transverse sinus, it drains a few of the interior occipital and cerebellar veins and connects with veins in the middle ear); and (9) the **inferior petrosal sinus** (which connects the cavernous sinus with the internal jugular vein and receives veins from the inner ear, the pons, the medulla, and the lower surface of the cerebellum). In addition, a number of veins drain blood into the sinuses from the cerebellum, the pons, and the medulla oblongata as well as the upper part of the spinal cord.

Disease of the intracranial veins and venous sinuses may obstruct the patency of the vein and cause inflammation of surrounding brain tissue. **Thrombotic occlusion** is the most common abnormal condition and may be caused by a number of factors such as infection, trauma, tendencies toward blood coagulation, and dehydration. However, the effects of cerebral venous thromboses may be limited by the fact that the sinuses do not contain valves and allow almost instantaneous shunting of blood from one area to another. Recovery is often rapid, again probably because of the excellent collateral channels for blood drainage. Nevertheless, a number of clinical symptoms and signs may result from venous occlusion and autopsy examinations have shown hemorrhagic areas of the cerebral cortex and adjacent white matter with such lesions. The hemorrhagic nature of these lesions contrasts with the pathological changes resulting from arterial occlusion, in which the involved area is usually bloodless.

Differential diagnosis of cerebral venous occlusion is difficult to achieve and may be confused with meningitis, abscess, or even arterial occlusion. Absence of focal signs, a high fever, and a stiff neck favor the diagnosis of meningitis; focal signs accompanied by severe headaches, stupor, or lateralized reflex or sensory changes suggest the presence of an abscess. Differentiation between venous and arterial occlusion may be aided by determination of factors which predispose to venous occlusion, such as paranasal sinusitis or middle ear infections or the presence of varicose veins and thrombophlebitis of the legs. In addition, weakness of the leg (in contrast to the arm) together with day-to-day variation in motor and sensory signs is more common in venous occlusion. Focal convulsions are also seen more frequently with venous lesions.

# A BRIEF REVIEW
# OF THE PHYSIOLOGY
# OF CEREBRAL CIRCULATION

According to Hachinski (1984), each minute the adult human brain requires about 1,000 ml of blood containing oxygen and glucose. If this circulation of blood is interrupted for six seconds, neuronal metabolism suffers; an interruption of two minutes causes brain activity to cease; and a five-minute interruption of blood supply begins to cause irreversible damage. The brain represents only one-fiftieth of body weight, but uses one-fifth of the resting cardiac output and has a priority claim on blood flow, sometimes at the expense of other organs in the body. The brain differs from other organs in that every part of the brain needs a continuous supply of blood or focal deficits may appear. Many other organs, which are relatively homogenous (e.g., kidney, lung, liver), may be able to sustain relatively large areas of impaired blood supply with little or no clinical deficit. These facts illustrate the high metabolic requirements of the brain and the special nature of this organ in a physiological sense. The internal carotid arteries provide approximately two-thirds of the total cerebral blood flow; the remaining one-third is delivered via the vertebral-basilar system. The frontal areas of the brain have a somewhat higher rate of blood flow than the parietal and temporal areas.

There have been various claims that blood flow to certain regions of the brain increases with particular perceptual or cognitive activities. Blood flow increases to a mild extent in sleep associated with slow waves on the EEG and increases quite markedly during REM (rapid eye movement) sleep. In coma, however, cerebral blood flow is decreased. Convulsions are associated with a greatly increased cerebral blood flow and oxygen consumption. In patients with complex partial seizures and epileptogenic foci, cerebral blood flow and glucose metabolism nearly doubles in the region of the focus. Between seizures the abnormal areas (foci) show a decreased glucose metabolism.

Among elderly individuals, cerebral blood flow tends to correlate with general physical and mental health and in some instances may be in the range of normality for young persons. On the average, however, cerebral blood flow, glucose metabolism, and oxygen consumption decrease with every decade of life beginning with the 20s. These changes are relatively mild and generalized in nature, although the frontal areas seem to show a somewhat greater decrease. The consistency of reduction of cerebral blood flow in the gray matter with advancing age was shown by Naritomi et al. (1979) when they obtained a Pearson product-moment coefficient of correlation of $-.70$ among 46 normal subjects ranging in age from the third to seventh decade. A greater degree of variability, and therefore a somewhat lower coefficient ($r = -.42$) was found among 14 subjects ranging in age from about 45 to 69 who showed evidence of risk factors for developing strokes.

Organs of the body are organized in a hierarchial fashion with respect to priority in receiving adequate blood supply. The brain, the heart, and the kidneys receive adequate perfusion even when other organs and skeletal muscles have an inadequate supply of blood. In addition, the brain receives a constant supply of about 1,000 ml per minute of the 5,000 ml supplied by the heart. This amount of blood to the brain remains constant regardless of extreme variations in cardiac output that may accompany exercise, anger, excitement, fright, or other conditions. In addition, the blood supply to the brain remains essentially constant regardless of gravitational changes that may occur during changes in bodily position and posture. This ability of the brain to adjust to varying circumstances and maintain its constant blood supply is called **autoregulation**.

Autoregulation is made possible by a number of mechanisms. The carotid arteries contract or dilate through muscular function in response to cardiac output and help to maintain constant blood flow. Biochemical and neurogenic mechanisms also play a role. Neurotransmitters, especially peptides, are probably also of significance in regulation of cerebral circulation. The cerebral arterioles are extremely sensitive to variations in carbon dioxide content of the blood and an increase in $CO_2$ may increase cerebral blood flow by as much as 50%; exhalation of $CO_2$ in excessive quantities may reduce blood flow by as much as 75%. Certain abnormal conditions may also impair respiratory mechanics, including extreme obesity, musculoskeletal diseases, and pulmonary diseases such as emphysema. When the volume of blood within the intracranial arteries and veins deviates from its normal level of about 100 ml, a corresponding adjustment in volume of cerebral spinal fluid occurs. An adjustment of this kind is necessary because the skull, surrounding the brain, is not compressible and some type of fluid volume balance is necessary to avoid increases or decreases in intracranial pressure. However, increases in intracranial pressure due to pathologic factors may cause decreases in cerebral blood content.

The anterior, middle, and posterior cerebral arteries interconnect in their terminal branches (leptomeningeal anasotomoses) and this extensive network of small arteries over the surface of the brain sends off arteries and arterioles that penetrate the brain and form capillary networks which nourish the gray and white matter. The muscle tone of these small peripheral arteries controls the arteriole blood pressure and represents one end of the system with respect to autoregulation of cerebral blood flow. The other end of the system is represented by contractions of the heart which provide the pumping force for initial circulation of blood. The capillary network is much more dense in the gray matter than the white matter. The gray matter receives three to five times as much blood and five to seven times as much oxygen as the white matter. The cell bodies (gray matter) have a higher metabolic rate than the axons and dendrites which constitute the bulk of the white matter.

A number of methods have been developed for measuring cerebral blood flow and cerebral metabolism. Kety and Schmidt (1948) devised a method utilizing nitrous oxide. A predetermined amount of nitrous oxide was inhaled by the subject, measured in venous blood at the jugular bulb, and compared with the amount of nitrous oxide in a peripheral artery. This comparison reflected the concentration of nitrous oxide in the carotid and vertebral arteries and served as a basis for calculating cerebral blood flow based on the relative differences. The differences in oxygen in arterial as compared with venous blood also provided a measure of cerebral metabolic rate of oxygen, taking into account a known and constant cerebral blood flow.

Lassen and Ingvar (1961) describe a procedure for measuring regional cerebral blood flow referred to as the *intra-arterial Xenon-133 method*. Either Xenon-133 or Krypton-87 (diffusible gamma-emitting gases) is injected into the internal carotid artery and the uptake and rate of clearance of radioactivity from the brain are monitored by a large number of detectors applied to the scalp. This procedure, done in conjunction with cerebral arteriography, is more accurate for measuring cortical cerebral blood flow rather than blood flow involving deeper brain structures.

Obrist, Thompson, Wang, and Wilkinson (1975) developed a technique for measuring cerebral blood flow using inhalation of Xenon-133. This method can determine the cerebral blood flow of both hemispheres simultaneously and has the advantage of being noninvasive and repeatable. Determination of regional blood flow continues to be a valuable technique in persons who have suffered cerebral infarcts, often showing areas of abnormalities even when computed tomography of the head is within normal limits. Computed tomography, however, has been studied with respect to cerebral blood flow by injecting a contrast medium that is carried by the blood. The distribution and density of the contrast medium is determined, but the measure principally derived is one of the time required for blood to flow through the brain. This procedure requires that numerous x-rays (brain "slices") be taken and the large dose of radiation is a disadvantage. In addition, the large doses of Xenon which are required may alter the normal cerebral circulation.

Positron emission tomography (PET) has also been studied with relation to estimating cerebral blood flow. The image provided by this procedure can be used to estimate regional cerebral blood flow as well as metabolism. However, PET scanning requires the availability of a cyclotron, a scanner, and an experienced and highly skilled team.

Nuclear magnetic resonance (NMR) appears to produce somewhat better imaging of white versus gray matter than is possible with computed tomography. This procedure is not invasive and does not require radiation. A magnetic field is applied to tissue which causes neutrons (atomic nuclei with an odd number of protons) to align their axis of rotation with the magnetic force. When the magnetic force is discontinued, the atoms return to their original position and emit energy. Tomographic computing permits an image to be formed. In addition to images of regional cerebral blood flow, brain water and inorganic substances which reflect metabolic activity may also be imaged.

Finally, it should be noted that drugs can affect cerebral circulation. The mechanisms include a direct effect on cerebral blood vessels or their innervation, effects on cerebral metabolism, and alteration of systemic blood pressure or respiration. General anesthetics and narcotics nearly always cause depression of cerebral metabolism and a decrease in blood flow. In moderate amounts ethyl alcohol appears to have no effect but severe intoxication leads to a decrease in cerebral blood flow. Lysergic acid diethylamide (LSD) appears to change neither cerebral metabolism or blood flow. Amphetamine, on the other hand, increases both cerebral metabolism and blood flow as does papaverine, a change that lasts for a few minutes.

# THE TELENCEPHALON

The **telencephalon** includes the cerebral cortex, corpus striatum and medullary center. The convoluted gray **cortex** (pallium) comprises about 40% of the weight of the human brain. The **corpus striatum** is a large mass of gray matter with motor functions situated near the base of each hemisphere. It consists of the caudate and lentiform nuclei. The **medullary center** of the hemisphere consists of white fibers which connect cortical areas of the same hemisphere, cortical areas of the two hemispheres, and the cortex with various subcortical centers.

The brain is the greatly modified and enlarged anterior portion of the CNS. The human brain is a relatively small structure, weighing about 1400 gm and constituting about 2% of the total body weight.

## THE MENINGES

The brain is surrounded by three tissue membranes (meninges) which provide additional protection for the central nervous system. The three layers enveloping the brain are (1) the dura mater; (2) the arachnoid; and (3) the pia mater. Fig. 2–15 illustrates the location of the meninges and their relationship to the surrounding structures.

The dura mater is attached to the **periosteum**, the internal surface of the bones enclosing the cranial cavity. The periosteum consists of collagenous connective tissue and contains the meningeal arteries, which supply blood to the underlying bone. The **middle meningeal artery** is the largest of these vessels. A fracture in the temporal region of the skull may tear a branch of the middle meningeal artery; the extravasated blood accumulates between the bone and the periosteum and forms an epidural hematoma.

The outermost layer of tissue surrounding the brain is the **dura mater** or pachymeninx (thick membrane). It extends downward to the level of the second sacral vertebra, where it ends as a blind sac. The dura mater is actually composed of two layers: (1) the outer or *periosteal* layer, which is the connective tissue of the skull bone; and (2) the inner or *meningeal* layer, which folds into a partition in several regions of the skull. The potential space between the two layers is called the **epidural layer**.

In a sagittal plane, four membranes formed by the folds of the dura mater can be identified: (1) the *falx cerebri*, the partition between the cerebral hemispheres in the midline; (2) the *falx cerebelli*, the division between the cerebellar hemispheres; (3) the *tentorium cerebelli*, located within the transverse fissure and separating the occipital lobe and the cerebellum; and (4) the *diaphragma sellae*, forming the roof of the sella turcica and separating the pituitary gland from the hypothalamus and the optic chiasm. The diaphragma sella contains an aperture for the infundibulum. Fig. 2–17 illustrates the membranes created by folds of dura.

The dura mater receives its blood supply from the small blood vessels of the periosteum. The smooth inner surface of the dura mater consists of simple squamous epithelial cells. A thin film of fluid occupies the potential **subdural space** between the dura and arachnoid. Because the cerebral veins crossing the subdural space have little supporting structure, they are most vulnerable to injury. Blood which accumulates here (secondary to cranial injury) is known as a *subdural hematoma*; it has no means of escaping and is trapped in the cranial vault.

The cranial dura mater has a plentiful supply of sensory nerve fibers, primarily from the trigeminal nerve (V). Most of these fibers terminate as nonencapsulated endings and are significant in certain types of headache. The dura lining the anterior cranial fossa is supplied by ethmoid branches of the ophthalmic division of the trigeminal nerve. Recurrent meningeal branches of the vagus nerve (X) innervate the posterior cranial fossa.

The veins draining the brain empty into the venous sinuses of the dura mater, from which blood flows into the internal jugular veins. The walls of the sinuses consist of dura mater and periosteum, lined by endothelium. The dural venous sinuses have been

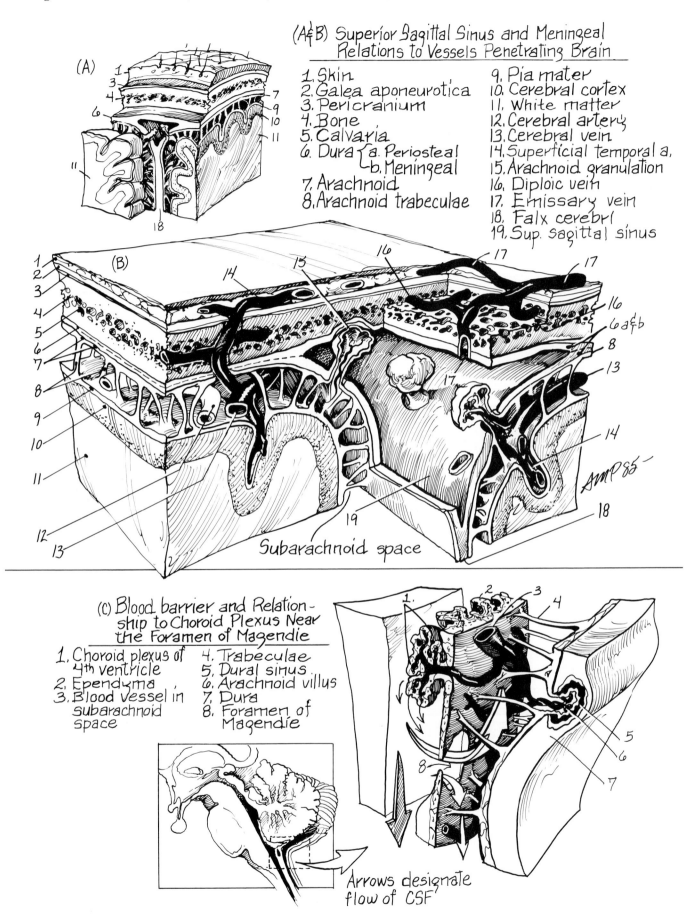

**Fig. 2-15.** *Detail of dura mater, arachnoid and pia mater and surrounding structures.*

(A)

**(A&B) Superior Sagittal Sinus and Meningeal Relations to Vessels Penetrating Brain**

1. Skin
2. Galea aponeurotica
3. Pericranium
4. Bone
5. Calvaria
6. Dura {a. Periosteal b. Meningeal
7. Arachnoid
8. Arachnoid trabeculae
9. Pia mater
10. Cerebral cortex
11. White matter
12. Cerebral artery
13. Cerebral vein
14. Superficial temporal a.
15. Arachnoid granulation
16. Diploic vein
17. Emissary vein
18. Falx cerebri
19. Sup. sagittal sinus

(B)

AMP 85

Subarachnoid space

**(c) Blood barrier and Relationship to Choroid Plexus Near the Foramen of Magendie**

1. Choroid plexus of 4th ventricle
2. Ependyma
3. Blood vessel in subarachnoid space
4. Trabeculae
5. Dural sinus
6. Arachnoid villus
7. Dura
8. Foramen of Magendie

Arrows designate flow of CSF

**Fig. 2-16.** *Detail of Foramen of Magendie, showing route of CSF.*

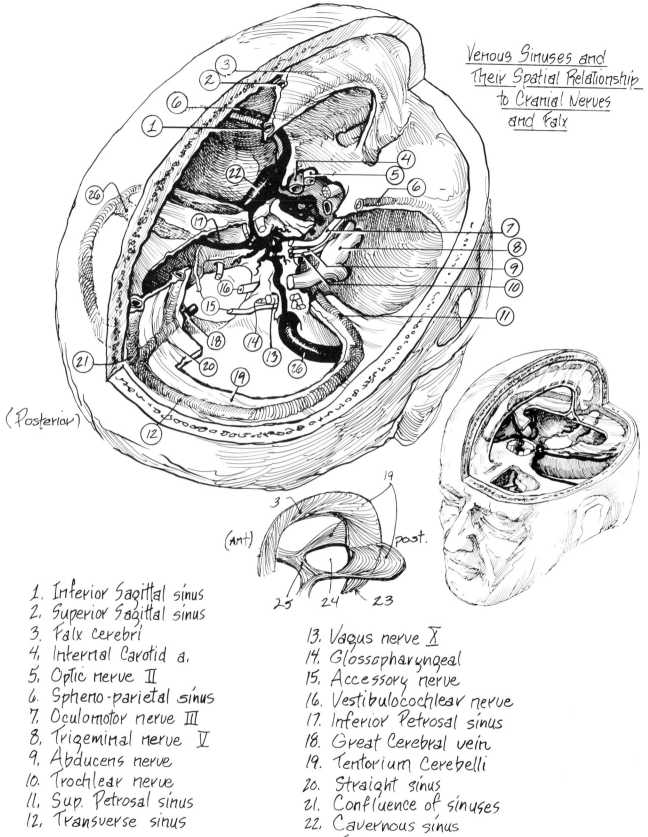

Venous Sinuses and Their Spatial Relationship to Cranial Nerves and Falx

(Posterior)

(Ant)

post.

Fig. 2-17. View from above. A large portion of the tentorium has been removed to expose the dura mater and its sinuses.

1. Inferior Sagittal sinus
2. Superior Sagittal sinus
3. Falx cerebri
4. Internal Carotid a.
5. Optic nerve II
6. Spheno-parietal sinus
7. Oculomotor nerve III
8. Trigeminal nerve V
9. Abducens nerve
10. Trochlear nerve
11. Sup. Petrosal sinus
12. Transverse sinus

13. Vagus nerve X
14. Glossopharyngeal
15. Accessory nerve
16. Vestibulocochlear nerve
17. Inferior Petrosal sinus
18. Great Cerebral vein
19. Tentorium Cerebelli
20. Straight sinus
21. Confluence of sinuses
22. Cavernous sinus
23. Falx cerebelli
24. Tentorial notch
25. Diaphragma sellae
26. Sigmoid sinus

described in more detail in another chapter of this book.

The dura mater has been used as a homograft in various conditions: the repair of thoracic wall and diaphragm defect, correction of transposition of the great arteries, and as a tracheal prosthesis. Cardiac heart valves constructed of homologous dura mater have been used for the correction of acquired or congenital valvular disease (Pansky & Allen, 1980).

The avascular **arachnoid** is a thin layer of meninges separated from the dura mater by a film of fluid in the potential subdural space; it is separated from the underlying pia mater by the **subarachnoid space**, which contains cerebrospinal fluid. The **arachnoid villi**, projections of the arachnoid tissue which extend through the dura into the superior sagittal sinus, absorb CSF and drain into the venous sinuses. These villi begin to appear at about the age of seven years and increase in size and number until adulthood. The arachnoid villi become hypertrophied with age, at which point they are called **arachnoid granulations** or **pacchionian bodies**. They may become sufficiently large to produce erosion or pitting of the cranial bones.

The **pia mater**, a membrane containing a network of small blood vessels, adheres to the surface of the brain. The larger arteries and veins entering and leaving the substance of the brain are surrounded by a sleeve of pia mater. The pia mater may serve as a barrier to harmful substances and organisms. The arachnoid membrane and pia mater are collectively referred to as the **leptomeninges**. An infectious disease of the nervous system that involves the meninges is called **meningitis**.

## THE CEREBRAL HEMISPHERES

The cerebrum is divided into left and right hemispheres. The two cerebral hemispheres make up the largest part of the brain and are partially separated from each other by the deep **longitudinal cerebral fissure**. As noted previously, the **falx cerebri**, a crescent-shaped double fold of dura mater, projects into the longitudinal cerebral fissure. Its anterior portion is often fenestrated.

The separation of the cerebral hemispheres is complete in the frontal and occipital regions; in the central region the fissure extends only to the **corpus callosum**, an extensive collection of nerve fibers which crosses the longitudinal cerebral fissure (Figs. 2–18 and 2–19). The corpus callosum is a major interhemispheric pathway connecting the cortex on one side with its corresponding or homologous area on the other side. The number of fibers in the corpus callosum has been estimated to be about 300 million.

The corpus callosum has four parts: (1) the **rostrum**; (2) the **genu**; (3) **the body**; and (4) the **splenium**. The genu contains fibers interconnecting rostral parts of the frontal lobes; the body contains fibers from the remaining parts of the frontal lobes and the parietal lobe. Fibers transversing the splenium relate regions of the temporal and occipital lobes. The splenium is reported to be generally larger in females than in males.

The numerous folds of the cerebral hemispheres substantially increase the surface area and therefore the volume of the cerebral cortex. The outer surface of the cerebral hemispheres contains many grooves or clefts, known as **sulci**. About two-thirds of the cortex forms the walls of the sulci and is therefore hidden from surface view. The elevated ridged portions of brain lying between the sulci are called convolutions, or **gyri**. The deeper grooves between some gyri are sometimes referred to as **fissures**. Some gyri are relatively constant in their location; others show a considerable variation. Fig. 2–20 shows the major sulci and gyri of the cerebral hemispheres.

The **lateral cerebral fissure** (fissure of Sylvius) separates the temporal from the frontal lobe. Caudally this fissure separates portions of the parietal and temporal lobes. The Sylvian fissure divides into three branches: (1) the *anterior horizontal ramus*, which ascends into the inferior frontal gyrus; (2) the *anterior ascending ramus*, which also ascends into the inferior frontal gyrus farther posteriorly; and (3) the *posterior ramus* (terminal ascending ramus), the main part of the lateral fissure, which continues backward and upward to terminate in the parietal lobe. The anterior

# Corpus Callosum and Surrounding Structures

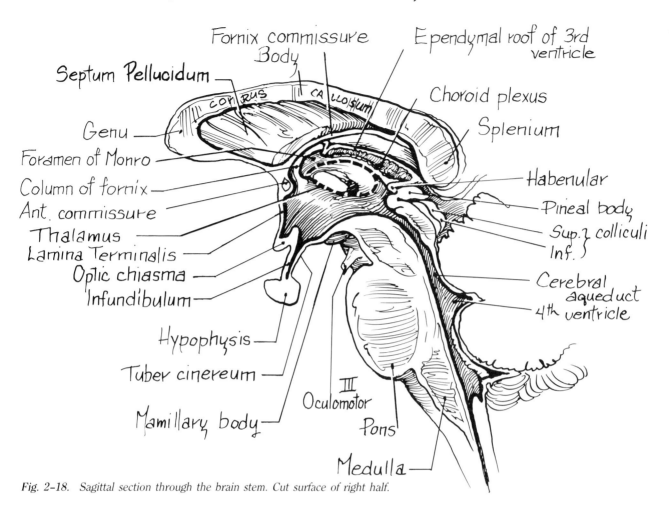

Fornix commissure
Body

Ependymal roof of 3rd ventricle

Septum Pellucidum

Choroid plexus

Splenium

Genu

CORPUS CALLOSUM

Foramen of Monro

Column of fornix

Ant. commissure

Thalamus

Lamina Terminalis

Optic chiasma

Infundibulum

Habenular

Pineal body

Sup. } colliculi

Inf. }

Cerebral aqueduct

4th ventricle

Hypophysis

Tuber cinereum

Mamillary body

III

Oculomotor

Pons

Medulla

**Fig. 2-18.** *Sagittal section through the brain stem. Cut surface of right half.*

1. Thalamus
2. Inf. horn of lat. ventricle
3. Hippocampus
4. Fimbria
5. Sup. colliculus
6. Inf. colliculus
7. Cerebellum
8. Column of fornix
9. Choroid plexus of lat. ventricle
10. Post. commissure
11. Pineal gland
12. Head of caudate nucleus
13. Corpus callosum
14. Septum pellucidum

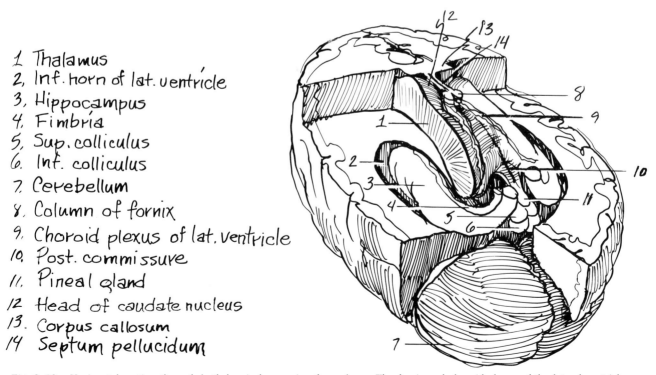

**Fig. 2-19.** *Horizontal section through both hemispheres, view from above. The fornix and choroid plexus of the lateral ventricles have been exposed.*

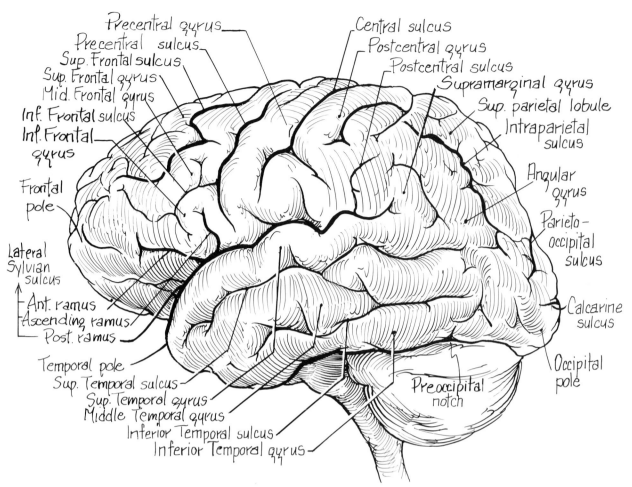

Precentral gyrus
Precentral sulcus
Sup. Frontal sulcus
Sup. Frontal gyrus
Mid. Frontal gyrus
Inf. Frontal sulcus
Inf. Frontal gyrus
Frontal pole
Lateral Sylvian sulcus
Ant. ramus
Ascending ramus
Post. ramus
Temporal pole
Sup. Temporal sulcus
Sup. Temporal gyrus
Middle Temporal gyrus
Inferior Temporal sulcus
Inferior Temporal gyrus
Central sulcus
Postcentral gyrus
Postcentral sulcus
Supramarginal gyrus
Sup. parietal lobule
Intraparietal sulcus
Angular gyrus
Parieto-occipital sulcus
Calcarine sulcus
Occipital pole
Preoccipital notch

**Fig. 2-20.** *Gyri and sulci of the left cerebral hemisphere, lateral view.*

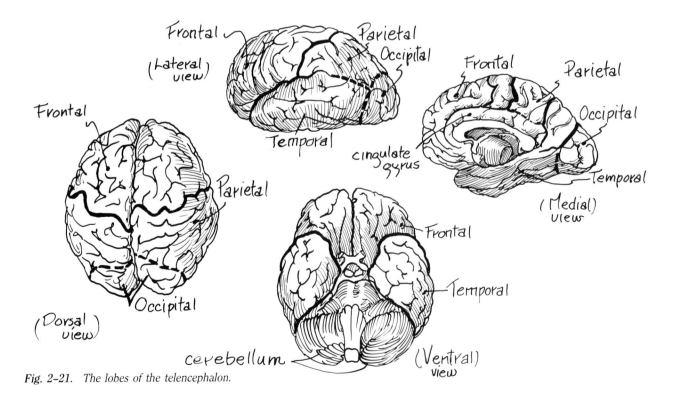

Frontal
(Lateral view)
Parietal
Occipital
Temporal
Frontal
Parietal
Occipital
cingulate gyrus
Temporal
(Medial) view
Frontal
Parietal
Occipital
(Dorsal) view
Frontal
Temporal
cerebellum
(Ventral) view

**Fig. 2-21.** *The lobes of the telencephalon.*

and ascending rami each measure about 2.5 cm; the posterior ramus is about 7.5 cm long.

The **central sulcus (fissure of Rolando)** separates the frontal and parietal lobes. It arises about the middle of the hemisphere, beginning near the longitudinal cerebral fissure and extends downward and forward to about 2.5 cm above the lateral cerebral fissure. This sulcus is an important landmark for the sensori-motor cortex because the general sensory area is immediately behind the sulcus and the motor area is directly in front of it. The central sulcus is about 2 cm deep; therefore, its walls constitute much of the sensorimotor cortex.

The **parieto-occipital fissure** passes along the medial surface of the posterior portion of the cerebral hemisphere, runs downward and forward as a deep cleft with much buried cortex, and joins the calcarine fissure.

The **calcarine fissure** begins on the medial surface, near the occipital pole, and extends forward to an area slightly below the splenium of the corpus callosum. The calcarine fissure is an important landmark for the visual cortex, most of which lies in the walls of the fissure.

The **cingulate sulcus** begins below the anterior end of the corpus callosum on the medial surface of the hemisphere, continues parallel to the corpus callosum, and finally curves up to the superior medial border a short distance behind the upper end of the central sulcus.

The **circular sulcus** (circuminsular fissure) surrounds the **insula**, or island of Reil and separates it from the adjacent frontal, parietal and temporal lobes.

The **septum pellucidum**, situated between the fornix and the corpus callosum, is a thin-walled structure containing scattered groups of neurons which separates the frontal horns of the lateral ventricles. It is composed of two thin sheets of tissue, which are sometimes separated by a space — the cavity of the septum pellucidum (cavum septi pellucidi) — which does not communicate with the ventricular system or the subarachnoid space.

## Main Divisions of the Cerebrum

Various sulci subdivide each cerebral hemisphere into four lobes: (1) frontal; (2) parietal; (3) occipital; and (4) temporal (Fig. 2–21). The lobes are named for the bones of the skull overlying them. Occasionally the insular and limbic lobes are included in this category; however, neither the limbic nor the insula is a true lobe. The **insula** is a cortical area buried in the lateral sulcus. The **limbic lobe** is a synthetic lobe on the medial aspect of the hemisphere consisting of portions of the frontal, parietal, occipital and temporal lobes which surround the upper part of the brain stem.

**Frontal Lobe.** The frontal lobe is the largest of all the lobes of the brain and comprises about one-third of the hemispheric surface. It extends from the frontal pole to the central sulcus (fissure of Rolando) behind and the lateral fissure at the side. The convexity of the frontal lobe has four principal gyri: (1) precentral; (2) superior frontal; (3) middle frontal; and (4) inferior frontal. The **precentral gyrus** passes anterior and parallel to the central sulcus. It is also referred to as the *motor cortex* and contains neurons whose axons give rise to corticospinal and corticobulbar (brainstem) tracts.

The **superior** and **middle frontal gyri**, located in front of the precentral gyrus, are concerned with control of body and eye movements. The **inferior frontal gyrus** includes *Broca's area*, a part of the brain which has been identified as being important in speech production.

The **orbital sulci and gyri** of the frontal lobe are located on the inferior surface of the hemisphere. It is believed that they give rise to pathways important in the expression of emotion. The **olfactory sulcus** lies beneath the olfactory tract on the orbital surface; lying medial to it is the gyrus rectus or **straight gyrus**.

**Parietal Lobe.** The parietal lobe extends from central sulcus to the parieto-occipital fissure and laterally to the level of the lateral cerebral fissure. There are two major sulci in the parietal lobe: (1) the **postcentral sulcus**, which extends behind and parallel to the lateral (Rolandic) fissure and consists of a superior and an inferior portion; and (2) the **inter-parietal sulcus**, a horizontal groove that sometimes unites with the postcentral sulcus. The **postcentral gyrus**, located between the central sulcus and the interparietal sulcus, is concerned with the appreciation of touch (*somesthesis*), the sense of position of the extremities (*kinesthesis*), vibratory sense, and other fine tactile discriminatory processes. For this reason it is frequently called the *sensory cortex*. The **superior parietal lobule** lies above the horizontal portion of the interparietal sulcus and the **inferior parietal lobule** lies below. They are important in the synthetic aspects of multiple sensory experiences brought to consciousness.

The supramarginal gyrus and angular gyrus are subdivisions of the inferior parietal lobule. The **supramarginal gyrus** arches above the ascending end of the posterior ramus of the lateral cerebral fissure. The **angular gyrus** arches above the end of the superior temporal sulcus and becomes continuous with the middle temporal gyrus. These gyri are concerned with the reception and organization of language functions.

**Occipital Lobe.** The occipital lobe is the pyramid-shaped posterior lobe situated behind the parieto-occipital sulcus. The **lateral occipital sulcus** extends transversely along the lateral surface, dividing the occipital lobe into a **superior** and **inferior gyrus**. The **calcarine sulcus** extends from the occipital pole to the splenium of the corpus callosum. The wedge-shaped region between the calcarine and parieto-occipital sulci and the paracentral lobule is the **precuneus**. Specialized neurons which receive visual information are located in the occipital lobe.

**Temporal Lobe.** The temporal lobe lies inferior to the lateral cerebral (Sylvian) fissure and extends back to the level of the parieto-occipital fissure. The **superior temporal sulcus** extends across the temporal lobe parallel to the lateral cerebral fissure. The **middle temporal sulcus** runs parallel to the superior temporal sulcus at a lower level. The **superior temporal gyrus** is the part of the lateral surface of the temporal lobe between the lateral cerebral fissure and the superior temporal sulcus. The **middle temporal gyrus** lies

between the superior and middle temporal sulci. The **inferior temporal gyrus** is below the middle temporal sulcus and extends posteriorly to connect with the inferior occipital gyrus.

The **transverse temporal gyri** (Heschl's gyri) occupy the posterior part of the superior temporal surface (the inferior border of the lateral cerebral fissure). These gyri constitute the *primary auditory cortex*. The **inferior temporal sulcus** extends along the inferior surface of the temporal lobe from the temporal pole in front to the occipital pole behind.

The anterior part of the temporal lobe has been referred to as the *psychic cortex*. When this area is electrically stimulated in a person who is conscious, there may be recall of music that has been heard, objects or places that have been seen or other experiences that occurred in the recent or distant past. A tumor in the temporal lobe may produce auditory or visual hallucinations that reproduce previous events.

**Insula.** The **insula** (island of Reil) is sometimes referred to as the *central lobe*. It is ovoid in shape and lies deep within the lateral cerebral fissure. As shown in Fig. 2–22, it can be exposed by separating the temporal and frontal lobes. The deep **circular sulcus** surrounds the insula. Several **short gyri**, formed by shallow sulci, occupy the anterior portion of the insula; a **long gyrus** occupies the posterior part. The **central sulcus** of the insula, which is approximately parallel to the central sulcus of the cerebrum, divides the insula surface into various posterior parts.

Angevine and Cotman (1981) report that stimulation of the human insula indicates that intra-abdominal sensation is represented here, along with some representation of visceral motility. They note, however, that the insula's concealed position and overlying vasculature (middle cerebral artery) greatly limit surgical exploration of this region.

## HISTOLOGY OF THE CEREBRAL CORTEX

**Types of Cortical Neurons.** Each cerebral hemisphere has a layer of gray matter, known as the **cortex** or **pallium**, which covers the white matter. The adult brain has approximately 1200 sq cm of cortex

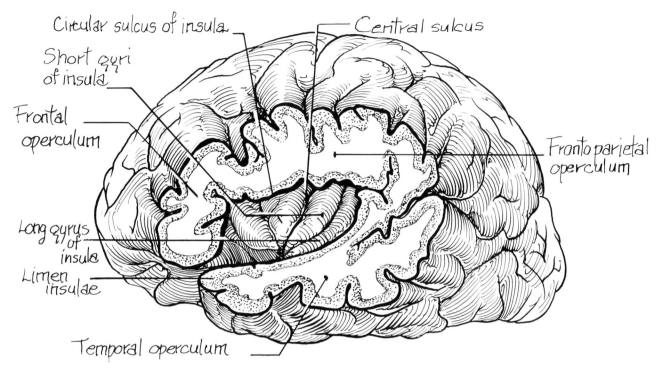

Circular sulcus of insula

Central sulcus

Short gyri of insula

Frontal operculum

Frontoparietal operculum

Long gyrus of insula

Limen insulae

Temporal operculum

Fig. 2–22. *Left hemisphere, lateral view. Portions of the frontal, parietal and temporal lobes have been removed to expose the insula.*

1. Corpus callosum
2. Head of caudate nucleus
3. Frontal horn of Lateral ventricle
4. External capsule
5. Insula
6. Claustrum
7. Internal capsule
8. Tail of caudate nucleus
9. Thalamus
10. Putamen
11. Globus pallidus

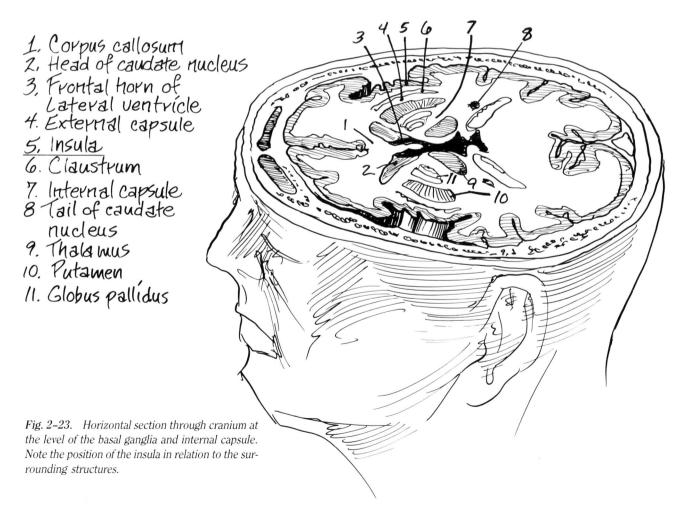

Fig. 2–23. *Horizontal section through cranium at the level of the basal ganglia and internal capsule. Note the position of the insula in relation to the surrounding structures.*

in each hemisphere. The cortex has a characteristic structure that consists of nerve cells and nerve fibers arranged in six layers and vertical columns (*see* Fig. 2–24). Except for the horizontal cells in layer I, most of the estimated 14 billion cortical neurons relay their activity in a vertical manner. The vertical cell axons and dendrites are arranged within the cortex in columns of neurons that have similar properties. In the sensory cortex, neurons within an individual column respond to the same stimulus. In the motor cortex, the activity of the neurons in a column is related to the activity of a single muscle or muscle group. A rich vascular supply and relative absence of myelinated nerve fibers give the cortex its characteristic gray appearance.

There are three types of cortical neurons, named according to the nature of their connection: (1) projection neurons; (2) association neurons; and (3) commissural neurons.

**Projection (efferent) neurons** transmit impulses from the cortex to a subcortical center, such as the thalamus, the corpus striatum, the brain stem or the spinal cord. These neurons originate from the giant pyramidal (Betz) cells in layer V or from spindle-shaped cells in layer IV.

**Association neurons** are small pyramidal cells which establish connections with other cortical nerve cells in the same hemisphere. They are found in the deep parts of layer III or in the superficial parts of layer V. They include the vast number of interneurons whose short axons do not leave the cortex, thereby providing for complex intracortical circuits. Axons of the remaining association neurons enter the white matter and terminate in another cortical area of the same hemisphere.

Axons of **commissural neurons** proceed to the homologous cortex of the opposite hemisphere. Most of the commissural fibers constitute the corpus callosum; a relatively small number connect cortical areas of the temporal lobes through the anterior commissure.

Classified on the basis of size and shape, five types of morphological variations among the cortical neurons can be established: (1) pyramidal cells; (2) stellate cells; (3) fusiform cells; (4) cells of Martinotti; and (5) horizontal cells of Cajal.

**Pyramidal cells** are the most numerous type of cell in the cortex. They derive their name from the triangular shape of their cell bodies. One type of pyramidal cell, the giant Betz cell, is found in the primary motor area of the frontal lobe (area 4). The pyramidal cell has an apical dendrite directed toward the surface of the cortex and several lateral dendrites. The dendritic branches bear large numbers of spines that make synaptic contact with axons of other neurons. The length of the axon, which arises from the base of the cell body or from one of the lateral dendrites, depends on the size of the cell.

**Stellate cells**, also known as granule cells, are polygonal or star-shaped. They have several short dendrites and the axon terminates on a neuron nearby. These cells are present in all cortical layers, but most numerous in layer IV and the primary sensory areas (areas 1, 2, 3, 17 and 41).

**Fusiform** or **polymorphic multiform cells** are located in the deepest cortical layer. The long axis of the cell body is perpendicular to the surface of the cortex. They are usually spindle-shaped but show a wide variation in their morphology. A dendrite extends from each end of the cell body; the deep dendrite is short, whereas the other one reaches into more superficial layers of the cortex. The axon enters the white matter as a projection, association or commissural fiber. The remaining cell types are intracortical association neurons.

**Cells of Martinotti** (ascending axon cells) are present throughout the cortex except in the most superficial (molecular) layer. Short dendrites arise from the small, polygonal cell body. The identifying feature of the cell of Martinotti is that the axon is directed toward the surface and ends in a more superficial layer, preferentially the external layer.

**Horizontal cells of Cajal** are restricted to the surface (molecular) layer. They are small neurons with fusiform cell bodies with large nuclei and scant cytoplasm. Horizontal cells have a dendrite extending

# Human Cerebral Cortex

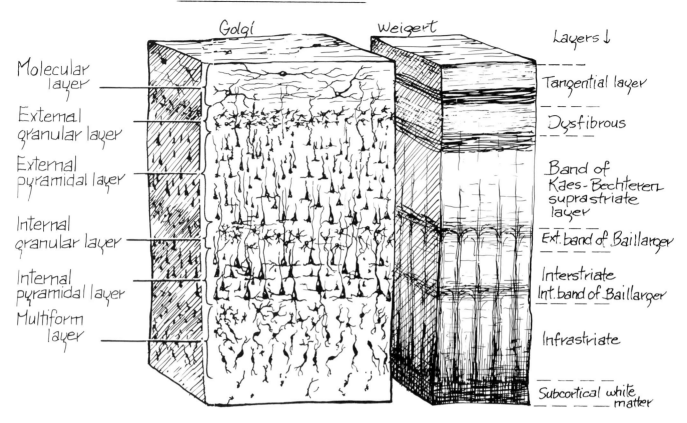

Golgi    Weigert    Layers ↓

Molecular layer — Tangential layer

External granular layer — Dysfibrous

External pyramidal layer — Band of Kaes-Bechterew suprastriate layer

Internal granular layer — Ext. band of Baillarger

Internal pyramidal layer — Interstriate Int. band of Baillarger

Multiform layer — Infrastriate

Subcortical white matter

# Cerebral Nerve Cells (cortex)

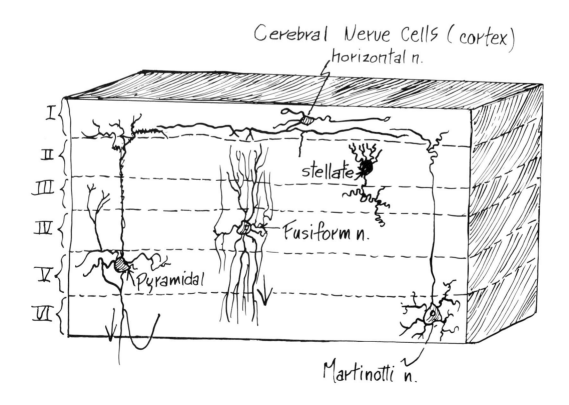

horizontal n.

I
II
III
IV
V
VI

stellate

Fusiform n.

Pyramidal

Martinotti n.

*Fig. 2-24.* *Histology of the cerebral cortex, showing the six layers and types of cortical neurons.*

from each end. The axon, which runs tangentially to the cortical surface, makes synaptic contact with branches of the apical dendrites of pyramidal neurons.

**Cortical Histology.** The thickness of the cortex varies from 4.5 mm in the primary motor area of the frontal lobe to 1.5 mm in the visual area of the occipital lobe. The cortex is generally thicker over the crest of a gyrus than in the depths of a sulcus. Six cell layers can be differentiated in the cortex: (I) molecular layer; (II) external granular layer; (III) external pyramidal layer; (IV) internal granular layer; (V) internal pyramidal layer; and (VI) multiform layer. These layers differ in the density of cell population and in the size and shape of constituent neurons. Histologic information about cortical nerve cells is obtained by using the *Golgi method*, which illustrates the neuronal relationships and their axonal and dendritic arborizations, and the *Weigert method*, which shows the course and distribution of myelin fibers.

I. The **molecular layer** (plexiform layer) is the superficial layer and consists predominantly of delicate neuronal processes, both dendrites and axons. Most of the dendritic branches come from pyramidal cells. The axons originate in cortex elsewhere in the same hemisphere, in that of the opposite hemisphere, and in the thalamus. Cells of Martinotti in any deeper layer also contribute axons to layer I. The infrequent horizontal cells of Cajal and scattered stellate cells intervene between some axons and dendrites. The molecular layer is essentially an important synaptic field of the cortex.

II. The **external granular layer** contains many densely packed neurons, both small pyramidal cells and stellate cells. The dendrites of many of these cells extend into the molecular layer; most of the axons terminate in deeper layers, and the remainder enter the medullary center. The external granular layer makes an important contribution to the complexity of intracortical circuits.

III. The **external pyramidal layer** contains neurons which are typical pyramidal cells that increase in size from the external to the internal borders of the layer. Apical dendrites extend into the synaptic field of layer

I; axons of the pyramidal cells enter the white matter and proceed to their destinations as projection, association, or commissural fibers.

Because layers I, II, and III have numerous stellate cells, it has been suggested that these three layers are important for association and higher functions such as memory, interpretation of sensory input and certain discriminative functions (Pansky & Allen, 1980).

IV. The **internal granular layer** consists of closely arranged stellate cells, many of which receive stimuli from fibers originating in the thalamus. It is a high density cell layer. The short axons of the stellate cells usually remain within layer IV and synapse with dendrites passing through the layer from cells in layers V and VI, with other stellate cells, and with cells of Martinotti. The internal granular layer is primarily a receptive layer. A large number of horizontal, myelinated nerve fibers (*external band of Baillarger*) from the thalamus end in this layer. Lateral geniculate fibers terminate primarily in this layer of area 17, where the prominent external band of Baillarger is called the *stripe of Gennari*.

V. The **internal pyramidal (ganglion) layer** contains medium- and large-sized pyramidal cells intermingled with scattered stellate cells and cells of Martinotti. The giant pyramidal cells (Betz cells) in the primary motor area of the cortex in the frontal lobe are situated in layer V. The internal pyramidal layer is primarily an efferent layer. Axons of pyramidal cells descend into white matter mainly as projection fibers. The *internal band of Baillarger* is formed by horizontal myelinated fibers in the deeper part of this layer.

VI. In the **multiform (fusiform) layer** there is a predominance of fusiform cells. A variety of stellate and small pyramidal cells are also present. Axons of the neurons in this layer are included among the projection, commissural, and association fibers in the white matter of the hemisphere. Like layer IV, the multiform layer is the origin of many cortical efferent fibers. All fibers entering or leaving the cortex must pervade this layer.

# THE CORPUS STRIATUM

The **corpus striatum** is a collection of gray matter located at the base of each cerebral hemisphere. During early development the corpus striatum is a single gray mass, but later becomes separated by the fibers of the internal capsule into two distinct cellular masses, the caudate nucleus and the lenticular nucleus. The lenticular nucleus is further divided into the putamen and globus pallidus. Figs. 2–25 to 2–27 show the locations of the various structures described in this section. The term **basal ganglia** is often used clinically to include the corpus striatum, the subthalamic nucleus and the substantia nigra. These three nuclei are grouped together because of their importance in certain motor disturbances (dyskinesia) characterized by purposeless involuntary movements.

The head of the **caudate nucleus** forms the lateral wall of the anterior horn of the lateral ventricle. Its body overlies the lateral part of the dorsal thalamus and its tail is located above the temporal horn of the lateral ventricle. The head of the caudate nucleus and the putamen are continuous with one another through a bridge of gray matter beneath the internal capsule.

The **lenticular** or **lentiform nucleus**, which resembles a Brazil nut in size and shape, is situated between the insula, the caudate nucleus, and the thalamus. It is divided into two parts by the **external medullary lamina** (a vertical plate of white matter): the putamen and the globus pallidus.

The **putamen**, located just beneath the insular cortex, is the larger and most lateral part of the basal ganglia. It is composed primarily of small medium-sized nerve cells.

The **globus pallidus** is the smaller, median triangular zone whose numerous myelinated fibers make it appear lighter in color. It is located between the internal capsule and the putamen. The caudate nucleus sends many fibers to the globus pallidus. The putamen and globus pallidus receive some fibers from the substantia nigra and the thalamus sends fibers to the caudate nucleus.

The amygdaloid body and claustrum are sometimes included as part of the basal ganglia. The **amygdaloid body** is a small, spherical gray mass of several small nuclei located in the roof of the terminal part of the inferior horn of the lateral ventricle. It represents the tail of the caudate nucleus. The amygdalas of both cerebral hemispheres are interconnected by white commissural fibers of the anterior commissure.

The **claustrum** is a thin layer of gray substance situated just beneath the insular cortex and separated from the more median putamen by the thin lamina of white matter known as the **external capsule**. The claustrum is separated from the insula by the **extreme capsule**, a thin layer of white matter. The function of the claustrum has not definitely been established, though connections with the frontal, parietal and temporal lobes have been identified.

The **internal capsule** is a broad band of white fibers separating the lenticular nucleus from the medial caudate nucleus and thalamus. In horizontal section, it presents a "V" appearance, with the apex, or **genu**, pointing medially. The anterior limb separates the lenticular from the caudate nucleus and contains (1) *thalamocortical* and *corticothalamic fibers*, which are reciprocal connections between the lateral thalamic nucleus and the frontal lobe; (2) *frontopontine fibers* from the frontal lobe to the pontine nuclei; and (3) fibers from the caudate nucleus to the putamen.

The posterior limb of the internal capsule, located between the thalamus and the lenticular nucleus, may be divided into three parts: (1) lenticulothalamic; (2) retrolenticular; and (3) sublenticular. The anterior two-thirds of the **lenticulothalamic** portion is divided into the corticobulbar tract and the corticospinal tract. The remaining one-third is the corticorubral tract, composed of fibers from the frontal lobe cortex to the red nucleus. The **retrolenticular part** contains fibers from the lateral nucleus of the thalamus to the postcentral gyrus. The **sublenticular part**, lying below the lenticular nucleus, contains (1) parietotemporopontine fibers from the temporal and parietal lobe cortex to the pontine nuclei; (2) auditory radiations from the medial geniculate body to Heschl's gyrus (the transverse tem-

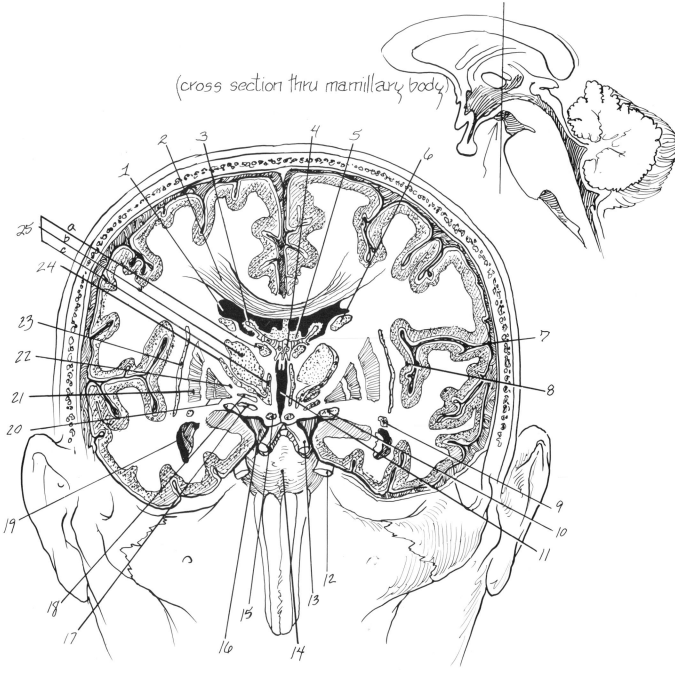

(cross section thru mamillary body)

1. Lateral ventricle
2. Corpus callosum
3. Choroid plexus
4. Tela choroidea
5. Body of fornix
6. Caudate nucleus
7. Lateral sulcus
8. Insula
9. Caudate nucleus (tail)
10. Optic tract
11. Third ventricle
12. Trigeminal nerve V
13. Oculomotor nerve III
14. Pons
15. Mamillary body
16. Crus cerebri
17. Substantia nigra
18. Subthalamic nucleus
19. Inferior horn of lat. ventricle
20. Globus pallidus
21. Putamen
22. Internal capsule
23. Claustrum
24. Reticular stratum (thalamus)
25. Thalamic nuclei ⎰ Ant. a
                    ⎱ Med. b
                      Lat. c

*Fig. 2-25. Frontal section through the cranium, illustrating the cerebrum above the cerebellar tentorium.*

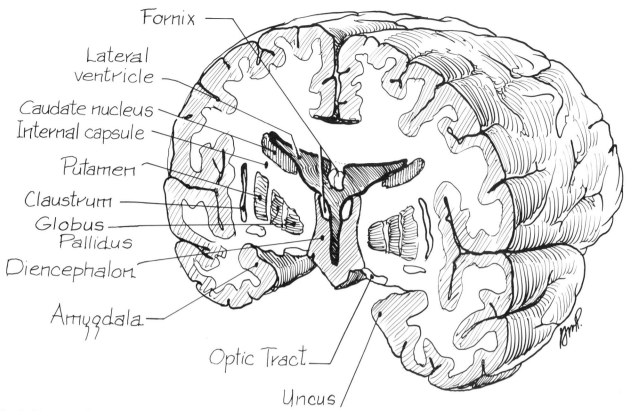

Fornix

Lateral ventricle

Caudate nucleus

Internal capsule

Putamen

Claustrum

Globus Pallidus

Diencephalon

Amygdala

Optic Tract

Uncus

Fig. 2–26. Frontal section through the telencephalon immediately behind the anterior commissure.

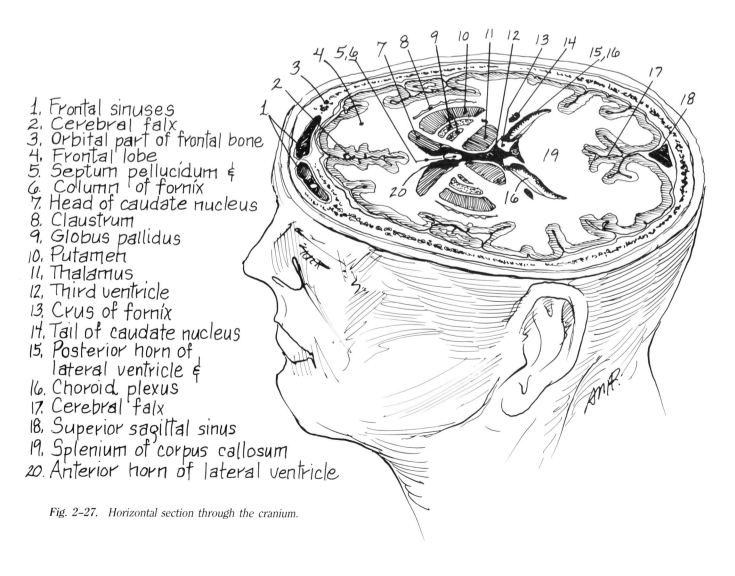

1. Frontal sinuses
2. Cerebral falx
3. Orbital part of frontal bone
4. Frontal lobe
5. Septum pellucidum &
6. Column of fornix
7. Head of caudate nucleus
8. Claustrum
9. Globus pallidus
10. Putamen
11. Thalamus
12. Third ventricle
13. Crus of fornix
14. Tail of caudate nucleus
15. Posterior horn of lateral ventricle &
16. Choroid plexus
17. Cerebral falx
18. Superior sagittal sinus
19. Splenium of corpus callosum
20. Anterior horn of lateral ventricle

Fig. 2–27. Horizontal section through the cranium.

poral gyrus); and (3) optic fibers from the lateral geniculate body to the calcarine cortex.

**Clinical Manifestations of Lesions Associated with the Corpus Striatum.** The corpus striatum is assumed to have motor functions because of the dyskinesia that results if it is involved in a pathological lesion. Several conditions have been identified with lesions of the corpus striatum: (1) Parkinson's disease; (2) Huntington's chorea; (3) Wilson's disease; (4) Sydenham's chorea (St. Vitus dance); and (5) dystonia musculorum deformans. Parkinson's disease, Huntington's chorea and Wilson's disease are described in detail in another section of this book. **Sydenham's chorea** is a disease that occurs principally in childhood. It is often associated with rheumatic fever and other infectious diseases caused by hemolytic streptococci. The disease is frequently characterized by *choreiform movements*, which are sudden, irregular and purposeless. The most common pathologic findings are scattered minute petechial lesions and capillary emboli in the corpus striatum.

**Dystonia musculorum deformans** is a condition characterized by *athetosis*. The typical signs of athetosis are slow, twisting, involuntary movements of the extremities. Sometimes referred to as "serpentine movements," they may occur at rest or during voluntary muscle movement. Dystonia musculorum deformans has been associated with lesions in the cerebral cortex, globus pallidus and thalamus.

## THE MEDULLARY CENTER

The white matter of the cerebral hemisphere constitutes the medullary center. It contains myelinated nerve fibers of many sizes running to and from all parts of the cortex as well as neuroglia. The medullary center is bounded by the cortex, the lateral ventricle, and the corpus striatum. The center of the cerebral hemisphere is composed of three types of myelinated nerves: (1) transverse fibers; (2) projection fibers; and (3) association fibers. The white matter extends from the cortex to the basal ganglia and the ventricular system. Figs. 2–28 and 2–29 show the location of the fibers in the medullary center.

**Transverse (Commissural) Fibers** interconnect the two cerebral hemispheres. The **corpus callosum** is the largest, and most of its fibers arise from various parts of one cerebral hemisphere and terminate in the corresponding area and in cortex closely related functionally with it in the opposite cerebral hemisphere. It is a broad transverse structure that forms the roof of the lateral and third ventricles. The corpus callosum measures about 10 cm long and 2.5 cm wide.

The **anterior commissure** is a band of white fibers that crosses the midline to connect the temporal lobes. It contains two parts: a rostral portion that joins both olfactory bulbs, and a remainder that connects the piriform areas of both cerebral hemispheres. The **hippocampal commissure**, or **commissure of the fornix**, joins the two hippocampi.

Afferent and efferent **projection fibers** connect the cerebral cortex with the lower portions of the brain and spinal cord. Near the upper part of the brain stem these fibers form the **internal capsule**, which is composed of two parts: the anterior limb and the posterior limb. The *anterior limb* partially separates two of the largest components of the basal ganglia; the larger and longer **posterior limb** contains fibers known as the optic radiation.

**Association fibers** are the most numerous of the fibers in the medullary center. They connect various cortical portions of the same cerebral hemisphere and are divided into long and short groups. *Short association fibers* connect adjacent gyri. Short association fibers located in the deeper portion of the cortex are known as **intracortical fibers**; those just beneath the cortex are called **subcortical fibers**. *Long association fibers* connect cortical regions in different lobes within the same hemisphere.

The **uncinate fasciculus** is a compact bundle which crosses the bottom of the lateral cerebral fissure and connects the inferior frontal lobe gyri with the anterior temporal lobe. The **cingulum**, the principal association bundle on the medial aspect of the hemisphere, is located within the white matter of the cingulate gyrus. It connects regions of the frontal and parietal lobes with the parahippocampal gyrus and adjacent temporal cortical regions.

The **arcuate fasciculus** connects the superior and middle frontal convolutions with the temporal lobe and temporal pole. The **superior longitudinal fasciculus** connects the temporal and occipital lobes and cortex of the frontal lobe, including the sensory and motor language areas of Wernicke and Broca. The **occipito-frontal fasciculus** extends backward from the frontal lobe and radiates into the temporal and occipital lobes.

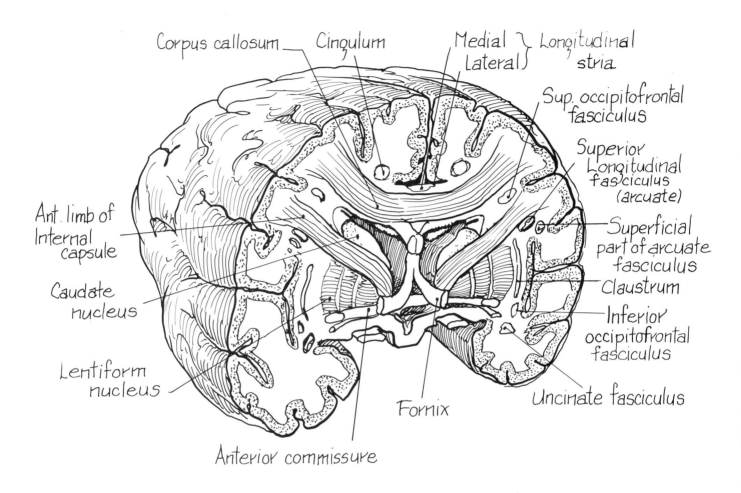

Corpus callosum    Cingulum    Medial ⎱ Longitudinal
                                Lateral ⎰  stria

Sup. occipitofrontal
      fasciculus

Superior
Longitudinal
fasciculus
(arcuate)

Ant. limb of
Internal
capsule

Superficial
part of arcuate
fasciculus

Caudate
nucleus

Claustrum

Inferior
occipitofrontal
fasciculus

Lentiform
nucleus

Uncinate fasciculus

Fornix

Anterior commissure

**Fig. 2–28.** *Coronal section through the cerebrum.*

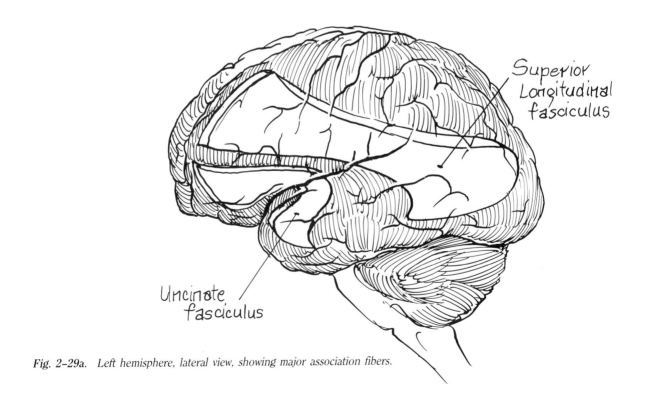

Superior
Longitudinal
fasciculus

Uncinate
fasciculus

**Fig. 2–29a.** *Left hemisphere, lateral view, showing major association fibers.*

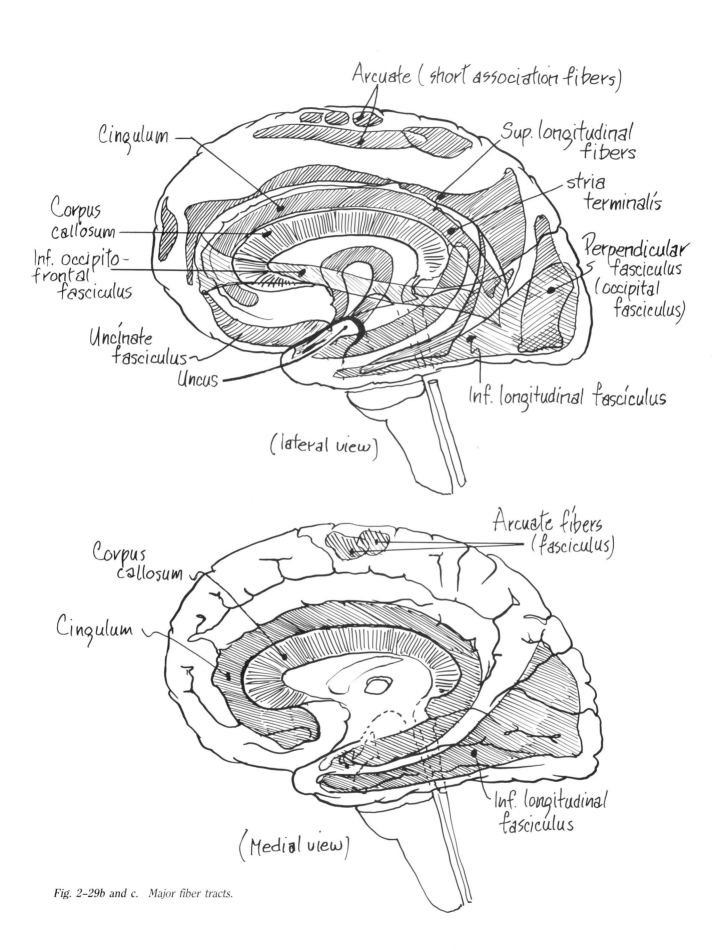

Arcuate (short association fibers)

Cingulum

Sup. longitudinal fibers

stria terminalis

Corpus callosum

Inf. occipito-frontal fasciculus

Perpendicular fasciculus (occipital fasciculus)

Uncinate fasciculus

Uncus

Inf. longitudinal fasciculus

(lateral view)

Arcuate fibers (fasciculus)

Corpus callosum

Cingulum

Inf. longitudinal fasciculus

(Medial view)

Fig. 2–29b and c. Major fiber tracts.

# CEREBRAL CORTICAL AREAS

Over the years several cytoarchitectural maps which divide the cerebrum into various areas have been proposed. The functions for some of these areas have been identified, mainly by electrically stimulating the area and observing the response elicited. Various investigators have mapped the areas of the cortex: In 1905 Campbell recognized some 20 cortical areas; in 1909 Brodmann extended the number to 52; Economo identified 109 areas in 1929; and the Vogts, in 1919, proposed more than 200 divisions of the cerebral cortex. For descriptive purposes Brodmann's map is still used (Fig. 2–30).

## THE PRIMARY MOTOR AREA (AREA 4)

The **primary motor area** is located on the anterior wall of the central sulcus and the adjacent portion of the precentral gyrus (Fig. 2–32). This area corresponds to the distribution of the giant pyramidal (Betz) cells, which control fine, highly skilled voluntary movements of skeletal muscles principally on the opposite side of the body. This area of cortex is unusually thick, measuring approximately 4.5 cm.

Area 4 receives afferent fibers from the premotor cortex (Area 6), somesthetic cortex (Areas 3, 2, and 1), the cerebellum, and the thalamic nuclei, a major center for motor and sensory interactions. Efferent fibers from the motor area extend to the reticular formation, red nucleus, pons, and other areas involved in the production of movement.

Electrical stimulation of the primary motor area elicits contraction of muscles that are primarily on the opposite side of the body. The response usually involves muscles that compose a functional group, although on occasion there is a contraction of a single muscle. The body is represented in the motor area as inverted, with a pattern similar to that of the somesthetic cortex (Fig. 2–32).

Destructive lesions of Area 4 produce contralateral flaccid paresis or paralysis of affected muscle groups.

Spasticity is more likely to occur if Area 6 is also ablated or if the lesion interrupts projection fibers in the medullary center or internal capsule.

## PREMOTOR AREA (AREA 6)

The **premotor area** is located anterior to the motor area in the frontal lobe. Histologically, Area 6 resembles Area 4 except that there are no Betz cells in Area 6. This area receives afferent fibers from the nuclei of the thalamus as well as other cortical areas.

This area controls the general muscular activity of the contralateral side of the body. While the primary motor area (area 4) is involved in the execution of movements and the maintenance of simple movements, the premotor area directs the primary motor area in its execution.

Portions of area 6 on the medial aspect of the hemisphere are considered to constitute part of the **supplementary motor area**. Stimulation of the supplementary motor area produces raising of the opposite arm, turning of the head and eyes and bilateral synergic contractions of the muscles of the trunk and legs.

Unilateral lesions of the supplementary motor area impair the performance of tasks in which bimanual coordination is required (Brazis, Masdeu, & Biller, 1985). Also, the hand contralateral to the lesion has a tendency to grasp when the palm is stimulated (*grasp reflex*) and may perform seemingly purposeful movements (such as reaching for an object or imitating what the other hand is doing) that are unwilled by the patient (*alien hand sign*) (Goldberg, Mayer, & Taglia, 1981).

Seizures originating in the supplementary motor area induce head turning to the opposite side and raising of the contralateral hand to the level of the head, in such a way that the patient seems to be performing a military salute (Brazis, Masdeu, & Biller, 1985).

## THE FRONTAL EYE FIELD (AREA 8)

The **frontal eye field** is located in Area 8 on the lateral surface of the hemisphere in front of the premotor area (Fig. 2–32). This area is responsible for

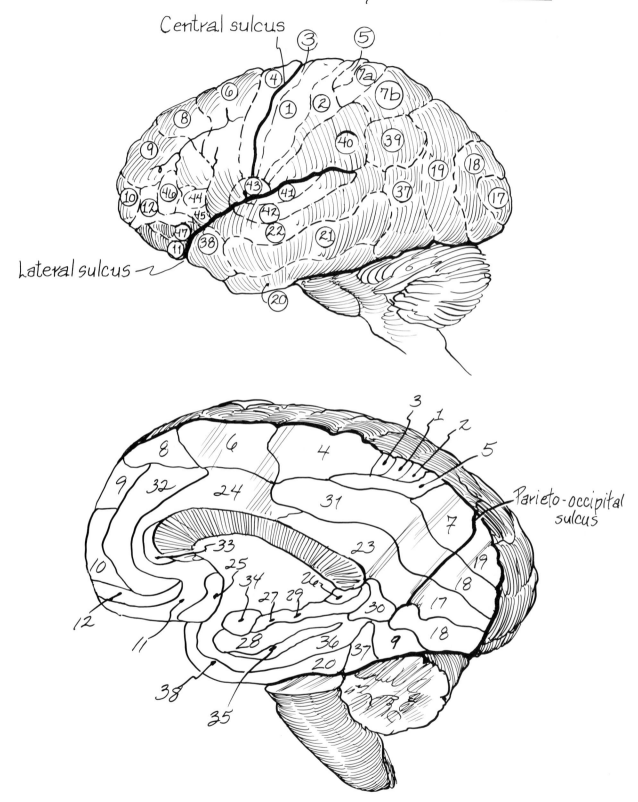

**Fig. 2–30.** *Brodmann's areas as shown in the left hemisphere. Above, lateral view; below, medial view.*

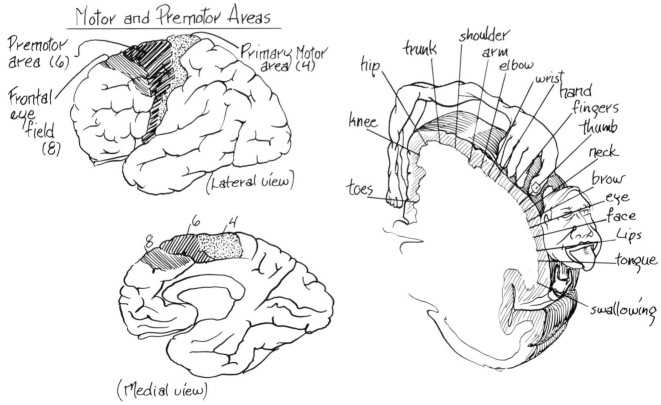

# Sensory Cortex and Somatosensory Areas

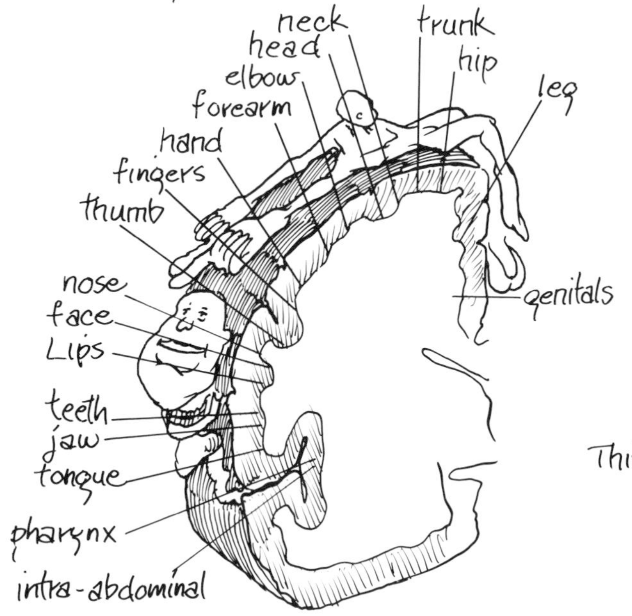

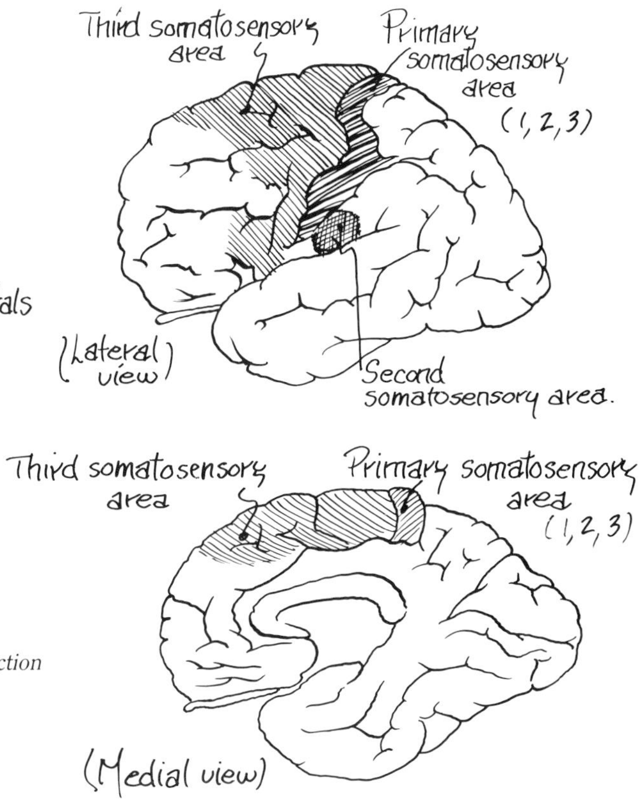

neck
head
elbow
forearm
hand
fingers
thumb
nose
face
Lips
teeth
jaw
tongue
pharynx
intra-abdominal
trunk
hip
leg
genitals

Third somatosensory area
Primary somatosensory area (1,2,3)
(Lateral view)
Second somatosensory area.

Third somatosensory area
Primary somatosensory area (1,2,3)
(Medial view)

*Fig. 2-31.* Sensory homunculus, drawn overlying a frontal section through the postcentral gyrus, and the somatosensory areas.

# Motor and Premotor Areas

Premotor area (6)
Frontal eye field (8)
Primary Motor area (4)
(Lateral view)

8  6  4
(Medial view)

hip
trunk
shoulder
arm
elbow
wrist
hand
fingers
thumb
neck
brow
eye
face
Lips
tongue
swallowing
knee
toes

*Fig. 2-32.* Motor and premotor areas and the motor homunculus, drawn overlying a frontal section through the precentral gyrus.

voluntary conjugate movements of the eyes. The eyes will deviate to the opposite side when Area 8 is stimulated. This cortical field is believed to be a center for voluntary eye movements not dependent upon visual stimuli. The conjugate eye movements are frequently called the "movements of command" since they can be elicited by instructing the patient to look to the left or right (Cogan, 1956).

If there is a destructive lesion in the frontal eye field, conjugate deviation of the eyes toward the side of the lesion will result. The patient is unable to voluntarily move his eyes in the opposite direction, but such a movement will occur spontaneously when he observes an object moving across his field of vision.

## THE PRIMARY SENSORY PROJECTION CORTEX (AREAS 3, 2, 1)

The **primary sensory projection cortex** (first somesthetic or general sensory area) is located in the postcentral gyrus on the lateral surface of the hemisphere. It has several functions: (1) to recognize the source, quality and severity of pain and temperature; (2) to appreciate light pressure and vibrations from bony prominences; and (3) to recognize fine discriminating touch and position and movement of body parts (proprioception and kinesthetic sense). The somesthetic area receives fibers from the posterior nucleus of the thalamus and conveys skin, muscle, joint, and tendon sense from the opposite side of the body. Fibers for cutaneous sensibility end preferentially in the anterior part of the area; fibers for deep sensibility end in the posterior part.

The pharyngeal region, tongue, and jaws are represented in the most ventral part of the somesthetic area, followed by the face, hand, arm, trunk and thigh (see Fig. 2–31). The extension of the somesthetic cortex on the medial surface of the hemisphere represents the remainder of the leg and the perineum. The functional importance of a particular part of the body and its need for sensitivity determine the size of the cortical area. Therefore, the area for the face (especially the lips) is disportionately large. The hand, and particularly the thumb and index finger,

are also assigned a large area. In addition to the main contralateral representation there is some ipsilateral representation of the face for touch.

Irritative lesions of this area produce paresthesias — e.g., numbness, formication, "electric shock," and "pins-and-needles" sensations — on the opposite side of the body, except in response to stimulation of the cortical area for the face. Evidence suggests that the face and tongue are represented bilaterally (Carpenter & Sutin, 1983). Sometimes a patient may report a sensation of movement in a particular part of the body, although no movement actually occurs. A sensation of pain is rarely produced by these lesions.

Destructive lesions produce objective impairment in sensibility — e.g., inability to localize or measure the intensity of painful stimuli and impaired perception of various forms of cutaneous sensation. In other words, a crude form of awareness persists for the sensations of pain, heat, and cold and there may also be minimal awareness of touch. The somesthetic cortex must be intact for any appreciation of the more discriminative sensations of fine touch and position and movement of the parts of the body. Lesions in this area render the patient unable to identify objects through touch (astereognosis). The more complicated the test, the more evident the sensory deficit becomes. The sensory deficit produced by a lesion in the first somesthetic area is contralateral and is in the part of the body represented in the affected region of the area.

Besides the first somesthetic area, there is some evidence that a **second somesthetic area** also exists, located in the dorsal wall of the lateral sulcus in line with the postcentral gyrus (Fig. 2–31). This area may also extend into part of the insula. Although contralateral representation predominates, there is some bilateral representation of the parts of the body. The secondary sensory area receives input from the intralaminar nuclei and the posterior complex of nuclei of the thalamus. Stimulation of the second somatic sensory area in the unanesthetized patient produces sensations in the extremities similar to those obtained by stimulating the primary somesthetic cortex. Consequently, this area is primarily involved in the less discriminative aspects of sensation. No clinical disorder has been ascribed to selective destruction of the second somesthetic area.

## THE SOMESTHETIC ASSOCIATION AREA (AREAS 5 AND 7)

The **somesthetic association cortex** is located primarily in the superior parietal lobule on the lateral surface of the hemisphere and in the precuneus on the medial surface. This association area receives afferent fibers from the first somesthetic area (Areas 3, 2, and 1) and sends efferent fibers to the nuclei in the lateral mass of thalamus. It is in the somesthetic association area that data pertaining to the general senses are integrated, permitting such abilities as the recognition (without the use of vision) of an object placed in the hand. An individual with a lesion in the somesthetic cortex will have awareness of the general senses (if the somesthetic area is intact) but will not be able to utilize his previous experience to appreciate the significance of the information being received.

## THE PRIMARY VISUAL RECEPTIVE CORTEX (AREA 17)

The **primary visual receptive cortex** is located in the occipital lobe in the cortex of the calcarine fissure and adjacent portions of the cuneus and lingual gyrus (Fig. 2–33). Much of Area 17 is not visible superficially because a considerable amount is located in the walls of the deep calcarine sulcus. This area is very thin, measuring approximately 1.5 mm. It is the site of lowest threshold for a response to electrical stimulation. Area 17 subserves movements of the eyes induced by visual stimuli, as in following moving objects.

Area 17 receives afferent fibers from the lateral geniculate nucleus of the thalamus via the geniculocalcarine tract. Part of this tract passes through the medullary center of the temporal lobe; therefore, a lesion that causes a defect in the visual field may be located in the temporal lobe, distant from the visual area of the occipital lobe.

Irritative lesions may produce visual hallucinations, such as flashes of light, rainbows, brilliant stars or bright lights. Destructive lesions may cause contralateral homonymous defects in the visual fields without destruction of macular vision. Cortex containing macular representation receives overlapping blood supply from the middle and posterior cerebral arteries.

A more detailed discussion of the functions of the visual cortex is found in a separate section of this book.

## THE VISUAL ASSOCIATION CORTEX (AREAS 18 AND 19)

The **visual association cortex** surrounds the visual area on the medial and lateral surfaces of the hemisphere (Fig. 2–33). The visual association cortex receives efferent fibers from Area 17; it has afferent connections with other cortical areas and with the pulvinar of the thalamus. This area has a variety of complex functions related to vision; it relates present visual experiences to those in the past, with recognition of what is seen and appreciation of its significance. Therefore, a lesion in Areas 18 and 19 may result in visual agnosia (inability to recognize objects in the opposite field of vision).

The visual and visual association cortex are connected to the superior colliculus of the midbrain through corticotectal fibers. This pathway originates in the retina and is responsible for the fixation of gaze and for tracking of a motor object in the field of vision.

## THE PRIMARY AUDITORY RECEPTIVE AREA (AREAS 41 AND 42)

A major part of the **primary auditory area** is concealed because it is located in the transverse temporal gyrus (Heschl's gyrus), which lies buried deep in the floor of the lateral cerebral fissure. It is a relatively thick layer of cortex, measuring approximately 3 mm. It receives the auditory radiation from the medial geniculate body of the thalamus, which conveys impulses from the cochlea of each ear. Impulses for low frequencies impinge on the anterolateral part of the auditory area and impulses for high frequencies impinge on the posteromedial part.

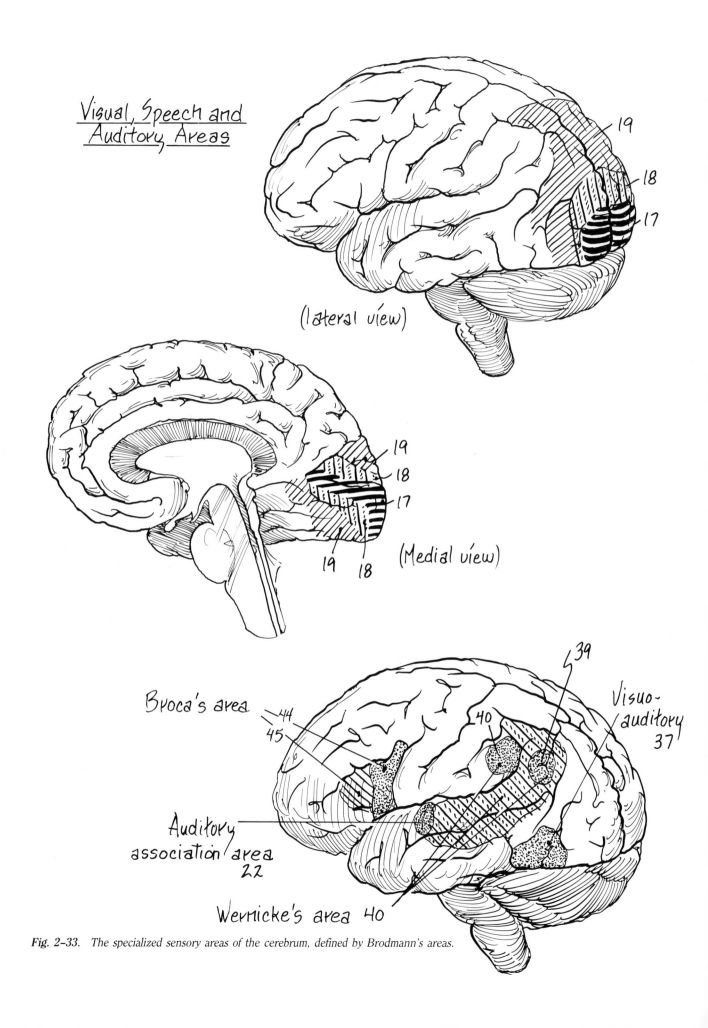

**Fig. 2–33.** *The specialized sensory areas of the cerebrum, defined by Brodmann's areas.*

A unilateral lesion of this area causes a mild loss in auditory acuity in both ears and the loss is greater in the opposite side. The impairment is slight because of the bilateral projection to the cortex and the deficit is difficult to detect by clinical tests. Electrical stimulation of the region near the primary auditory receptive area in humans causes buzzing and roaring sensations.

## THE AUDITORY ASSOCIATION CORTEX (AREA 40)

The **auditory association cortex** is located behind the auditory area, near the lateral sulcus. This area receives fibers from areas 41 and 42 and has connections with areas of the parietal, occipital and insular cortex. In the left hemisphere this region is known as *Wernicke's area* and is important in language comprehension (*see* Fig. 2–33).

Lesions of area 40 in the dominant hemisphere (or bilateral lesions) produce *word deafness* or *sensory aphasia*. Although patients with these lesions can hear, they cannot interpret the meaning of sounds, especially speech. This form of sensory aphasia is usually associated with lesions in the posterior part of area 40.

## THE OLFACTORY RECEPTIVE AREA (AREA 28)

The **olfactory receptive area** is located in the uncus and adjacent portions of the parahippocampal gyrus of the temporal lobe. Destruction of the olfactory pathways or cortex produces anosmia. Unilateral anosmia may be of important diagnostic significance in localizing intracranial neoplasms, especially meningiomas of the sphenoid ridge or olfactory groove.

Irritative lesions may cause olfactory hallucinations known as *uncinate fits*, characterized by sensations of peculiar odors and tastes and often associated with a dreamy state. Uncinate fits may also occur as an epileptic aura.

## THE GUSTATORY AREA (AREA 43)

The **gustatory** or taste area is located in the dorsal wall of the lateral sulcus and extends into the insula. Taste buds send efferent fibers to the gustatory nucleus in the brain stem. Efferent fibers from the gustatory nucleus ascend ipsilaterally in the central tegmental tract and terminate in the medial part of the ventral posterior nucleus of the thalamus. Thalamocortical fibers complete the pathway. Stimulation of the parietal operculum and adjacent insular cortex in conscious patients produces gustatory sensations.

## THE PREFRONTAL CORTEX (AREAS 9, 10, 11, AND 12)

The **prefrontal area** is the region that envelopes the frontal pole. It receives projections from the dorsomedial nuclei of the thalamus, which in turn have connections with the hypothalamus; this forms a system that involves affective reactions to present situations on the basis of past experience. This part of the cerebral cortex also receives connections from the anterior portions of the temporal lobe and the parietal and occipitotemporal association areas, thereby gaining access to contemporary sensory experience and to the data received from past experience. Persons with disease or damage in the prefrontal area (as may occur with craniocerebral trauma, tumor, or other conditions) may exhibit a variety of symptoms. These patients are often noted to lack judgment and insight and may have a feeling of euphoria. Frequently their personal hygiene deteriorates and their speech is uncharacteristically vulgar.

## THE POSTERIOR PORTION OF THE ORBITAL SURFACE (AREA 47)

Area 47 and the contiguous portion of the anterior half of the insula produce pronounced autonomic effects upon electrical stimulation; inhibition of respiration and alteration of blood pressure may also be readily induced.

## THE ANTERIOR CINGULATE AREA (AREA 24)

Upon stimulation of the **anterior cingulate area** (Area 24), which lies on the medial aspect of the cerebral hemisphere, pronounced autonomic effects and inhibition of skeletal muscle tone may occur.

# THE VENTRICLES

The **ventricles** are interconnected cavities in the brain which contain cerebrospinal fluid. There are four ventricles: two paired lateral ventricles (the left and right ventricles), the third ventricle and the fourth ventricle (Figs. 2–34 and 2–35). Each ventricle contains a choroid plexus, which produces cerebrospinal fluid.

**The Lateral Ventricles.** The two lateral ventricles, the largest of the ventricles, are C-shaped cavities contained within the cerebral hemispheres. Each of the lateral ventricles is connected with the third ventricle via a **foramen of Monro** (interventricular foramen). These foramina serve as a basic reference point and are of great importance in radiographic studies. The lateral ventricles are continuous with the ependyma of the third ventricle. Each lateral ventricle is composed of four parts: (1) the *anterior (ventral) horn*, which is located in the frontal lobe; (2) the *body*, located in the parietal lobe; (3) the *inferior (temporal) horn*, contained in the temporal lobe; and (4) the *posterior (occipital) horn*, located in the occipital lobe.

The cerebrospinal fluid is produced mainly by the **choroid plexuses** of the lateral, third and fourth ventricles. The choroid plexuses in the lateral ventricles are the largest and most important. The choroid plexus of the lateral ventricle is a vascular process of the pia mater projecting into the ventricular cavity. It forms a semipermeable filter between arterial blood and the cerebrospinal fluid. The choroid plexus of each lateral ventricle extends from the interventricular foramen (where it is joined with the plexus of the opposite lateral ventricle) to the end of the inferior horn. The surface area of the choroid plexuses of the two lateral ventricles combined is about 40 sq cm. The arteries to the plexus consist of (1) the anterior choroidal artery, a branch of the internal carotid artery, which enters the plexus at the inferior horn of the ventricle; and (2) the posterior choroidal artery, a branch of the posterior cerebral artery.

**The Third Ventricle.** The third ventricle is a narrow vertical chamber between the two lateral ven-tricles. The roof of the third ventricle is formed by a thin layer of ependyma. The brain wall is exceptionally thin in this area and susceptible to trauma. The lateral walls are formed mainly by the medial surfaces of the two thalami. The lower lateral wall and the floor of the ventricle are formed by the hypothalamus and subthalamus. The following structures may be found in the floor of the third ventricle (from anterior to posterior end): the optic chiasm, infundibulum, tuber cinereum, mammillary bodies, and subthalamus.

Three openings communicate with the third ventricle: the two interventricular foramina (of Monro) at the anterior end communicate with the lateral ventricles, and the cerebral aqueduct (of Sylvius) opens into the caudal end of the third ventricle. Two choroid plexuses extend side by side in the roof of the third ventricle from the interventricular foramina to the caudal extremity of the roof.

**The Fourth Ventricle.** The fourth ventricle is a cavity overlying the pons and medulla. It is continuous with the central canal of the upper cervical spinal cord below and the cerebral aqueduct (of Sylvius) above. The aqueduct of Sylvius, which connects the third and fourth ventricles, is about 1.5 cm long and 1 mm — 2 mm in diameter. The **tela choroidea** is a vascular connective tissue derived from the pia mater that covers the brain. The tela choroidea invaginates into the cavity of the fourth ventricle to form the choroid plexus of the fourth ventricle.

Three small apertures, a median foramen (of Magendie) and two lateral foramina (of Luschka), allow the passage of cerebrospinal fluid into the subarachnoid space that surrounds and protects the brain and spinal cord. Because these are the only communications between the ventricular and subarachnoid spaces, their blockage can produce a type of hydrocephalus. Under normal circumstances, the CSF is eventually reabsorbed into the bloodstream through **arachnoid villi** which empty into the venous sinuses of the outermost brain membrane, the dura mater, as well as through similar structures along the dorsal roots of the spinal nerves.

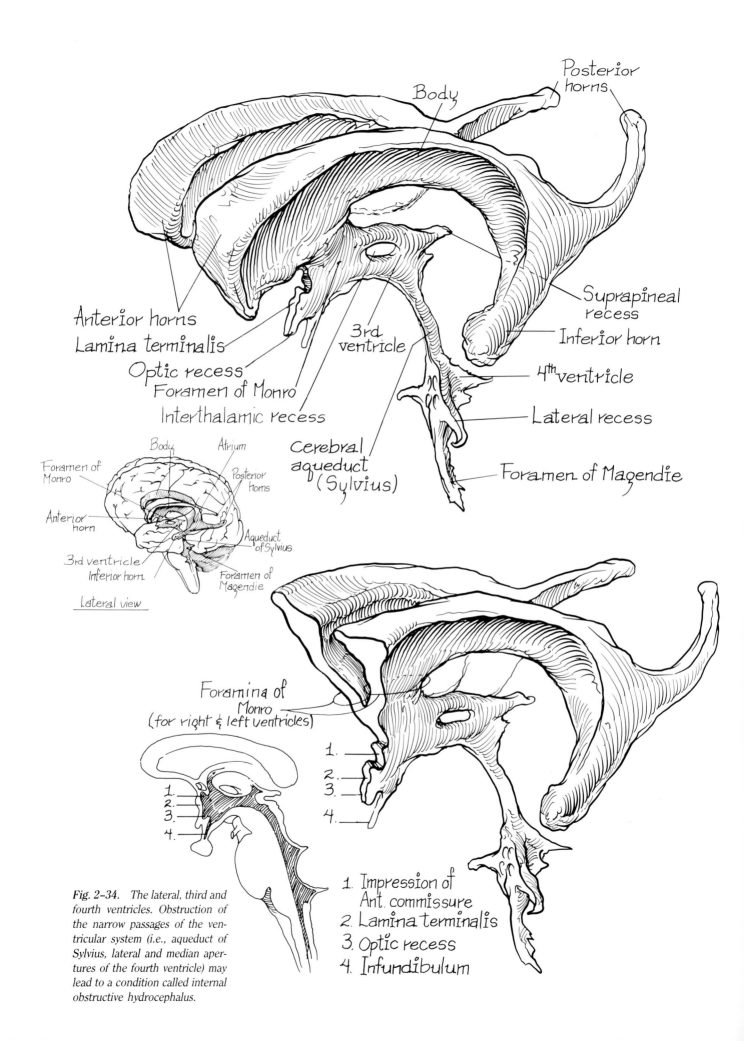

Posterior horns

Body

Anterior horns
Lamina terminalis
Optic recess
Foramen of Monro
Interthalamic recess

3rd ventricle

Cerebral aqueduct (Sylvius)

Suprapineal recess
Inferior horn
4th ventricle
Lateral recess
Foramen of Magendie

Foramen of Monro
Body
Atrium
Posterior horns
Anterior horn
3rd ventricle
Inferior horn
Aqueduct of Sylvius
Foramen of Magendie

Lateral view

Foramina of Monro
(for right & left ventricles)

1.
2.
3.
4.

1. Impression of Ant. commissure
2. Lamina terminalis
3. Optic recess
4. Infundibulum

*Fig. 2-34. The lateral, third and fourth ventricles. Obstruction of the narrow passages of the ventricular system (i.e., aqueduct of Sylvius, lateral and median apertures of the fourth ventricle) may lead to a condition called internal obstructive hydrocephalus.*

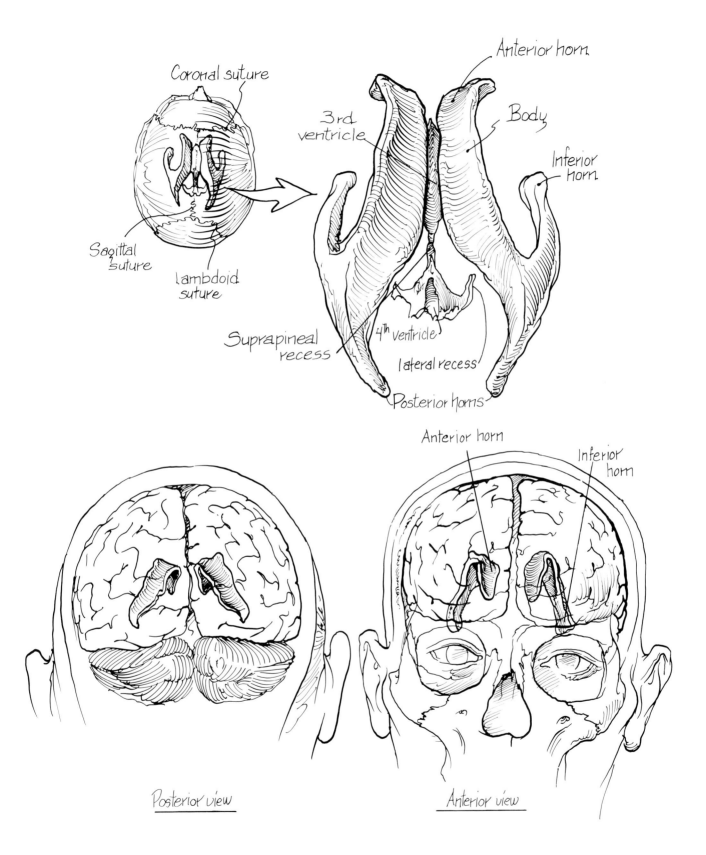

**Fig. 2-35.** *Superior, posterior and anterior views of the ventricles. Normally, the anterior horns do not extend beyond the coronal suture; the posterior horns do not extend beyond the lambdoid suture.*

The volume of CSF in the body varies from 80 ml-150 ml, including fluid in both the ventricles and arachnoid space. Research indicates that the average normal ventricular system has a capacity of 15 ml-40 ml. The rate of production of cerebrospinal fluid is thought to be sufficient to effect a total replacement several times daily.

# THE VISUAL PATHWAY

The rods and cones of the retina are visual receptors which react specifically to photic stimulation. A photochemical reaction occurs when light falls on the rods and cones, causing membrane potential changes through which nerve impulses are conducted from the retinae backward through the optic nerves. The cones have a higher threshold of excitability and are stimulated by light of relatively high intensity; they are responsible for color discrimination and sharp visual definition. The rods respond to low intensities of illumination and subserve night vision. It is estimated that there are some 7 million cones and 100 million rods in each eye (Carpenter & Sutin, 1983). There is a point-to-point projection from the retina to the lateral geniculate nucleus of the thalamus and from this nucleus to the visual cortex (areas 17, 18 and 19) of the occipital lobe. This pathway is known as the **geniculostriate system.**

For the purpose of describing the retinal projection, each retina is divided into nasal and temporal halves by a vertical line that passes through the fovea. A horizontal line, also passing through the fovea, divides each half of the retina into upper and lower quadrants (*see* Fig. 2–36). The inner layers of the retina in the macular area are pushed far apart, forming the **fovea centralis,** a small central pit composed of closely packed cones, where vision is sharpest and color discrimination most acute (Chusid, 1979). Close to the posterior pole of the eye, the retina shows the **macula lutea,** a small, circular, yellowish area. The macula represents the retinal area for central vision; the retinal image of any object is always focused on the macula.

The optic nerves enter the cranial cavity through the optic foramina and unite to form the **optic chiasm.** The fibers in front of the optic chiasm are known as **optic nerves;** fibers behind the chiasm are called **optic tracts.** Fibers from the right halves of the two retinae terminate in the right lateral geniculate nucleus, at the extreme lateral margin of the thalamus, and the visual information is then relayed to the visual cortex of the right hemisphere. The converse is true for the left halves of the retinae.

The partial crossing of optic nerve fibers in the optic chiasma is a requirement for binocular vision. Within the chiasm fibers from the nasal or medial half of each retina decussate and join uncrossed fibers from the temporal or lateral half of the retina to form the optic tract. Most of the fibers of each tract synapse in the lateral geniculate body, although a small number of fibers continue as the brachium of the superior colliculus to the superior colliculus and pretectal area. The superior colliculus is concerned with the coordination of eye and head movements needed to bring an object of interest into the center of the visual field. The pretectal region is concerned with the pupillary light reflex.

The lateral geniculate body gives rise to the **geniculocalcarine tract,** which passes through the internal capsule and forms the **optic radiations,** which terminate in area 17 of the occipital lobe. Some of the fanlike geniculocalcarine fibers radiate forward over the temporal horn of the lateral ventricle. These fibers, which constitute the **temporal** or **Meyer's loop** of the geniculocalcarine tract, terminate in the visual cortex below the calcarine sulcus. A temporal lobe lesion involving Meyer's loop causes a defect in the upper visual field on the side opposite the lesion. A lesion in the parietal lobe, on the other hand, may involve geniculocalcarine fibers that proceed to the visual cortex above the calcarine sulcus; the result is then a defect in the lower visual field on the side opposite the lesion.

The **primary visual cortex** occupies the upper and lower lips of the calcarine sulcus on the medial surface of the cerebral hemisphere. The area is much larger than suggested by the usual cortical maps because of the depth of the calcarine sulcus. The primary visual cortex (area 17) is also known as the **striate area** because a cross-section of the cortex contains a horizontal stripe of white matter within the gray matter (*Gennari's line*). The **visual association cortex** (areas 18 and 19), located adjacent to area 17, is involved

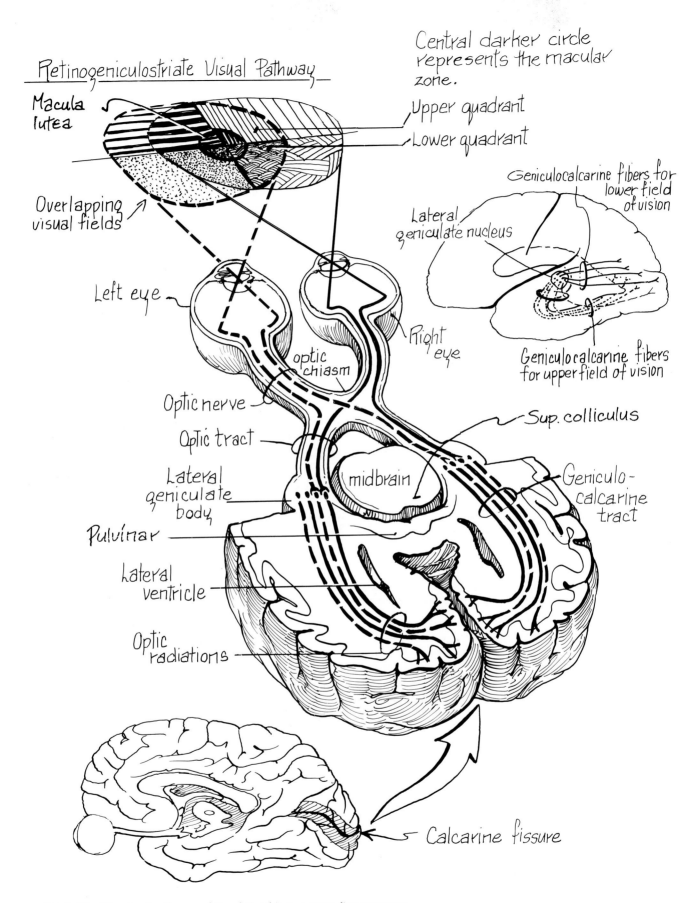

Retinogeniculostriate Visual Pathway

Macula lutea

Overlapping visual fields

Left eye

optic chiasm

Optic nerve

Optic tract

Lateral geniculate body

Pulvinar

Lateral ventricle

Optic radiations

Central darker circle represents the macular zone.

Upper quadrant

Lower quadrant

Lateral geniculate nucleus

Right eye

Geniculocalcarine fibers for lower field of vision

Geniculocalcarine fibers for upper field of vision

Sup. colliculus

midbrain

Geniculo-calcarine tract

Calcarine fissure

**Fig. 2–36.** *The visual pathway and its relationship to surrounding structures.*

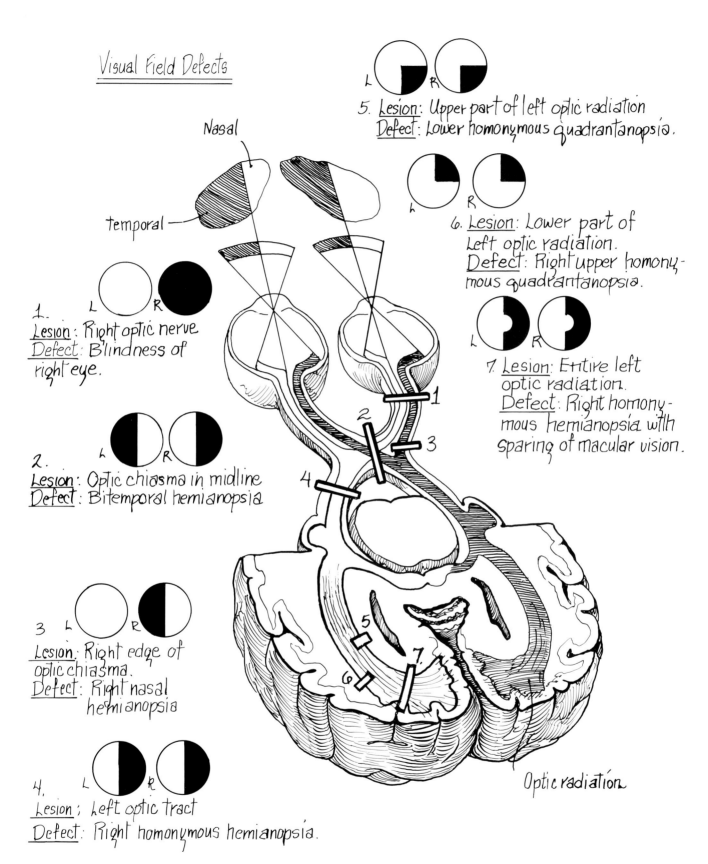

Visual Field Defects

Nasal

temporal

1.
Lesion: Right optic nerve
Defect: Blindness of
right eye.

2.
Lesion: Optic chiasma in midline
Defect: Bitemporal hemianopsia

3
Lesion: Right edge of
optic chiasma.
Defect: Right nasal
hemianopsia

4.
Lesion: Left optic tract
Defect: Right homonymous hemianopsia.

5. Lesion: Upper part of left optic radiation
Defect: Lower homonymous quadrantanopsia.

6. Lesion: Lower part of
Left optic radiation.
Defect: Right upper homony-
mous quadrantanopsia.

7. Lesion: Entire left
optic radiation.
Defect: Right homony-
mous hemianopsia with
sparing of macular vision.

Optic radiation.

Fig. 2-37. Visual field defects that result from various lesions along the visual pathway.

in recognition of objects, perception of color and depth, and other complex aspects of vision such as visual fixation.

In addition to receiving the fibers of the geniculocalcarine tract, the primary visual cortex projects upon the lateral geniculate nucleus and is thus able to modulate its input of sensory information. The primary and association cortices of the occipital lobe also receive some visual information from the pulvinar.

# VISUAL DEFECTS CAUSED BY INTERRUPTION OF THE PATHWAY

The nature of the visual defect depends upon the location and extent of the injury. Fig. 2–37 illustrates some of the common lesions with the visual pathway.

A visual defect is said to be *homonymous* when it is restricted to a single visual field, either right or left. Homonymous defects are caused by lesions on one side anywhere behind the optic chiasm, such as the optic tract, optic radiation, or visual cortex. Complete destruction of any of these structures results in a loss of the whole opposite field of vision and is known as *homonymous hemianopsia*; partial injury may produce quadrantic homonymous defects, also called *quadrantanopsia*.

Lesions of the chiasm frequently involve the crossing fibers from the nasal portions of the retina and result in loss of the two temporal fields of vision (*bitemporal hemianopsia*). Injury of one optic nerve will produce blindness in the corresponding eye with loss of the pupillary light reflex.

# THE DIENCEPHALON

The diencephalon and telencephalon together constitute the cerebrum; the **diencephalon**, an ovoid mass of gray matter, forms the central core and the **telencephalon** forms the cerebral hemispheres. Only the ventral aspect of the diencephalon is exposed to view; most of the diencephalon is surrounded by the two hemispheres. The diencephalon is divided into symmetrical halves by the third ventricle. In most (but not all) human brains, the two halves of the diencephalon are connected at a small area called the **massa intermedia** or **interthalamic adhesion**. The diencephalon is divided into four major parts or regions on each side: (1) the epithalamus; (2) the thalamus; (3) the hypothalamus; and (4) the subthalamus.

## THE EPITHALAMUS

The **epithalamus** is located dorsomedial to the thalamus and adjacent to the roof of the third ventricle. It consists of six structures: (1) the pineal body; (2) the posterior commissure; (3) the habenular commissure; (4) the habenula; (5) the tela choroidea; and (6) the stria medullaris thalami (Figs. 2–38 and 2–39). Its structures are concerned with autonomic responses to olfactory stimuli and to emotional changes.

The **pineal body** is a small mass attached to the roof of the third ventricle in the region of the posterior commissure. Also known as the **epiphysis**, it is shaped like a pine cone and measures about 5 mm x 7 mm in size. Microscopically, it consists of glial cells (astrocytes) and parenchymal cells (pinealocytes). The pineal body is attached to the diencephalon by the pineal stalk. At their proximal ends the laminas of the stalk are separated, forming the **pineal recess** of the third ventricle.

The **habenular commissure**, located in the dorsal wall of the stalk, contains fibers of the **stria medullaris thalami** that terminate in the opposite habenular nuclei. The ventral wall of the pineal stalk is attached to the **posterior commissure**, a bundle of white fibers that crosses the midsagittal plane at the point where the third ventricle becomes continuous with the cerebral aqueduct. The posterior commissure contains fibers connecting the two superior colliculi. The **tela choroidea** is a membrane which forms most of the roof of the third ventricle.

The pineal gland appears to be a rudimentary gland whose functions in the adult are not fully known. The pineal gland secretes melatonin, which aids in the regulation of the secretion of gonadotropins and melanocyte-stimulating hormones, which contain endorphins, important substances in pain control. There is some evidence that pineal hormones also influence pituitary cells that produce the growth (somatotrophic) hormone (STH), the thyroid-stimulating hormone (TSH) and the adrenocorticotrophic hormone (ACTH). These secretions of the pineal gland which alter hypothalamic functions have their effect after they enter the general circulation or the cerebrospinal fluid. Daily fluctuations in pineal serotonin and melatonin are rhythmic in response to the cycle of photic (light) input. It is known that the pathway originates in the retina, and that sympathetic innervation has an inhibitory effect on the gland. Because of these rhythmic changes in pineal activity, it has been suggested that this gland may function as a biological clock that delivers signals that regulate both physiological and behavioral processes. These fluctuations, called **circadian rhythms**, have a period of exactly 24 hours in the presence of environmental cues. Without such cues they only approximate the 24-hour cycle.

The pineal body lies in the midline of the body. After about the age of 20 years, granules of calcium and magnesium salts appear and later solidify to form larger particles (*corpora arenacea* or *brain sand*). These calcified deposits are visible on x-ray and are a useful landmark for the radiologist. A shift of the pineal gland to one side may represent a shift of brain structures due to a mass lesion on the opposite side or an atrophic lesion on the same side.

The pineal gland is sometimes the site of primary neoplasms. A pineal tumor which develops around

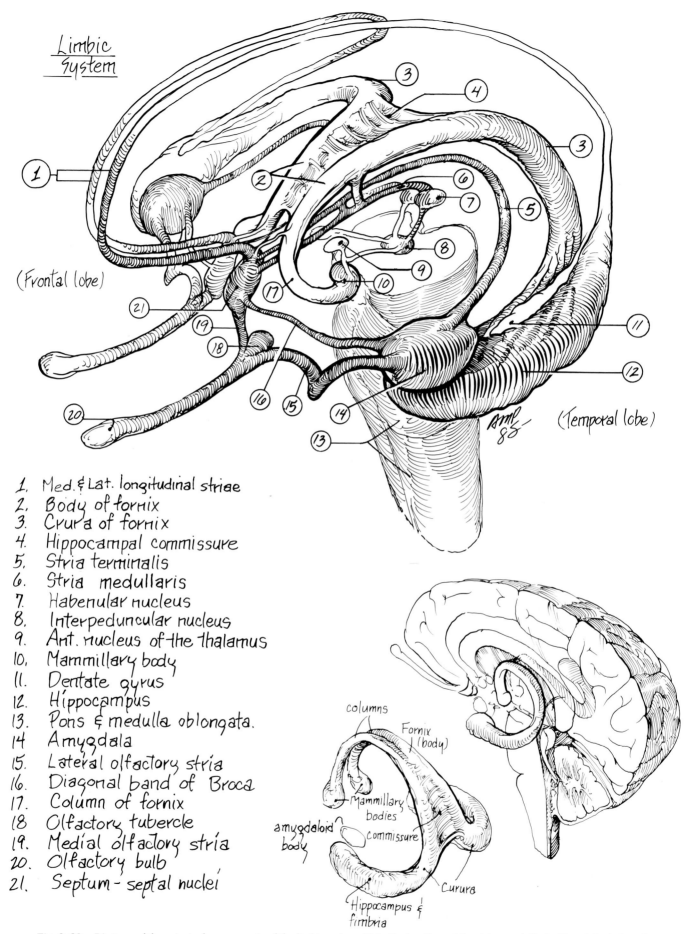

# Limbic System

(Frontal lobe)

(Temporal lobe)

1. Med. & Lat. longitudinal striae
2. Body of fornix
3. Crura of fornix
4. Hippocampal commissure
5. Stria terminalis
6. Stria medullaris
7. Habenular nucleus
8. Interpeduncular nucleus
9. Ant. nucleus of the thalamus
10. Mammillary body
11. Dentate gyrus
12. Hippocampus
13. Pons & medulla oblongata.
14. Amygdala
15. Lateral olfactory stria
16. Diagonal band of Broca
17. Column of fornix
18. Olfactory tubercle
19. Medial olfactory stria
20. Olfactory bulb
21. Septum - septal nuclei

**Fig. 2–38.** *Diagram of the principal components of the limbic system. Note the location of the striae medullaris (6) and the habenular nucleus (7). two of the structures which comprise the epithalamus.*

the age of puberty may alter the age of onset of pubertal changes. Puberty may be early if the tumor is of a type that destroys parenchymatous cells; puberty may be delayed if the tumor is derived from parenchymatous cells.

The **habenula** or **habenular trigone** is a small depressed area of gray matter located anterior to the superior colliculi. It is an important link between forebrain and midbrain structures. It consists of (1) the *habenular nuclei*, which receive afferent fibers from the stria medullaris thalami, which runs along the dorsomedial border of the thalamus; (2) the *habenular commissure*, which joins the habenular nuclei; and (3) the *habenulopeduncular tract*, which is comprised of nerve fibers from the habenular nucleus to the interpeduncular ganglion of the mesencephalon. The habenular nuclei constitute a portion of the limbic system pathway through which basic emotional drives and the sense of smell can influence the viscera.

## THE THALAMUS

Each cerebral hemisphere contains a thalamus — a large, ovoid gray mass located on either side of the third ventricle (Fig. 2–39). Because it receives sensory information, correlates it, and sends reports on to the cortex for further analysis, the thalamus has been referred to as the "gateway to the cerebral cortex" (Angevine & Cotman, 1981). The thalamus measures about 3 cm anteroposteriorly and 1.5 cm in the other two directions. It comprises about four-fifths of the diencephalon. In about 70% of human brains the thalami of both sides often fuse in the midline of the third ventricle to form the **interthalamic adhesion** or **massa intermedia**, a short bar of gray matter.

The thalamus is the major source of afferent fibers to the cortex. Major ascending pathways of the auditory, visual and somatosensory systems have their final subcortical relays here. The rostral end (the anterior tubercle) of the thalamus lies close to the midline and forms the posterior limit of the interventricular foramen. The posterior end is broader; its prominent medial portion is known as the **pulvinar** and the lateral oval swelling is called the **lateral geniculate body**. The dorsal surface is separated from the more laterally placed caudate nucleus by the **stria terminalis** and the **terminal vein**. The superior surface is separated from the medial surface by a slender white strand, the **stria medullaris**.

The **thalamic radiation** (geniculostriate pathway) is composed of the tracts emerging from the lateral surface of the thalamus which then enter the internal capsule and terminate in the cerebral cortex. The **external medullary lamina** is a vertical sheet of white matter that divides the gray matter of the thalamus into lateral, medial, and anterior portions.

The 30 thalamic nuclei can be classified into five major groups:

**(1) Anterior nuclear group.** This group of nuclei lies beneath the dorsal surface of the most rostral part of the thalamus, where it forms a distinct swelling, the **anterior tubercle**. The **internal medullary lamina**, consisting mainly of fibers passing from one thalamic nucleus to another, separate this group from the rest of the thalamus. The anterior nuclear group receives fibers from the mammillary bodies via the mammillothalamic tract and projects to the cingulate cortex of the cerebrum.

**(2) Nuclei of the Midline.** These are groups of cells located just beneath the lining of the third ventricle and in the massa intermedia. They receive fibers conveying sensory information from the reticular formation and have connections with the hypothalamus and dorsomedial thalamic nuclei. It is believed that the midline nuclei participate in visceral and affective responses to certain modalities of sensation.

**(3) Medial Nuclei.** These include most gray substance medial to the internal medullary lamina (**intralaminar nuclei**), the **dorsomedial nucleus**, which projects to the frontal cortex anterior to the motor cortex, and the nucleus of the **centrum medianum**, which connects with the corpus striatum. The intralaminar nuclei receive afferent fibers from the central group of nuclei of the reticular formation of the brain stem, through which data from most of the sensory systems are relayed. Although some fibers from the intralaminar nuclei pass directly to the cerebral cortex,

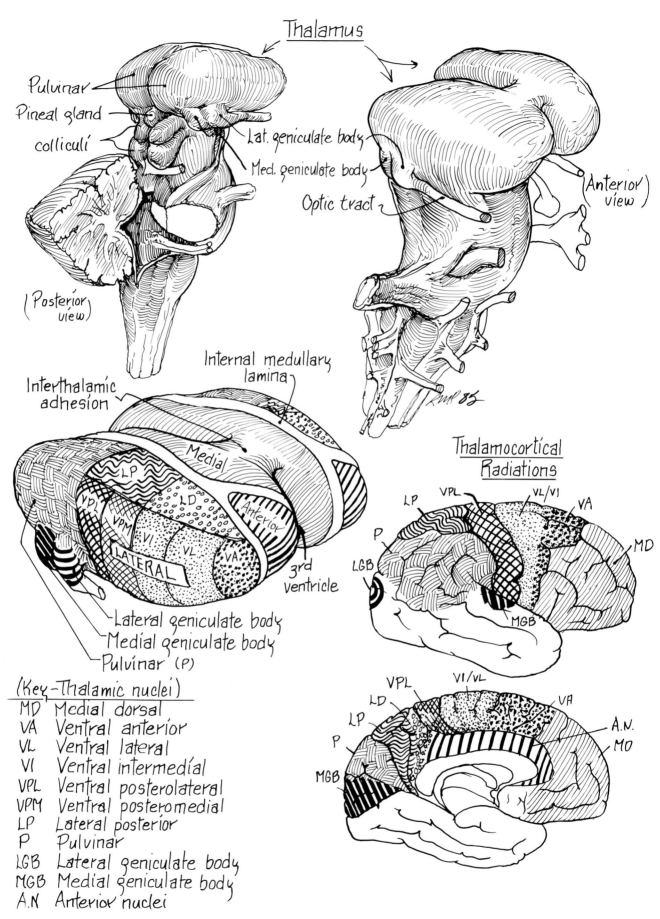

Thalamus

Pulvinar
Pineal gland
colliculi

Lat. geniculate body
Med. geniculate body
Optic tract

(Anterior view)

(Posterior view)

Interthalamic adhesion

Internal medullary lamina

Medial

LP
LD
Anterior
VPL
VPM
VI
VL
VA
LATERAL

3rd ventricle

Lateral geniculate body
Medial geniculate body
Pulvinar (P)

Thalamocortical Radiations

LP    VPL    VL/VI    VA
P
LGB
MGB
MD

VPL    VI/VL
LD
LP
P
MGB
VA
A.N.
MO

(Key-Thalamic nuclei)

| | |
|---|---|
| MD | Medial dorsal |
| VA | Ventral anterior |
| VL | Ventral lateral |
| VI | Ventral intermedial |
| VPL | Ventral posterolateral |
| VPM | Ventral posteromedial |
| LP | Lateral posterior |
| P | Pulvinar |
| LGB | Lateral geniculate body |
| MGB | Medial geniculate body |
| A.N | Anterior nuclei |

**Fig. 2-39.** Diagrams showing (1) the thalamus and its relationship to surrounding structures and (2) the principal thalamocortical projections.

the main projection is to surrounding parts of the thalamus (i.e., to the lateral nuclear mass and the dorsomedial and anterior nuclei), which in turn project to widespread areas of cortex. This is the anatomical basis for the important effect of the reticular system on levels of consciousness and degrees of alertness. It also provides for vague awareness of sensory stimulation without specificity or discriminative qualities but with emotional responses, especially to painful stimuli. The intralaminar nuclei, through thalamic nuclei having abundant cortical projections, constitute the key generator of much of the activity of the cerebral cortex shown in the electroencephalogram (Barr & Kiernan, 1983).

The dorsomedial nucleus constitutes part of a system that contributes to those aspects of the emotions generally considered as "moods" or "feeling tone." Depending on the nature of the present sensory input and past experience, the mood may be that of well-being or malaise, euphoria or depression. Visceral changes may accompany changes in mood through reciprocal connections between the dorsomedial thalamic nucleus and the hypothalamus (Barr & Kiernan, 1983).

There is also some evidence that the dorsomedial thalamic nucleus appears to play a role in memory. In Korsakoff's syndrome, characterized by amnesia, the degenerative changes in the brain follow a variable pattern. The lesions are typically in regions surrounding the third ventricle, and the dorsomedial nucleus is reported as being most consistently affected (Barr & Kiernan, 1983).

The projection of the dorsomedial nucleus of the anterior portion of the thalamus to the frontal lobe is the site of surgical section in frontal lobotomy and leukotomy. If the frontal pole of the cerebral hemisphere is removed, degeneration of the dorsomedial nucleus subsequently occurs. Prefrontal lobotomy and lesions in the dorsomedial nucleus of the thalamus modify the patient's reaction to chronic pain, but it is doubtful that these procedures eliminate pain.

**(4) Lateral Nuclear Mass.** This constitutes a large part of the thalamus anterior to the pulvinar between the internal and external medullary laminae. This mass includes (a) a *reticular nucleus*, a thin sheet of nerve cells between the external medullary lamina and the internal capsule, which receives collateral branches of thalamocortical and corticothalamic fibers; (b) an *anterior ventral nucleus*, which connects with the corpus striatum; (c) a *ventrolateral nucleus*, which projects to the cerebral motor cortex; (d) a *posterolateral ventral nucleus*, which projects to the postcentral gyrus and receives fibers from the medial lemniscus and the spinothalamic and trigeminal tracts; and (e) a *dorsolateral nucleus* and a *posterolateral nucleus*, which project to the parietal lobe cortex.

Through its inputs which arise from the deep cerebellar nucleus, the globus pallidus, and the substantia nigra, the ventrolateral nucleus of the thalamus makes important contributions to the initiation of movement, the control of muscle tone and the regulation of cortical reflexes (Carpenter & Sutin, 1983).

**(5) Posterior Nuclei.** These include the pulvinar and medial and lateral geniculate bodies, including (a) the *pulvinar nucleus*, a large nucleus in the posterior portion of the thalamus that connects with the parietal and temporal lobe cortices via projection fibers and may serve to integrate auditory, visual and somatic impulses; (b) the *medial geniculate body*, which lies on the auditory pathway, lateral to the midbrain under the pulvinar, and receives acoustic fibers from the lateral lemniscus and inferior colliculus and projects fibers (via the acoustic radiation) to the primary auditory area (area 41) of the temporal lobe (Heschl's gyrus); and (c) the *lateral geniculate body* which lies lateral to the medial geniculate body and projects to the visual cortex of the occipital lobe. At this site, and in the surrounding association cortex, there is awareness of visual stimuli accompanied by discriminative and mnemonic aspects of vision.

**Function of the Thalamus.** The thalamus (rather than the sensory cortex) may be the crucial structure for the perception of some types of sensation, and the sensory cortex may function to give finer detail to the sensation. All sensory impulses, with the sole exception of the olfactory stimuli, terminate in the gray masses of the thalamus. From there they are projected to specific cortical areas by the thalamocortical radiations. The thalamus is concerned not only with general and specific types of awareness, but with certain emotional connotations that accompany, or are associated with, most sensory experiences. Other data suggest that some thalamic nuclei serve as integrative centers for motor functions, since they receive the principal efferent projections from the cerebellum and the corpus striatum (Carpenter & Sutin, 1983).

The thalamus receives its blood supply from the internal carotid and vertebral systems of arteries. Cerebrovascular disease is the most common cause of discrete thalamic pathology. Infarcts are more common than hemorrhages (Brazis, Masdeu & Biller, 1985). A lesion caused by vascular occlusion in this area will produce variable symptoms, depending on the nuclei involved. However, due to the small size of the thalamus, several of the nuclei and even several of the different functional regions are usually affected simultaneously, even by fairly discrete lesions.

The **thalamic syndrome** (thalamic apoplexy, Dejerine-Roussy syndrome) is a disturbance of the sensory experiences subserved by the thalamus due to a lesion in the posterior thalamic region. Thalamic syndrome is characterized by immediate hemianesthesia. Later, the threshold to touch, pain, heat, and cold is raised on the side of the body opposite the lesion; when the threshold is reached, the sensations are disagreeable and unpleasant. This phenomenon is sometimes referred to as *thalamic hyperpathia*. The syndrome usually appears during the phase of recovery from a thalamic infarct; thalamic pain rarely occurs with tumors. The pains are persistent and greatly aggravated by emotional stress and fatigue and are described as burning, drawing, pulling, swelling, or tension. Pain may be spontaneous or may occur in response to a stimulus (such as a pinprick) and persist after the stimulus has been removed. The pain may become intractable to analgesics.

Following an acute thalamic lesion (even a unilateral lesion), the patient may be transiently unable to stand or even sit, despite normal strength of the limbs when tested against resistance (Winfield, 1960). Neglect to use the limbs contralateral to the lesion (*thalamic neglect*) may convey a posture similar to the one demonstrated by patients with athetosis: flexion at the wrist and metacarpophalangeal joints and hyperextension at the interphalangeal joints. The thumb is either abducted or pushed against the palm (Martin, 1969).

Lesions in the anterior region of the thalamus may produce a variety of non-sensory deficits. As noted previously, motor disturbances may occur if the lesion involves areas of the thalamus through which the cerebellar and basal ganglia pathways pass.

The **ventrolateral nucleus** of the anterior portion of the thalamus projects to the primary motor and sensory areas of the cerebral hemispheres (areas 1, 3, 4, and 6). This nucleus is a relay on the path from the red nucleus. Thalamotomy by interruption of the ventrolateral nucleus of the thalamus has been used in the treatment of parkinsonism as well as dystonia musculorum deformans.

## THE HYPOTHALAMUS

The hypothalamus is the principal autonomic center of the brain; it influences both the sympathetic and parasympathetic divisions of the nervous system. These dual activities are integrated into coordinated responses which maintain adequate internal conditions in the body. In addition, neurosecretory cells in the hypothalamus synthesize hormones that reach the blood stream via the neurohypophysis or influence the hormonal output of the adenohypophysis through a special portal system of blood vessels. The hypothalamus also plays a major role in the organization of goal-seeking behavior such as feeding, drinking, mating and aggression and is important for maintaining a constant internal environment (homeostasis).

The hypothalamus lies below or ventral to the thalamus and forms the floor and part of the inferior lateral walls of the third ventricle. It is a small structure, weighing only about 4 g. The shallow **hypothalamic sulcus** on the wall of the third ventricle divides the hypothalamus from the thalamus. The hypothalamus includes a number of well-defined structures: (1) the **mammillary bodies**, two adjacent pea-sized white masses inferior to the gray matter of the floor of the third ventricle and rostral to the posterior perforated substance; (2) the **tuber cinereum**, a funnel-shaped structure between the mammillary bodies and the optic chiasm; (3) the **infundibulum**, a hollow process extending downward from the undersurface of the tuber cinereum to which the posterior lobe of the **hypophysis** (pituitary gland) is attached; and (4) the **optic chiasm** and **optic tracts**. Fig. 2–40 illustrates the major structures of the hypothalamus and their relationship to the surrounding structures.

The lower portion of the infundibulum is continuous with the neural lobe of the hypophysis. The enlarged upper portion of the infundibulum, the median eminence, the infundibular stem and the neural lobe of the hypophysis constitute the **neurohypophysis**. The hypophysis receives its blood supply from two sets of arteries, both of which arise from the internal carotid artery.

Each half of the hypothalamus may be divided, from front to back, into three regions: **supraoptic** (anterior), **tuberal** (middle), and **mammillary** (posterior). Anterior to the hypothalamus, between the optic chiasm and the anterior commissure, is a region referred to as the **preoptic area**.

**(1) Supraoptic or Anterior Region.** The supraoptic region is the most rostral portion of the hypothalamus. It contains the following structures: (a) The **paraventricular nucleus**, a flat sheet of large cells lying close to the lining of the third ventricle in the lateral wall of the hypothalamus; (b) The **supraoptic nucleus**, which straddles the lateral portions of the optic chiasm and extends along the anterior part of the tuber capillaries, consists of several well-defined clusters of nerve cell bodies. The paraventricular and supraoptic nuclei have an abundant supply of capillaries. (c) The **anterior hypothalamic area**, an indistinctly bounded

group of cells between the supraoptic and paraventricular nuclei; and (d) The **lateral hypothalamic area**, a long narrow zone which begins just behind the lateral preoptic area and extends into the intermediate and caudal regions of the hypothalamus.

**(2) The Tuberal or Middle Region.** This area is a mass of gray matter at the base of the hypothalamus and contains several small nuclei: (a) the **dorsomedial nucleus**, located in the dorsomedial portion of the lateral wall of the ventricle; (b) the **ventromedial nucleus**, located ventral to the dorsomedial nucleus; (c) the **infundibular** or **arcuate nuclei**, located in the floor of the hypothalamus near the infundibulum; and (d) the **lateral hypothalamic area**, located lateral to the other three nuclei in this region.

**(3) The Mammillary or Posterior Region.** This area contains the following nuclei: (a) the **mammillary nuclei**, located within the mammillary bodies; (b) the **posterior nucleus**, located dorsal to the mammillary nuclei; and (c) the **lateral nuclear area**, extending through all three nuclear groups of the hypothalamus.

**Afferent Connections**

The hypothalamus receives input from many parts of the limbic system and the reticular formation as well as other nuclei in the brain stem. Afferent connections to the hypothalamus that have been described include the following: (1) The **medial forebrain bundle**, a large, somewhat diffuse tract located mainly in the septal or medial olfactory area, which sends fibers to the hypothalamic nuclei. Other fibers from this bundle continue through the hypothalamus to the raphe nuclei of the reticular formation of the midbrain and pons. The afferent fibers from this tract are related to the sense of smell and the basic emotional drives. Many fibers join this tract and others leave it in all areas through which the tract travels. (2) The **fornix**, a large, compact bundle of axons which brings fibers from the hippocampal formation in the temporal lobe to the mammillary bodies. (3) The **stria terminalis**, a small slender, compact bundle of fibers from the amygdala. This tract is also related to smell and emotional drives. (4) The **pallidohypothalamic fibers**,

# Hypothalamus

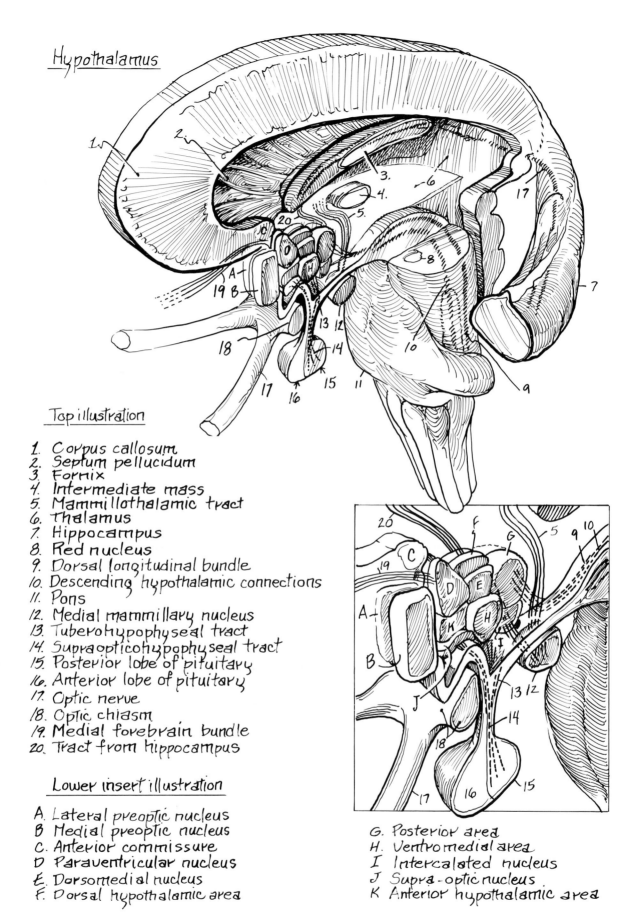

## Top illustration

1. Corpus callosum
2. Septum pellucidum
3. Fornix
4. Intermediate mass
5. Mammillothalamic tract
6. Thalamus
7. Hippocampus
8. Red nucleus
9. Dorsal longitudinal bundle
10. Descending hypothalamic connections
11. Pons
12. Medial mammillary nucleus
13. Tuberohypophyseal tract
14. Supraopticohypophyseal tract
15. Posterior lobe of pituitary
16. Anterior lobe of pituitary
17. Optic nerve
18. Optic chiasm
19. Medial forebrain bundle
20. Tract from hippocampus

## Lower insert illustration

A. Lateral preoptic nucleus
B. Medial preoptic nucleus
C. Anterior commissure
D. Paraventricular nucleus
E. Dorsomedial nucleus
F. Dorsal hypothalamic area

G. Posterior area
H. Ventromedial area
I. Intercalated nucleus
J. Supra-optic nucleus
K. Anterior hypothalamic area

Fig. 2-40. The hypothalamic nuclei.

which lead from the lenticular nucleus to the ventromedial hypothalamic nucleus. (5) The **inferior mammillary peduncle**, which sends fibers from the tegmentum of the midbrain into the hypothalamus.

### Efferent Connections

Efferent pathways arising from cells of the hypothalamus include (1) the **hypothalamicohypophyseal tract**, from the supraoptic nuclei to the neurohypophysis; (2) the **mammilotegmental tract** to the tegmentum of the midbrain; (3) the **hypothalamic-thalamic tracts**, including the tract from the mammillary nuclei to the anterior thalamic nuclei; (4) the **periventricular system**, including the dorsal fasciculus of Schutz to the lower brain levels; and (5) the **tuberohypophyseal tract**, from the tuberal portion of the hypothalamus to the posterior pituitary.

**Hypothalamic-Pituitary Relationships.** The hypothalamus is believed to have diversified activities. It functions as the primary control center for the visceral system and integrates activity for consciousness, visceral, limbic and endocrine systems. The hormonal control of the pituitary is determined by two factors: (1) the direct influence of hormones in the blood on pituitary cells; and (2) the preoptic area and the supraoptic and tuberal areas of the hypothalamus. These areas influence the pituitary through the production of polypeptides produced in the neurons and transported to their terminals. The supraoptic nucleus serves as an osmoreceptor; the secretory activity of its cells is influenced by the osmolarity of the blood flowing through its abundance of vessels. If the osmotic pressure is slightly elevated, its cells will propagate impulses with greater frequency. Impulses arriving at the neurohemal terminals causes release of antidiuretic hormone (vasopressin) into the capillary blood of the neurohypophysis. Resorption of water from the collecting tubules is then accelerated, and the osmolarity of the blood returns to normal, restoring homeostasis with respect to water balance (Barr & Kiernan, 1981).

Cells in the supraoptic and paraventricular nuclei produce the peptide hormones oxytocin and vasopressin (antidiuretic hormone). Cells in the tuberal area produce peptide-releasing hormones, which influence the pituitary to synthesize and secrete thyroid-stimulating hormone (TSH), follicle-stimulating hormone (FSH), luteinizing hormone (LH), growth hormone (GH), adrenocorticotrophic hormone (ACTH), and prolactin. These substances, collectively referred to as *trophic hormones*, have a stimulating effect on their target organs. TSH affects the function of the thyroid hormone. FSH promotes growth of ovarian follicles and spermatogenesis. LH promotes ovulation and converts the ruptured ovarian follicle into a corpus luteum. ACTH acts primarily on the adrenal cortex, stimulating its growth and its secretion of corticosteroids. Prolactin stimulates and sustains lactation during the postpartum period.

### Clinical Features of Hypothalamic Dysfunction

Barr and Kiernan (1981) provide an instructive example with respect to the role of the hypothalamus in maintaining homeostasis. They point out that certain hypothalamic cells act as a thermostat, monitoring the temperature of blood flowing through the capillaries and initiating the responses necessary to maintain a normal body temperature. Thermosensitive neurons in the parasympathetic region of the anterior hypothalamus respond to an increase in temperature of the blood. Mechanisms that promote heat loss, such as cutaneous vasodilation and sweating, are activated. A lesion in the anterior hypothalamus may therefore result in hyperthermia in a hot environment or under states of high metabolic rate. Sustained hyperthermia occurs only as a consequence of an acute process (trauma, bleeding) (Brazis, Masdeu & Biller, 1985).

Cells in the sympathetic region, especially the posterior hypothalamic nucleus, respond to a lowering of blood temperature. Responses such as cutaneous vasoconstriction and shivering are triggered for conservation and production of heat, and a lesion in the posterior hypothalamus interferes with temperature regulation in a cold environment. A lesion in the posterior part of the hypothalamus may not only destroy cells involved in conservation and production of heat but may also interrupt fibers running caudally from the heat-dissipating region. This results in a serious impairment of temperature regulation in either a cold or hot environment. The most common causes include Wernicke's encephalopathy, head trauma, craniopharyngioma, glioblastoma multiforme, surgery, hydrocephalus, and infarction (Martin, Reichlin, & Brown, 1977).

Lesions of the hypothalamic region may produce a variety of other symptoms, including diabetes insipidus (lateral area); obesity (ventromedial area); aphagia and emaciation (lateral area); sexual dystrophy; and hypersomnia (posterior area). Tumors of the adenohypophysis may produce symptoms due to their mass effect outside the pituitary or increased or decreased hormonal secretions. As the tumors expand they may compress the optic chiasm or tract and also cause headaches due to traction of the meninges about the diaphragma sella.

In 1 of 7 patients with a pituitary tumor the presenting complaint is headache. It is usually bitemporal or bifrontal, and behind the eyes (Martin, Reichlin, & Brown, 1977). The visual field defects typically take the form of a bitemporal hemianopsia, although the visual symptoms vary with the growth pattern of the tumor (Carpenter & Sutin, 1983). Endocrine pathology resulting from hypersecretion depends on the type of cell involved. The most commonly observed syndromes involve cells producing excess prolactin (amenorrhea-galactorrhea), growth hormone (acromegaly) and ACTH (Cushing's disease). Diabetes insipidus may be caused by destruction of the neurohypophysis, the supraoptic nuclei or the tract connecting these structures. Production of antidiuretic hormone ceases, and the patient consumes more fluids (polydipsia) and passes excessive quantities of sugar-free urine of low specific gravity (polyuria). Specialized vesicular bodies in the supraoptic nuclei are sensitive to small changes in the osmotic pressure of blood from the internal carotid artery.

Emotions are also considered to be in the realm of hypothalamic activities since it is part of the limbic system. When caused by hypothalamic lesions, rage and fear occur in episodic outbursts, usually triggered by a threatening stimulus (such as restraint or delay in feeding), and are part of a fully coordinated behavioral response with an intense autonomic component (Plum & Van Uitert, 1978). Between outbursts, the behavior is normal and the patient may realize the inappropriateness of his behavior and apologize for his actions. Lesions of the orbitofrontal cortex or temporal lobe may also result in attacks of rage.

## Subthalamus

The **subthalamus** is the zone of brain tissue that lies between the tegmentum of the midbrain and the dorsal thalamus. Also known as the "ventral thalamus," it is the smallest part of the diencephalon. The hypothalamus lies medial and rostral to the subthalamus; lateral to it lies the internal capsule. The **red nucleus** and **substantia nigra** extend into its caudal part from the midbrain.

The **subthalamic nucleus**, or body of Luys, is a cylindrical mass of gray matter located on the inner surface of the peduncular portion of the inner capsule. It has the shape of a thick biconvex lens. It receives a rich blood supply from branches of the posterior communicating, posterior cerebral and anterior choroidal arteries. It has no visible or prominent external structures but is an important subcortical station for voluntary muscle activities. The subthalamic nucleus receives fibers from the globus pallidus, forming a part of the efferent descending path from the corpus striatum.

A lesion in the subthalamic nucleus causes **hemiballismus**, a motor disturbance on the side of the body opposite side the lesion. The condition is characterized by involuntary movements, beginning suddenly and having great force and rapidity. The movements are purposeless and generally of a throwing or flailing type, although they may be choreiform or jerky. The spontaneous movements occur most severely at proximal joints of the limbs, especially at the arms. The muscles of the face and neck are sometimes involved (Barr & Kiernan, 1981).

# THE BRAIN STEM

The brain stem consists of the medulla oblongata, the pons and the midbrain. These three regions have certain fiber tracts in common and each region includes nuclei of cranial nerves. We will consider each of these three structures in this chapter.

## THE MIDBRAIN

The **midbrain**, measuring about 2.5 cm long, is the smallest of the major subdivisions of the brain stem. Located between the pons and the diencephalon, the midbrain contains sensory and motor pathways and nuclei for two cranial nerves. The midbrain also includes two important motor nuclei, the *red nucleus* and the *substantia nigra* (*see* Fig. 2–43). The midbrain is traversed by the cerebral aqueduct, the small tubular passage connecting the third and fourth ventricles.

The dorsal portion of the midbrain, the **tectum** (or roof), measures about 1.5 cm long. It contains four rounded elevations, the corpora quadrigemina. The ventrolateral portions of the midbrain contain the two cerebral peduncles. As shown in Fig. 2–47 the **corpora quadrigemina** consist of four rounded eminences arranged in pairs, the superior colliculi and the inferior colliculi. The two pairs are separated from each other by a **cruciate sulcus**.

The **superior colliculi** are larger and darker than the inferior colliculi. They are associated with the voluntary control of ocular movements and with movement of the eyes and head in response to visual and other stimuli (e.g., turning of the eyes and head toward the source of an unexpected sound). The superior quadrigeminal brachium extends laterally from them and connects with the **lateral geniculate body**. The superior colliculi are interconnected by the **commissure of the superior colliculi**. The **inferior colliculi** act as relay nuclei on the auditory pathway to the

thalamus and then to the cerebral cortex. Fibers connecting the inferior colliculus with the specific thalamic nucleus for hearing (medial geniculate nucleus) form an elevation known as the **inferior brachium**. The trochlear nerve (IV), smallest of the cranial nerves, emerges from the posterior surface of the inferior colliculi.

The **cerebral peduncles** converge from the lower surface of the cerebral hemispheres toward the midline, entering the pons on its upper surface. The interpeduncular fossa is the depressed area between the peduncles that contains the **interpeduncular ganglion**, the terminus for the retroflex bundle of Meynert from the habenular ganglion. The ventral portion of each peduncle is known as the **base**. The corticospinal tract occupies the middle three-fifths of the base, the fronto-pontine tract is located in the medial fifth, and the temporopontine tract is in the lateral fifth. Corticobulbar fibers accompany the corticospinal tract.

The **substantia nigra** is a broad layer of pigmented gray substance separating the ventral portion, or base, from the tegmentum. It extends from the upper surface of the pons to the hypothalamus. The substantia nigra projects to and receives fibers from the corpus striatum. The importance of the substantia nigra is manifest most clearly when considering the symptoms of paralysis agitans (Parkinson's disease). The most consistent pathological finding in Parkinson's disease is degeneration of the melanin-containing cells in the pars compacta of the substantia nigra.

The **tegmentum** is the dorsal portion of the cerebral peduncle. The **lateral lemniscus**, containing ascending fibers of the special sensory path of hearing, is located in the lateral part of the tegmentum posterior to the anterolateral system. Just ventral to the lateral lemniscus is a group of fibers containing the **spinothalamic** and **spinotectal tracts**. The **medial lemniscus** forms, with the trigeminal lemniscus, a triangular bundle medial to the spinothalamic tract. The **medial longitudinal fasciculus** is in the dorsomedial part close to the central gray substance.

The **rubrospinal tract** arises in the posterior portion of the red nucleus and decussates early in the

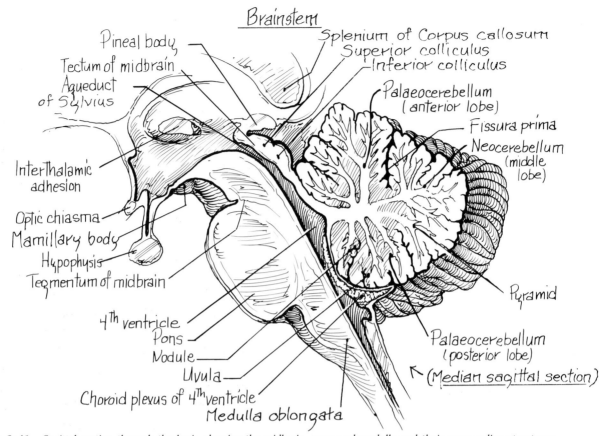

**Brainstem**

Pineal body
Tectum of midbrain
Aqueduct of Sylvius
Interthalamic adhesion
Optic chiasma
Mamillary body
Hypophysis
Tegmentum of midbrain
4th ventricle
Pons
Nodule
Uvula
Choroid plexus of 4th ventricle
Medulla oblongata

Splenium of Corpus callosum
Superior colliculus
Inferior colliculus
Palaeocerebellum (anterior lobe)
Fissura prima
Neocerebellum (middle lobe)
Pyramid
Palaeocerebellum (posterior lobe)
(Median sagittal section)

*Fig. 2-41. Sagittal section through the brain showing the midbrain, pons and medulla and their surrounding structures.*

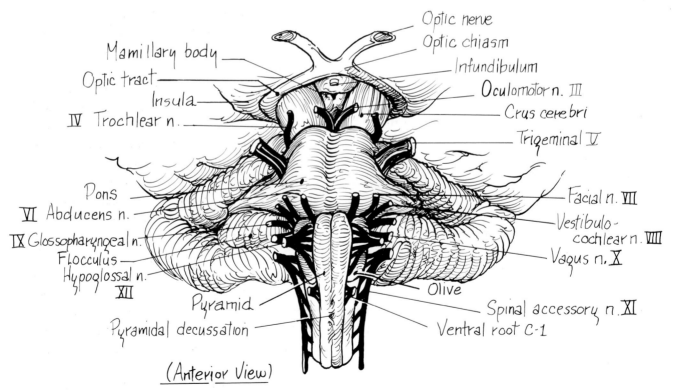

Mamillary body
Optic tract
Insula
IV Trochlear n.
Pons
VI Abducens n.
IX Glossopharyngeal n.
Flocculus
Hypoglossal n. XII
Pyramid
Pyramidal decussation
(Anterior View)

Optic nerve
Optic chiasm
Infundibulum
Oculomotor n. III
Crus cerebri
Trigeminal V
Facial n. VII
Vestibulo-cochlear n. VIII
Vagus n. X
Olive
Spinal accessory n. XI
Ventral root C-1

*Fig. 2-42. Drawing of the anterior aspect of the midbrain, pons and medulla.*

ventral tegmental decussation (decussation of Forel). The **superior cerebellar peduncles** enter the tegmentum and decussate beneath the central gray matter at the level of the inferior colliculus.

The **nucleus of the trochlear nerve** (IV) is situated in the ventral part of the central gray substance at the level of the inferior colliculus. The **nucleus of the oculomotor nerve** (III) lies rostral to the nucleus of the trochlear nerve in the ventral part of the central gray substance beneath the superior colliculus. The **nucleus of the mesencephalic root of the trigeminal nerve** (V) lies in the dorsolateral surface of the central gray substance. The **central periaqueductal gray matter** is continuous posteriorly with the gray substance of the third ventricle. The nucleus of Ardschewitsch lies in the ventrolateral section of this area. The **reticular formation of the midbrain** is continuous with that of the pons and reticular nucleus of the thalamus, zona incerta, and the lateral hypothalamic area.

The **red nucleus**, the large ovoid mass in the anterior part of the tegmentum at the level of the superior colliculus, extends upward into the posterior portion of the subthalamic area. The nucleus has a pinkish hue in a fresh specimen because it is more vascular than the surrounding tissue. Fibers leave this nucleus to go to the reticular formation nuclei, the ventrolateral nucleus of the thalamus and the rubrospinal tract. Afferent fibers to the nucleus proceed from the superior cerebellar peduncle, globus pallidus and frontal cortex.

**Clinical Features of Midbrain Dysfunction.** Symptoms that may arise from destructive lesions of the midbrain are usually a reflection of the structure involved. Destruction of the corpora quadrigemina causes paralysis of upward movements of the eyes. Destruction of the third and fourth cranial nerve nuclei gives rise to the classic syndromes of paralysis of these nerves. Destruction of the red nucleus, the substantia nigra, or reticular substance (which may occur in encephalitic states) may give rise to involuntary movements and rigidity. Destruction of the cerebral peduncle gives rise to spastic paralysis of the contralateral side resulting from destruction of the corticospinal tract.

Cats with experimentally produced lesions of the periaqueductal gray substance resemble behavior of humans with akinetic mutism. A cataleptic state comparable to flexibilitas cerea (waxy flexibility of movements) may occur following destruction of portions of the tegmentum of the midbrain in cats. A syndrome of "obstinate progression" occurs in cats with destructive lesions of the interpeduncular area. These animals continue to push and attempt to walk against interposed resistance, such as a restraint or wall (Chusid, 1979).

Irritative lesions of the midbrain may conceivably occur but are not well recognized. In animals, electrical stimulation produces definite reactions: stimulation of the quadrigeminal region may produce dilatation of pupils and conjugate movement of the eyes to the opposite side. Stimulation of the ventral surface may give rise to slow tonic movements of the extremities. Stimulation of the red nucleus may cause involuntary movements of the extremities in decorticate primates.

Clinical syndromes may be correlated to the portions of the midbrain involved. Lesions of the ventral portion of the midbrain may produce clinical features of Weber's syndrome. Lesions of the tegmentum may produce the clinical picture of Benedikt's syndrome. Disorders or lesions involving the superior colliculi of the tectum, or roof, of the midbrain may produce Parinaud's syndrome.

**Weber's syndrome** is characterized by ipsilateral ophthalmoplegia and contralateral hemiplegia. The ophthalmoplegia results from oculomotor nerve or nucleus interruption; the hemiparesis results from involvement of the cerebral peduncle and its corticospinal tract.

**Benedikt's syndrome** is characterized by ipsilateral ophthalmoplegia and contralateral hyperkinesia such as tremor, chorea and athetosis. It results from a lesion of the tegmentum that destroys the oculomotor nerve and the red nucleus on one side of the midbrain.

**Parinaud's syndrome** consists of conjugate ocular paralysis in the vertical plane, resulting in paralysis of upward gaze. It is associated with lesions or disorders of the quadrigeminal plate of the midbrain, especially the superior colliculi, as occurs when this area is compressed by a pineal body tumor. Section of the posterior commissure can produce Parinaud's syndrome.

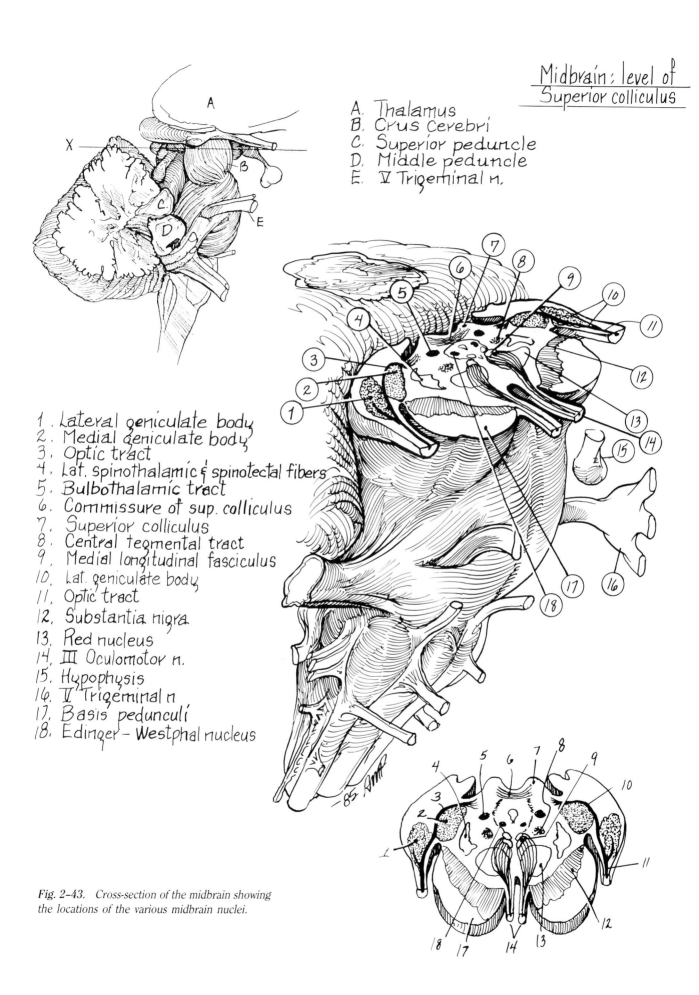

A. Thalamus
B. Crus Cerebri
C. Superior peduncle
D. Middle peduncle
E. V Trigeminal n.

1. Lateral geniculate body
2. Medial geniculate body
3. Optic tract
4. Lat. spinothalamic & spinotectal fibers
5. Bulbothalamic tract
6. Commissure of sup. colliculus
7. Superior colliculus
8. Central tegmental tract
9. Medial longitudinal fasciculus
10. Lat. geniculate body
11. Optic tract
12. Substantia nigra
13. Red nucleus
14. III Oculomotor n.
15. Hypophysis
16. V Trigeminal n
17. Basis pedunculi
18. Edinger-Westphal nucleus

Fig. 2-43.  Cross-section of the midbrain showing
the locations of the various midbrain nuclei.

# THE PONS

The **pons** is the region of the brain stem between the midbrain and the medulla lying in front of the cerebellum (Fig. 2–41). It is a large mass which consists of two distinct parts: the **dorsal** portion, which has features shared with the rest of the brain stem (and therefore includes both sensory and motor tracts) and the **ventral** portion, which provides extensive connections between the two cerebral hemispheres. These connections are important for maximal efficiency of motor activities. The pons is separated from the medulla by a groove through which the abducens, facial and acoustic nerves emerge. The word "pons" means "bridge" and refers to the prominent ventral bulge (or bridge) between the cerebellar hemispheres.

**External Structure.** The pons is about 3.0 cm long. Its anterior surface is covered by a band of thick, transverse fibers, which constitutes the pons proper. The **basal sulcus**, which is a shallow furrow extending along the midline, coincides with the course of the basilar artery.

The anterior limits of the pons are marked by the **middle cerebellar peduncles** that appear on both sides of the midline. Also known as the **brachia pontis**, this pair of peduncles attach the pons to the overlying cerebellum. It is in this area that the facial nerve (VII) and the vestibulocochlear nerve (VIII) are attached to the brain stem. The trigeminal nerve (V), one of the largest cranial nerves, penetrates the brachium pontis near the middle of the lateral surface of the pons.

The posterior surface of the pons forms the rostral floor of the fourth ventricle. Like the medulla, the pons receives its blood supply from the anterior and posterior spinal arteries and from branches of the vertebral, basilar and posterior inferior cerebellar arteries.

**Internal Structure.** The pons can be divided into two parts: (1) the **dorsal portion** or **tegmentum** and (2) the **basilar portion**. The basilar, or ventral, portion contains (a) a thick superficial layer, the **superficial transverse fibers**, which give rise to the brachia pontis; (b) **deep transverse fibers**, which lie dorsal to the corticospinal tract and also contribute to the brachium pontis; and (c) **longitudinal fasciculi**, which lead from the cerebral peduncles to the pons.

The longitudinal fasciculi consist of (1) the **corticospinal tract**, which occupies the middle three-fifths of the cerebral peduncle, enters the pons and breaks up into small bundles and then becomes relatively compact again as it leaves the pons; (2) the **corticobulbar fibers**, which originate in the medial portion of the cerebral peduncle, enter the pons, and pass dorsally toward the cranial nerve nuclei; (3) the **frontopontine tract** (Arnold's bundle), which originates from area 6 of the cerebral cortex and then traverses the anterior limb of the internal capsule and medial fifth of the cerebral peduncle to terminate in ipsilateral pontine nuclei; and (4) the **parietotemporopontine tract** (Turck's bundle), which leads from the parietal and temporal cortex through the posterior limb of the internal capsule and the lateral fifth of the cerebral peduncle, terminating in the ipsilateral pontine nuclei. Figs 2–44 and 2–45 illustrate the afferent and efferent fiber tracts of the pons.

The **pontine nuclei** are small collections of nerve cells profusely scattered among the transverse and longitudinal fiber bundles. Data from the cerebral cortex, in which most neural events underlying volitional movements occur, are made available to the cerebellar cortex through the relay in the pontine nuclei. Activity in the cerebellar cortex influences motor areas in the frontal lobe of the cerebral hemisphere through a pathway that includes the dentate nucleus of the cerebellum and the ventral lateral nucleus of the thalamus. The circuit linking the cerebral and cerebellar cortices provides for precision and efficiency of voluntary movements (Barr & Kiernan, 1981).

The dorsal, or tegmental, portion of the pons consists mainly of the rostral continuation of the gray substance and the reticular formation of the medulla and midbrain. It contains cranial nerve nuclei, ascending and descending tracts and reticular nuclei (Fig. 2–46).

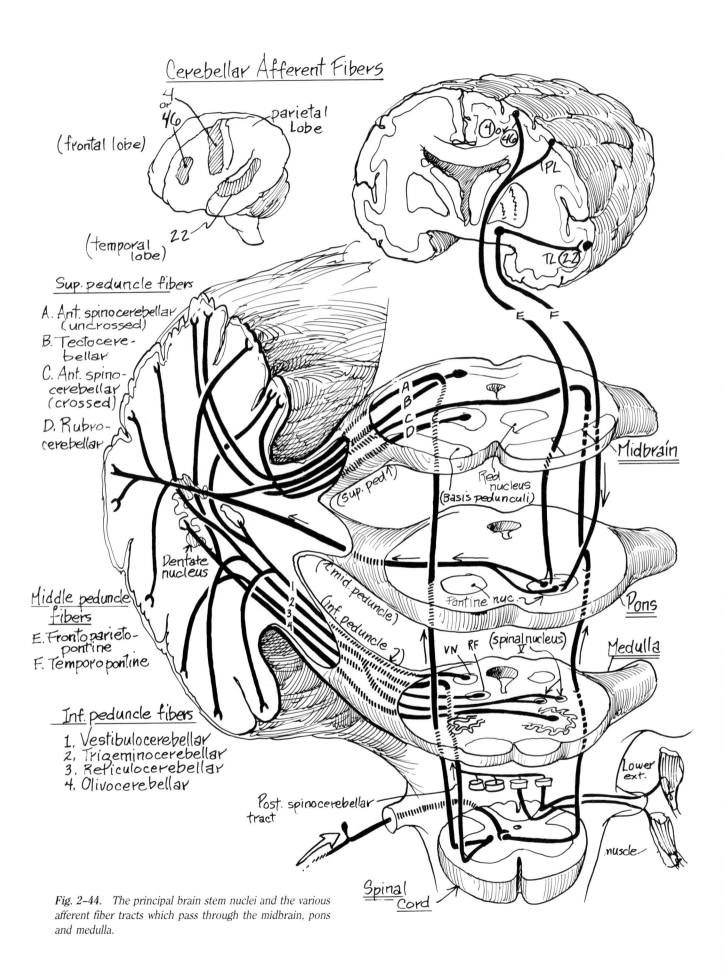

**Cerebellar Afferent Fibers**

(frontal lobe)

4 or 46

parietal Lobe

22

(temporal lobe)

PL

4 or 46

TL 22

E F

**Sup. peduncle fibers**

A. Ant. spinocerebellar (uncrossed)

B. Tectocere-bellar

C. Ant. spino-cerebellar (crossed)

D. Rubro-cerebellar

A
B
C
D

Midbrain

(Sup. Ped.)

Red nucleus (Basis pedunculi)

Dentate nucleus

**Middle peduncle fibers**

E. Fronto parieto-pontine

F. Temporo pontine

(mid. peduncle)

(Inf. peduncle)

Pontine nuc.

Pons

1
2
3
4

VN RF (spinal nucleus) V

Medulla

**Inf. peduncle fibers**

1. Vestibulocerebellar
2. Trigeminocerebellar
3. Reticulocerebellar
4. Olivocerebellar

Lower ext.

Post. spinocerebellar tract

muscle

Spinal Cord

*Fig. 2-44.* *The principal brain stem nuclei and the various afferent fiber tracts which pass through the midbrain, pons and medulla.*

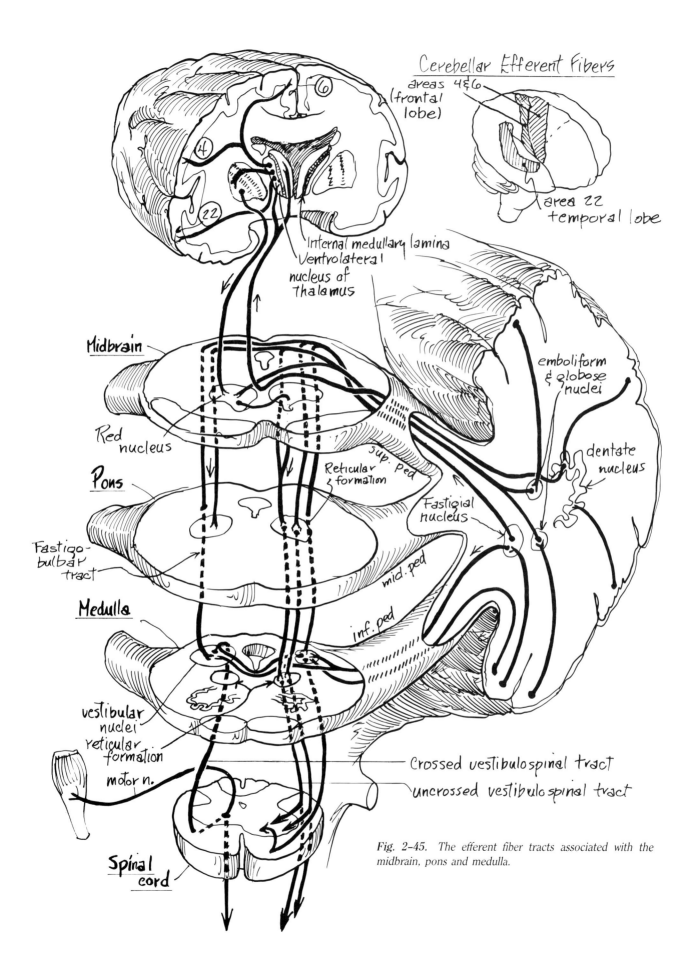

areas 4&6
(frontal lobe)

area 22
temporal lobe

Internal medullary lamina
Ventrolateral
nucleus of
Thalamus

Midbrain

emboliform
& globose
nuclei

Red
nucleus

sup. ped

dentate
nucleus

Reticular
formation

Pons

Fastigial
nucleus

Fastigo-
bulbar
tract

mid. ped

Medulla

inf. ped

vestibular
nuclei
reticular
formation
motor n.

Crossed vestibulospinal tract
uncrossed vestibulospinal tract

Spinal
cord

Fig. 2-45. The efferent fiber tracts associated with the
midbrain, pons and medulla.

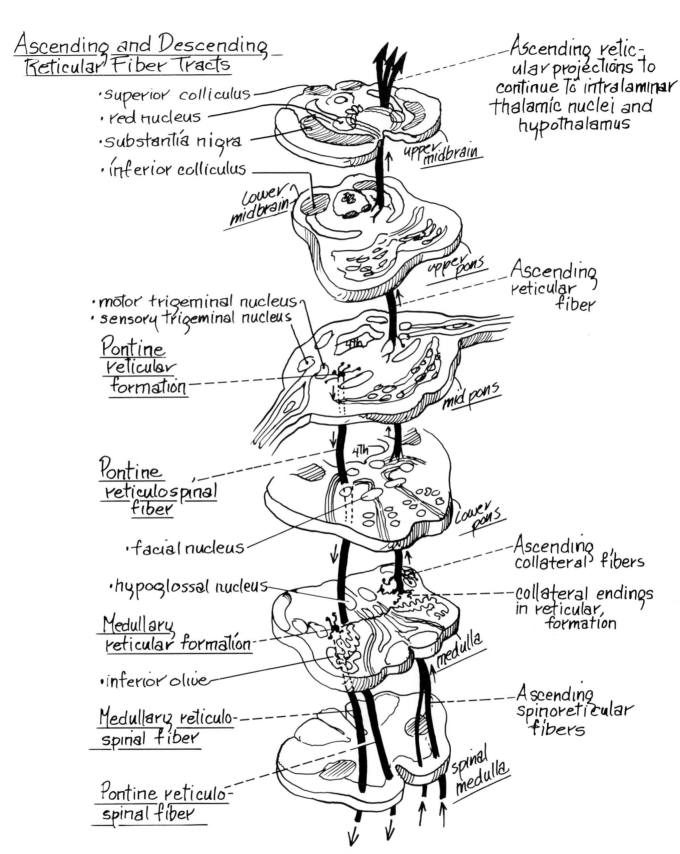

## Ascending and Descending Reticular Fiber Tracts

- superior colliculus
- red nucleus
- substantia nigra
- inferior colliculus

Ascending reticular projections to continue to intralaminar thalamic nuclei and hypothalamus

upper midbrain

Lower midbrain

upper pons

Ascending reticular fiber

- motor trigeminal nucleus
- sensory trigeminal nucleus

### Pontine reticular formation

4th

mid pons

### Pontine reticulospinal fiber

4th

Lower pons

- facial nucleus

Ascending collateral fibers

collateral endings in reticular formation

- hypoglossal nucleus

### Medullary reticular formation

- inferior olive

medulla

Ascending spinoreticular fibers

### Medullary reticulospinal fiber

### Pontine reticulospinal fiber

spinal medulla

**Fig. 2-46.** *The principal nuclei of the midbrain, pons and medulla and the ascending and descending reticular fiber tracts associated with the brain stem.*

Cranial Nerve Nuclei in the Pons. The **nucleus of the abducens nerve (VI)** is a rounded gray cellular mass located in the dorsomedial area just beneath the floor of the fourth ventricle. Its fibers pass ventrally between lateral bundles of the corticospinal fibers to exit at the groove separating the pons and the medulla. These fibers innervate the lateral rectus muscle of the orbit.

Lesions of the abducens nerve in the brain stem or in its long intracranial course cause medial strabismus and ipsilateral paralysis of the lateral rectus muscle, manifested by an inability to direct the affected eye laterally. Because contraction of the medial rectus muscle on the affected side is unopposed, the eye is strongly adducted. The contralateral eye is unaffected and can move in all directions. The patient has diplopia (double vision) on attempting to gaze to the side of the lesion; two images are seen side by side. This is called *horizontal diplopia*. Diplopia results because light reflected by an object in the visual field does not fall upon corresponding points of the two retinae (Carpenter & Sutin, 1983).

The **nucleus of the facial nerve (VII)** is a pear-shaped gray mass in the lateral part of the reticular formation immediately dorsal to the superior olivary nucleus. Its fibers run dorsomedially toward the floor of the fourth ventricle, make an acute compact bend at the medial side of the abducens nucleus, and then turn laterally through the pons to exit at the lower border between the olive and the inferior cerebellar peduncle. The fibers of the facial nerve innervate a thin sheet of branchiomeric muscles underneath the skin of the face. These are the muscles that control facial expression.

The signs of facial nerve lesion depend not only on the severity of the lesion, but also on where the facial nerve is affected in its passage through the facial canal. A complete lesion of the motor part of the facial nerve as it emerges from the stylomastoid foramen produces paralysis of all ipsilateral facial movements (*Bell's palsy*). The patient with this type of lesion is unable to wrinkle his forehead, close his eye, show his teeth, purse his lips, or whistle on the affected side. The corner of the mouth droops on the side of the lesion. Although corneal sensation is present, the corneal reflex is lost on the side of the lesion because the motor fibers participating in this reflex are destroyed.

In addition to the paralysis of facial muscles, there is a loss of taste sensation in the anterior two-thirds of the tongue and in the palate of the affected side, together with impairment of secretion by the submandibular, sublingual and lacrimal glands. Sounds may seem abnormally loud (*hyperacusis*) because of paralysis of the stapedius muscle.

Aberrant regeneration of preganglionic parasympathetic fibers may occur, since the cell bodies lie within the central nervous system. In this aberrant regeneration, fibers previously synapsing upon postganglionic neurons of the submandibular ganglion establish new relationships with cells of the pterygopalatine ganglion. This results in lacrimation (*crocodile tears*) when aromas and taste sensations cause stimulation of cells in the superior salivary muscle.

The **motor nucleus of the trigeminal nerve (V)** and the **main sensory nucleus of the trigeminal nerve** are located close together in the dorsolateral portion of the reticular formation. The sensory nucleus is located more laterally, and the tracts that arise from it are functionally comparable to the posterior columns of the spinal cord. The **nucleus of the descending spinal tract of the trigeminal nerve** is a continuation of the substantia gelatinosa rolandi of the spinal cord, and the spinal tract is functionally similar to the spinothalamic tract.

**Trigeminal neuralgia** (*tic douloureux*) results from a lesion of the trigeminal nerve. The condition is characterized by paroxysms of pain in the distributions of one of the trigeminal divisions, usually with periods of remission and exacerbation. The pain is usually of sudden onset and may be initiated by merely touching the skin of the face. The cause of tic douloureux is unknown.

The sensory and motor nuclei of the trigeminal nerve may be affected by areas of degeneration in the brain stem, or the intracranial portion of the nerve may be affected by trauma, tumor growth or another lesion. A lesion of the motor fibers will cause paralysis and eventual atrophy of the muscles of mastication. The mandible deviates to the affected side because of the unopposed action of the contralateral lateral pterygoid muscle.

The **nuclei of the vestibular nerve (VIII)** make up a diamond-shaped mass of gray matter in the floor and lateral wall of the fourth ventricle in the pons and the medulla. The **superior vestibular nucleus** (nucleus of Bechterew) is situated in the angle of the floor and lateral wall of the fourth ventricle just behind the trigeminal motor nucleus. The **medial vestibular nucleus** (nucleus of Schwalbe), the largest of the vestibular nuclei, occupies part of the area acoustica of the rhomboid fossa. Fibers pass from it to the medial longitudinal fasciculus, cranial nerve nuclei, and cerebellum. The connections established through the medial longitudinal fasciculus are important in coordinating movements of the eyes with movements of the head.

The **caloric test** (caloric irrigation) is used when there is a reason to suspect a tumor of the vestibulocochlear nerve or a lesion interrupting the vestibular pathway in the brain stem. The procedure causes nystagmus if the vestibular pathway for the side tested is intact.

Labryinthine irritation or disease may cause vertigo, nausea, vomiting, pallor, a cold sweat, and nystagmus. Paroxysms of labyrinthine irritation constitute Meniere's disease, the cause of which is poorly understood. The **lateral vestibular nucleus** (nucleus of Deiters) is next to the inferior cerebellar peduncle and gives rise to the fibers of the vestibular tract. The **inferior vestibular nucleus**, or nucleus of the descending tract of the vestibular nerve, extends from the lateral nucleus to the cuneate nucleus in the medulla and lies medial to the inferior cerebellar peduncle and dorsal to the spinal trigeminal tract.

**Nuclei of the cochlear nerve (VIII)** (acoustic nuclei) include the **dorsal cochlear nucleus**, located on the dorsolateral surface of the inferior cerebellar peduncle, and the **ventral cochlear nucleus**, located in the ventrolateral region of the inferior cerebellar peduncle at the level of the entrance of the auditory fibers. Destruc-tion of the cochlear nerve or the cochlear nuclei causes complete deafness on the same side.

**Other Clinical Manifestations Associated with Lesions of the Pons.** Certain clinical syndromes are characteristically associated with lesions of the pons. Lesions of the more ventral portion of the inferior pons may produce alternating abducent hemiplegia, Millard-Gubler syndrome, or Foville's syndrome.

**Millard-Gubler syndrome** is a crossed paralysis, affecting the limbs on one side of the body and the face on the opposite side. There is also paralysis of the outward movement of the eye. This syndrome is due to infarction of the pons involving the sixth and seventh cranial nerves and the fibers of the corticospinal tract.

**Foville's syndrome** is similar to the Millard-Gubler syndrome, except that in addition to paralysis of the outward movement of the eye there is paralysis of conjugate movement.

Lesions of the lateral pons are often associated with tumors in the pontocerebellar angle and may produce a characteristic picture. Lesions of the ventral portion of the mid-pons may produce alternating trigeminal hemiplegia. More extensive lesions of the inferior pons may produce the clinical features of **Raymond-Cestan syndrome**, which includes alternating abducent hemiplegia characterized by ipsilateral lateral rectus muscle paresis and contralateral hemiplegia resulting in nystagmus. It may occur with softening of the paramedian area of the pons resulting from involvement of the abducens nerve and corticospinal tract.

Bilateral ventral pontine lesions (due to infarction, tumor, hemorrhage, trauma, etc.) may result in **locked-in syndrome** (Brazis, Masdeu & Biller, 1985). Also known as **deefferentation**, this condition is characterized by (1) quadraplegia (due to bilateral corticospinal tract involvement); and (2) aphonia (due to involvement of the corticobulbar fibers destined to the lower cranial nerves). Since the reticular formation is not injured, the patient is completely awake. The vertical eye movements and blinking reflexes are intact. Some patients with this condition have been able to communicate with others by using a "Morse code" with their eye movements.

# THE MEDULLA OBLONGATA

The **medulla oblongata** (myelencephalon), the pyramid-shaped structure between the spinal cord and the pons, is the most caudal segment of the brain stem. Measuring about 3 cm long, it represents an expanded continuation of the upper cervical spinal cord. Although the spinal cord seems to pass imperceptibly into the medulla, internally there is a rather abrupt and extensive rearrangement of the gray matter and white matter. The nuclei of the medulla initiate and regulate many vital functions, which will be described below.

The central canal of the spinal cord continues through the caudal half of the medulla and then, at a point called the **obex**, flares open into the wide cavity of the fourth ventricle. Thus, the rostral part of the medulla occupies the floor of the fourth ventricle. The roof of the ventricle is formed by the **tela choroidea** and **choroid plexus**, a thin sheet of ependyma and pia mater with blood vessels between them.

Two longitudinal grooves can be identified on the anterolateral aspect of the medulla: (1) the **ventrolateral sulcus**, which extends along the lateral border of the pyramid; and (2) the **dorsolateral sulcus**. The rootlets of the hypoglossal nerve (XII) exit from the ventrolateral sulcus. Radicles of the bulbar accessory nerve (XI), vagus nerve (X) and glossopharyngeal nerve (IX) are attached along the dorsolateral sulcus. The spinal portion of the accessory nerve (XI) arises from the gray matter of spinal cord segments C-2 to C-5. The prominent oval swelling of the lateral area of the medulla between the ventrolateral and dorsolateral sulci is the **olive**, which marks the position of the inferior olivary nucleus.

Certain gray nuclear areas located within the substance of the medulla receive afferent fibers from various sources and project to the cerebellum. These nuclei initiate and regulate many vital activities, including breathing, swallowing, heart rate, waking and sleeping. Seven of the twelve cranial nerves are attached to the medulla or the junction of the medulla and pons. The **hypoglossal nucleus** is located near the ventrolateral portion of the central canal in the lower half of the medulla; its upper part lies a short distance from the midline under an eminence called the **hypoglossal trigone** (see Fig. 2–47). The root fibers of the hypoglossal nerve gather on the ventral surface of the nucleus. Injury to the hypoglossal nerve (XII) produces a lower motor neuron paralysis of the ipsilateral half of the tongue with loss of movement, loss of tone, and atrophy of the muscles. The genioglossus muscle effects protrusion of the tongue; when the tongue is protruded, it will deviate to the side of the lesion because of the unopposed protrusor action of the contralateral genioglossus muscle.

The **dorsal motor nucleus of the vagus nerve** (X), the largest of the parasympathetic nuclei in the brain stem, lies along side the hypoglossal nucleus. It contains neurons that form an important part of the parasympathetic division of the autonomic nervous system. The **vestibular nuclei** receive afferent fibers from the vestibulocochlear nerve (VIII). This nerve brings information to the brain regarding movement and position of the head in space.

The **nucleus ambiguus** lies in the anterolateral part of the reticular formation. Its fibers innervate the glossopharyngeal (IX), vagus (X) and bulbar accessory (XI) nerves, which control the muscles of the pharynx and larynx, thus controlling swallowing and vocalization. The nucleus ambiguus also contains parasympathetic neurons whose axons end in the cardiac ganglia and control the heart rate. The accessory nerve is motor, whereas the glossopharyngeal and vagus nerves are mixed (having both motor and sensory components).

The spinal portion of the accessory nerve supplies the sternocleidomastoid and upper parts of the trapezius muscles. Weakness of the upper part of the trapezius muscle can be tested by having the patient shrug his shoulders against resistance.

A unilateral lesion of the vagus nerve is followed by ipsilateral paralysis of the soft palate, pharynx and larynx, which results in hoarseness, dyspnea and dysphagia. Anesthesia of the pharynx and larynx results in an ipsilateral loss of the cough reflex. Bilateral lesions of the vagus nerve are usually fatal unless immediate precautions are taken to prevent asphyxia, resulting from complete laryngeal paralysis.

The **reticular formation**, containing scattered groups of cells, is a continuation of the reticular substance of the spinal cord that extends upward through the medulla, pons, midbrain and thalamus. In the medulla, there are five major reticular nuclei: (1) the **lateral reticular nucleus**, located near the surface of the medulla and projecting into the cerebellum; (2) the **paramedian nucleus**, which lies adjacent to the midline of the medulla and also projects into the cerebellum; (3) the **ventral reticular nucleus**; (4) the **parvicellular nucleus**; and (5) the **magnocellular nucleus**. These nuclear groups carry out vital functions, such as the control of blood pressure and respiration.

**Clinical Findings in Lesions of the Medulla.** The medulla receives its blood supply from the anterior and posterior spinal arteries and branches of the vertebral, basilar and posterior inferior cerebellar arteries. Complete or partial thrombosis of the basilar artery may occur suddenly and is accompanied by severe headache, vomiting, and loss of consciousness. Insufficiency of the basilar arterial system is characterized by varying signs and symptoms occurring in transient episodes over a period of months or years. The most common symptoms of basilar artery insufficiency are vertigo, dysarthria, dysphagia, diplopia, nystagmus and varying degrees of paresis on one or both sides of the body (Gillian, 1964).

Lesions of the brain stem produce symptoms referable to involvement of the motor and sensory pathways passing through it and particularly to involvement of the nuclei of the cranial nerves that lie within it.

Clinical syndromes may be related to the portion of the medulla involved. Lesions of the ventral portion of the upper medulla may produce hypoglossal hemiplegia alternans (alternating hypoglossal hemiplegia) whereas lesions of the dorsolateral area of the upper medulla may produce Wallenberg's syndrome, often associated with posterior inferior cerebellar artery disease. It has also been described with medullary neoplasms (usually metastases) abscess, and hematoma (secondary to rupture of an arteriovenous malformation).

**Wallenberg's syndrome** is characterized by ipsilateral loss of temperature and pain sensations of the face and contralateral loss of these sensations of the extremities and trunk. Ipsilateral ataxia, dysphagia, dysarthria, nystagmus, vomiting, and vertigo may also occur. Occasionally, hiccups (due to involvement of the medullary respiratory centers) and diplopia (secondary to involvement of the lower pons) have also been reported (Brazis, Masdue & Biller, 1985). Involvement of the more central area of the upper medulla may produce a variety of clinical pictures depending upon the cranial nuclei and other structures involved.

Integration of reflexes concerned with swallowing, vomiting, respiration and cardiovascular control occurs in the medulla. The respiratory center in the medulla is composed of an inspiratory and an expiratory portion. Electrical stimulation of the ventral reticular portion of the medulla in animals produces forced, deep inspiration. Similar stimulation of the reticular formation lying more dorsally and rostrally may produce expiration. Cardiovascular reflexes essential for maintenance of blood pressure, vasopressor and vasodilator reflexes, and some cardiac reflexes require an intact medulla. **Cheyne-Stokes respiration**, with periodic breathing characterized by intense hyperventilation alternating with apnea, is believed to be due to increased respiratory sensitivity to $CO_2$ (resulting from bilateral descending motor system dysfunction at higher levels) and moderate arterial oxygen desaturation.

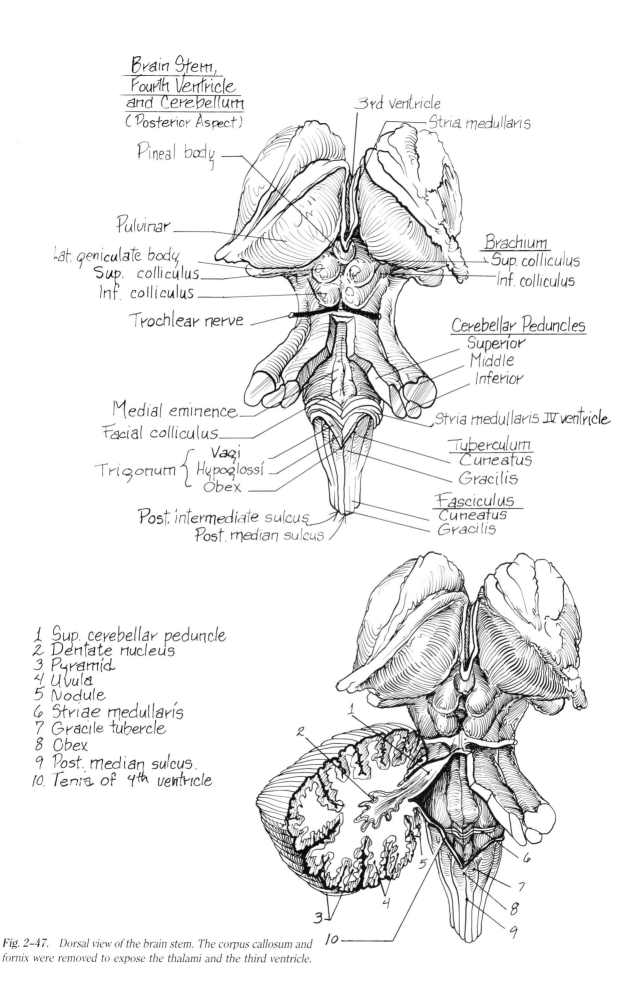

Brain Stem,
Fourth Ventricle
and Cerebellum
( Posterior Aspect )

Pineal body

3rd ventricle

Stria medullaris

Pulvinar

Lat. geniculate body
Sup. colliculus
Inf. colliculus

Trochlear nerve

Brachium
Sup. colliculus
Inf. colliculus

Cerebellar Peduncles
Superior
Middle
Inferior

Medial eminence
Facial colliculus

Vagi
Trigonum { Hypoglossi
Obex

Stria medullaris IV ventricle

Tuberculum
Cuneatus
Gracilis

Fasciculus
Cuneatus
Gracilis

Post. intermediate sulcus
Post. median sulcus

1 Sup. cerebellar peduncle
2 Dentate nucleus
3 Pyramid
4 Uvula
5 Nodule
6 Striae medullaris
7 Gracile tubercle
8 Obex
9 Post. median sulcus.
10. Tenia of 4th ventricle

**Fig. 2–47.** *Dorsal view of the brain stem. The corpus callosum and fornix were removed to expose the thalami and the third ventricle.*

# RETICULAR FORMATION

Physiologists differ with regard to the anatomical delineation of the reticular formation. Broadly defined, it is a substantial region of the lower brain stem (medulla through midbrain) in which the groups of neurons and bundles of fibers present a complicated netlike appearance; clearly circumscribed nuclei and tracts are absent. The reticular formation is a combination of both gray and white matter (*see* Fig. 2–49).

It is important to realize that the *ascending reticular activating system*, to be considered later in this section, is not identical with the reticular formation. This system includes large parts of the reticular formation, together with parts of the diencephalon and telencephalon.

The reticular formation receives data from most of the sensory systems and has efferent connections (direct and indirect), with all levels of the central nervous system. Each reticular neuron may receive input from over 4000 other nerve cells, many of which lie at a great distance along the neuraxis (Angevine & Cotman, 1981). In this way, the reticular formation samples much of the activity in the CNS and can use this information to modulate overall nervous activity. The reticular formation is organized in such a way that all of the varied sensory input that it receives is selectively filtered. Only certain patterns of sensory input will trigger the reticular activating system to alert the cerebral cortex (CIBA, 1983). The reticular formation makes significant contributions to several functions, including the sleep-arousal cycle, the motor system of the brain and spinal cord, and the regulation of visceral functions. The parts of the reticular formation differ from one another in their cytoarchitecture, connections, and physiological functions. Aggregations of neurons, called nuclei even though they are not clearly circumscribed, are physiologically similar to most of the other nuclei of the central nervous system.

## Nuclei of the Reticular Formation

Three of the reticular formation nuclei — the lateral reticular nucleus, the paramedian reticular nucleus, and the reticulotegmental nucleus — project to the cerebellum. Termed the **precerebellar reticular nuclei**, they are functionally quite separate from the rest of the reticular formation.

The **noncerebellar reticular nuclei** are classified into three longitudinally arrayed groups: (1) the **raphe nuclei**, located in the midline of the brain stem, are interspersed among bundles of decussating myelinated axons; (2) the **central group** of nuclei — the *ventral reticular nucleus* and the *gigantocellular reticular nucleus* in the medulla, and the *caudal* and *oral pontine reticular nuclei*; and (3) the **lateral group** of reticular nuclei, including the *parvicellular reticular nucleus* in the medulla and caudal half of the pons, the *cuneiform* and *subcuneiform nuclei* in the midbrain, and the *pedunculopontine nucleus* in the midbrain.

Most of the dendrites of neurons of the central group of reticular nuclei have long axons that branch out in a complex manner. The long axons run rostrally and caudally, with many collateral branches that synapse with the dendrites of other reticular neurons. Terminal branches of the axons end in other nuclei of the reticular formation in more remote regions, such as the thalamus and spinal cord.

The functional organization of the reticular formation can best be understood by dividing it into three systems: (1) the ascending reticular activating system; (2) the reticulobulbar system (concerned with motor and visceral functions; and (3) a system involving the raphe nuclei.

**The Ascending Reticular Activating System (RAS).** As previously mentioned, the reticular activating system includes part of the reticular formation as well as the "nonspecific" thalamic nuclei (midline, intralaminar and reticular). Specifically, the RAS extends from the superior half of the pons through the midbrain to the posterior portion of the hypothalamus and to the thalamic reticular formation.

The ascending reticular activating system consists of the sensory input to the reticular formation and transmission to certain "specific" thalamic nuclei, from which activity spreads to the cerebral cortex. In this way activation of the RAS alerts the cerebral cortex to be more receptive to incoming signals.

When the cortex is stimulated by way of the reticular formation during sleep, the electrical activity of the cortex, as seen on the electroencephalogram, changes from the large wave pattern of sleep to the small wave pattern of the waking state. This is referred to as **desynchronization** or **arousal reaction**. When someone is awake, stimuli reaching the cortex through the activating system sharpen attentiveness and create optimal conditions for perception of sensory data conveyed through more direct pathways. Cutaneous stimuli appear to be especially important in maintaining consciousness whereas visual, acoustic, and mental stimuli have a special bearing on alertness and attention.

Sleep is not merely the absence of wakefulness; it is an active, ongoing process. It is thought that slow-wave sleep is produced by a center in the reticular formation of the medulla. It does this by depressing the activity of the RAS. As the center in the medulla inhibits the RAS it simultaneously activates the sleep center in the pons. This pontine sleep center is responsible for the generation of paradoxical (or REM) sleep.

The reticular activating system is of considerable pharmacological interest because general anesthetics are thought to suppress transmission through the polysynaptic pathway in the brain stem. Similarly, the reticular formation of the the brain stem may be a site of action of tranquilizing drugs. Prolonged coma results from serious damage to the reticular formation. Damage to the RAS, described in animals by Moruzzi and Magoun (1949), induces a state in which the animal becomes unresponsive and its EEG shows sleep patterns despite vigorous sensory stimulation.

The medial longitudinal fasciculus, which connects the abducens and oculomotor nuclei, and the oculomotor and trochlear nuclei themselves are situated amid the neurons of the pontine and midbrain portions of the RAS. Thus, when unresponsiveness is caused by brainstem lesions, their location can often be determined by the abnormal patterns of ocular motility (Brazis, Masdeu, & Biller, 1985).

**The Reticulobulbar System.** Groups of neurons in the reticular formation regulate visceral functions through connections with nuclei of the autonomic outflow, and, in the case of respiration, with motor neurons in the phrenic nucleus and and thoracic region of the spinal cord. Respiratory and cardio-vascular regions, commonly referred to as "centers," have been identified by electrical stimulation within the brain stem in experimental animals. Maximal inspiratory responses are obtained from the gigantocellular reticular nucleus in the medulla, whereas expiratory responses are evoked by stimulation of the parvicellular reticular nucleus, also in the medulla. A pneumotaxic center in the pontine reticular formation controls normal respiratory rhythm. Stimulation of the ventral and gigantocellular reticular nuclei in the medulla has a depressor effect on the circulatory system, with slowing of the heart rate and lowering of blood pressure. The opposite effects are produced by stimulation of the parvicellular reticular nucleus in the medulla. Damage to the brain stem is life-threatening because of the presence of these centers that control vital functions.

**The Raphe Nuclei.** The raphe nuclei are several groups of cells located along the midline of the medulla, pons and midbrain. Afferent fibers to the raphe nuclei of the midbrain and pons come from various parts of the hypothalamus and limbic system. Many of the neurons of the raphe nuclei synthesize serotonin, a substance that they probably use as a neurotransmitter.

From a clinical viewpoint, the most interesting aspects of raphe nuclei are the indirect input from the periaqueductal gray matter and the projection from the nucleus raphe magnus to the spinal dorsal horn. Electrical stimulation of either the periaqueductal gray matter or the nucleus raphe magnus produces an inhibitory action upon sensory neurons and results in loss of the ability to experience pain from sites of injury or disease; the former procedure has been used

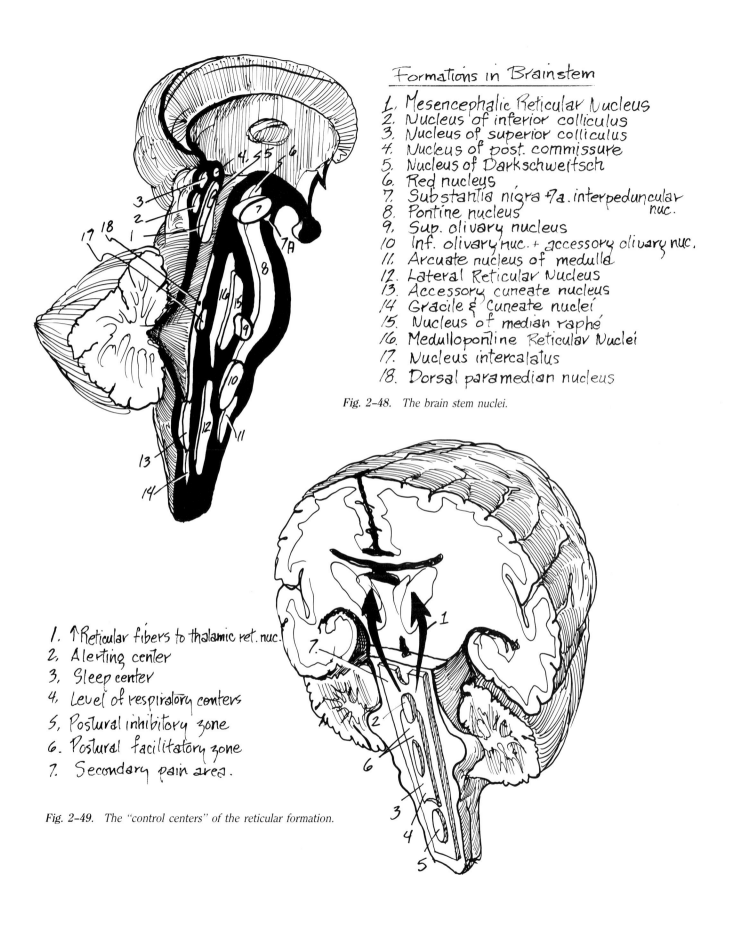

## Formations in Brainstem

1. Mesencephalic Reticular Nucleus
2. Nucleus of inferior colliculus
3. Nucleus of superior colliculus
4. Nucleus of post. commissure
5. Nucleus of Darkschweitsch
6. Red nucleus
7. Substantia nigra 7a. interpeduncular nuc.
8. Pontine nucleus
9. Sup. olivary nucleus
10. Inf. olivary nuc. + accessory olivary nuc.
11. Arcuate nucleus of medulla
12. Lateral Reticular Nucleus
13. Accessory cuneate nucleus
14. Gracile & Cuneate nuclei
15. Nucleus of median raphé
16. Medullopontine Reticular Nuclei
17. Nucleus intercalatus
18. Dorsal paramedian nucleus

*Fig. 2-48. The brain stem nuclei.*

1. ↑Reticular fibers to thalamic ret. nuc.
2. Alerting center
3. Sleep center
4. Level of respiratory centers
5. Postural inhibitory zone
6. Postural facilitatory zone
7. Secondary pain area.

*Fig. 2-49. The "control centers" of the reticular formation.*

clinically in the management of otherwise intractable pain. The analgesic effect requires the integrity of the raphe spinal tract in the dorsolateral funiculus of the spinal cord; it is antagonized by the administration of drugs, such as naloxone, that are known to be competitive antagonists of morphine and related opiates.

It has been postulated that the analgesic action of opiates used medicinally is produced in the periaqueductal gray matter and in the dorsal horn, where the drugs mimic the action of naturally occurring peptides known as enkephalins. These peptides, which are pharmacologically similar to morphine, occur in nerve terminals in the periaqueductal gray matter and in the dorsal horn, as well as in some other parts of the central nervous system. Other opiatelike peptides, the endorphins, have been found in other parts of the brain and in the pituitary gland.

Surgical section of the ventrolateral spinal cord has also been done for the relief of intractable pain. Occasionally, a condition known as *Ondine's curse* has occurred after this surgical procedure. In this condition, there is a loss of automatic breathing during sleep, probably due to reticulospinal tract interruption.

# THE CEREBELLUM

The **cerebellum** is the largest part of the hindbrain. It is located in the posterior fossa of the skull behind the pons and medulla and receives data from most of the sensory systems and the cerebral cortex. It eventually influences motor neurons supplying the skeletal musculature. The function of the cerebellum is to produce changes in muscle tonus in relation to equilibrium, locomotion and posture, as well as nonstereotyped movements based on individual experience. The cerebellum operates at a subconscious level (Barr & Kiernan, 1983).

The cerebellum is separated from the overlying cerebrum by an extension of dura mater, the **tentorium cerebelli**. The cerebellum has an ovoid shape, with its widest diameter along the transverse axis. Fig. 2–41 shows the cerebellum in relation to its surrounding structures.

The surface of the cerebellum contains many sulci and furrows. Because of the extensive folding of the cerebellar surface in the form of thin transverse **folia** (long gyri), 85% of the cortical surface is concealed. Therefore, there is a large cortical area, about three-fourths as extensive as that of the much larger cerebrum. Numerous deep fissures divide the cerebellum into several lobes. The numerous shallower sulci within each lobe separate the individual folia from each other. (Fig. 2–50 and 2–51.)

The cerebellum is composed of two large lateral masses, the **cerebellar hemispheres**. A midline portion, the **vermis**, connects the hemispheres. The inferior surface of the vermis is subdivided into the nodule, uvula, pyramid and tuber. Each hemisphere has three lobes.

(1) The **flocculonodular lobe** (archicerebellum) includes the **nodulus**, which is the inferior part of the vermis, and the attached **flocculi** (small appendages in the posterior inferior region). This part of the cerebellum has connections with the vestibular nuclei; the function of the flocculonodular lobe is to keep the individual oriented in space. A lesion in this area will result in trunk ataxia, swaying, and staggering.

(2). The **posterior lobe** (neocerebellum) makes up the greater part of the cerebellum. It is located between the anterior lobe and the flocculonodular lobe. The neocerebellum consists of the main bulk of the cerebellar hemispheres and part of the vermis. It receives connections from the cerebrum and is involved in muscular coordination of phasic movements. A lesion in this area will produce intention tremors and the inability to perform rapidly changing movements.

(3) The **anterior lobe** (paleocerebellum), which consists of most of the vermis and the anterior aspect of the cerebellar hemispheres, is involved in the regulation of muscle tone.

Several laminae project from the white matter into the cortical folia. On cross-section this can be seen quite distinctly and has been termed the *arbor vitae cerebelli*. On histological section, the cerebellum shows three cortical layers. From the surface to the white matter of the folium, these are: (1) the molecular layer; (2) the layer of Purkinje cells; and (3) the granule layer (Fig. 2–52).

The **molecular layer** contains relatively few nerve cells; it is largely a synaptic layer, composed of profusely branching dendrites of Purkinje cells and, in the deepest layer, axons of the granule cells. In transverse section it presents a finely punctate appearance. The two types of cell bodies in the molecular layer are the *basket cell* and the outer (superficial) *stellate cell*.

The **Purkinje cell layer** consists of a single row of bodies of Purkinje cells arranged side by side between the molecular layer and the granular layer. It is estimated that there are approximately 15 million Purkinje cells in the cerebellum. These flask-shaped cells have a profuse dendritic branching in the molecular layer, in a plane transverse to the folium. This allows maximal opportunity for a Purkinje cell to receive stimuli from a very large number of granule cells, and also allows a granule cell to contact many Purkinje cells.

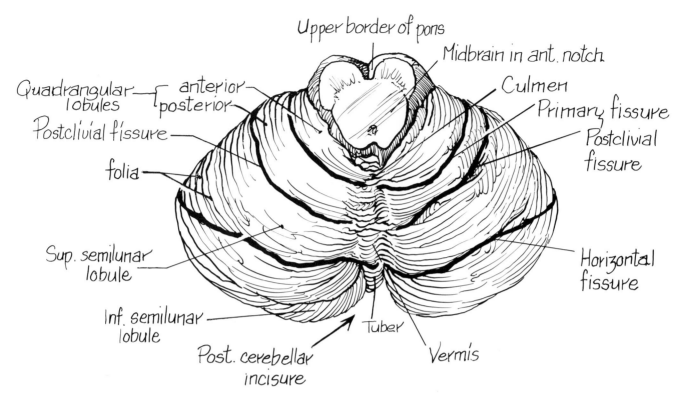

Upper border of pons
Midbrain in ant. notch
Quadrangular lobules
anterior
posterior
Culmen
Primary fissure
Postclivial fissure
Postclivial fissure
folia
Sup. semilunar lobule
Horizontal fissure
Inf. semilunar lobule
Tuber
Post. cerebellar incisure
Vermis

**Fig. 2-50.** *Posterior view of the cerebellum.*

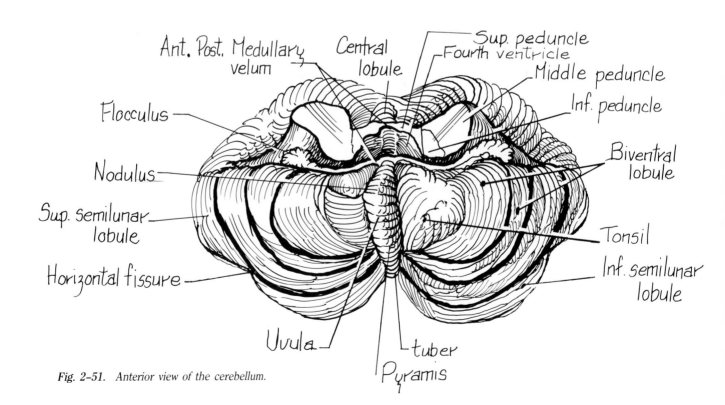

Ant. Post. Medullary velum
Central lobule
Sup. peduncle
Fourth ventricle
Middle peduncle
Flocculus
Inf. peduncle
Nodulus
Biventral lobule
Sup. semilunar lobule
Horizontal fissure
Tonsil
Inf. semilunar lobule
Uvula
tuber
Pyramis

**Fig. 2-51.** *Anterior view of the cerebellum.*

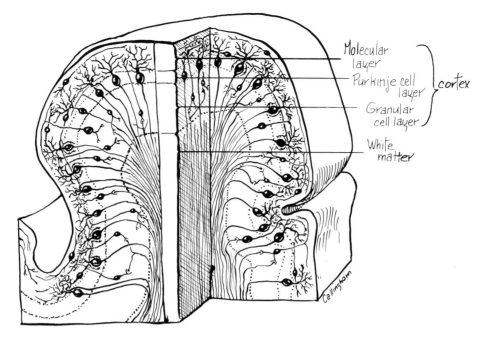

Molecular
layer

Purkinje cell
layer

cortex

Granular
cell layer

White
matter

Callingham

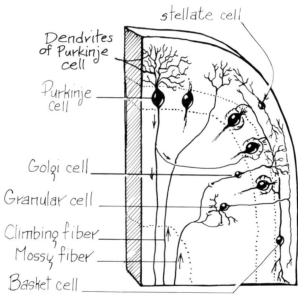

stellate cell

Dendrites
of Purkinje
cell

Purkinje
Cell

Golgi cell

Granular cell

Climbing fiber

Mossy fiber

Basket cell

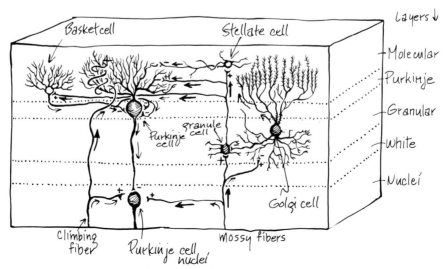

Basket cell

Stellate cell

Layers ↓

Molecular

Purkinje

Granular

White

Nuclei

granule
cell

Purkinje
cell

Golgi cell

Climbing
fiber

Purkinje cell
nuclei

mossy fibers

**Fig. 2–52.** *The layers of the cerebellar cortex and its associated nerve cells.*

The **granule cell layer** consists of closely packed small multipolar neurons, from which axons extend into the molecular layer. *Golgi type II cells* are found in this layer of the cerebellar cortex.

The cerebellum has two types of incoming (afferent) fibers, and both are excitatory. The **mossy fibers** arise from the pontine, medullary and spinal nuclei. The other type of afferent fiber is the **climbing fiber**. It comes to the cerebellum primarily from the inferior olivary nucleus.

Each cerebellar hemisphere has a connection to the rest of the nervous system through three bundles of nerve fibers: the superior, middle, and inferior peduncles. The **superior peduncle** is the bridge between the midbrain and the cerebellum. It is the main efferent pathway to the cerebellum. The **middle cerebellar peduncle** is the bridge between the pons and the cerebellum. It is entirely afferent. The **inferior peduncle** coordinates information between the medulla and cerebellum. It is predominantly an efferent pathway.

The internal structure of the cerebellum is characterized by a layer of gray matter and an internal mass of white matter (the medullary center) in which are located the **cerebellar nuclei** (Fig. 2–53).

The **dentate nucleus** is the most prominent of the cerebellar nuclei. It is slightly medial to the center of the white substance of each cerebellar hemisphere. It receives some fibers from the neocerebellar portion of the posterior lobe and some from the anterior lobe. It sends fibers by the superior cerebellar peduncle to the red nucleus and the ventrolateral nucleus of the thalamus.

The **emboliform nucleus** is an elongated mass just anteromedial to the hilum of the dentate nucleus. It receives fibers from the paleocerebellum and sends fibers by way of the superior cerebellar peduncle to the red nucleus. The **globus nucleus** is composed of small groups of cellular masses between the emboliform and fastigial nuclei. The nearly spherical **fastigial nucleus** lies close to the midline just over the roof of the fourth ventricle in the anterior portion of the vermis. It is larger than either the globose or emboli-form nuclei. It receives fibers from the flocculonod-ular lobe and sends fibers to the vestibular and reticular nuclei via the uncinate fasciculus.

Each half of the cerebellum is supplied by one superior and two inferior cerebellar arteries which pass, respectively, to the superior and inferior surfaces of the cerebellum.

**Clinical Manifestations Associated with Lesions of the Cerebellum.** Disorders of the cerebellum may result from vascular occlusion, tumors, or other pathological conditions. The vestibular portion of the cerebellum may be invaded by a tumor, typically a *medulloblastoma* occurring in childhood. The resulting disorder of cerebellar function is known as the **archi-cerebellar syndrome**. The patient is unsteady, walks on a wide base, and sways from side to side. At first, the clinical signs are limited to disturbances of equilibrium; as the tumor invades other parts of the cerebellum other signs will appear.

The clinical signs of destructive lesions of the corpus cerebelli (main mass of the cerebellum) or its major afferent and efferent pathways are commonly referred to as the **neocerebellar syndrome**. In many instances the paleocerebellum is also involved. It should be recalled that the cerebrum functions mainly with the contralateral cerebellar hemisphere in producing skilled voluntary movements. Therefore, while cerebral lesions produce contralateral disturbances (hemiparesis or hemiparalysis), cerebellar lesions will have ipsilateral effects (hemiataxia) (Angevine & Cotman, 1981).

In the neocerebellar syndrome the symptoms may vary in their degree of severity. *Ataxic movements*, irregular and lacking coordination, are frequently manifested. *Vertigo* frequently accompanies the ataxia. There may be a tendency to lean and fall to the side of the lesion (*pleurothotonos*).

The patient may show signs of *dysmetropsia*, a defect in the visual appreciation of the measure of size of objects. This is also known as the "past-pointing phenomenon." In performing the finger-to-nose test, the patient's finger will shoot past the nose onto the cheek.

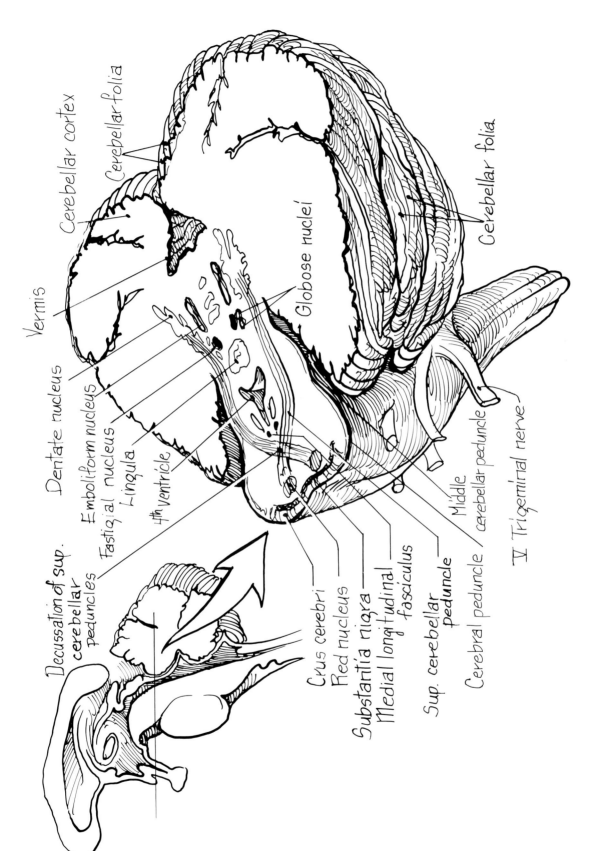

Cerebellar cortex

Cerebellar folia

Cerebellar folia

Vermis

Globose nuclei

Dentate nucleus

Emboliform nucleus

Fastigial nucleus

Lingula

4th ventricle

Decussation of Sup. cerebellar peduncles

Crus cerebri

Red nucleus

Substantia nigra

Medial longitudinal fasciculus

Sup. cerebellar peduncle

Cerebral peduncle

Middle cerebellar peduncle

V Trigeminal nerve

**Fig. 2-53.** Cross-section through the cerebellum and brain stem at the level of the superior cerebellar peduncle, showing the brain stem and cerebellar nuclei.

Rapidly alternating movements (such as flexion and extension of the fingers or pronation and supination of the forearm) are performed in a clumsy manner (dysdiadochokinesia).

*Hypotonia* of the muscles may be present, characterized by a tendency of the muscles to tire easily. The limbs may also appear "floppy" and show decreased resistance to passive movement. *Cerebellar tremor* is typically a terminal tremor, occurring at the end of a particular movement. This is also known as *intention or kinetic tremor* because it is not present at rest. It is most evident in the upper extremities because it is masked by weight-bearing in the lower extremities. Cerebellar tremor is frequently contrasted with the tremor seen in Parkinson's disease, which is a *rest tremor*. This indicates that the tremor occurs in the absence of voluntary and associated movements.

The *rebound phenomenon of Holmes* or lack of cheek reflex may also be seen. When the examiner flexes the patient's arm against resistance and then suddenly releases it, the arm will strike the patient's own body or face.

Occasionally a patient with cerebellar disease will demonstrate *cerebellar fits*. These are not actually seizures but episodes of decerebrate rigidity that are usually seen with large midline cerebellar masses.

# Section III

# Diagnostic Methods in Neurology

# THE NEUROLOGICAL EXAMINATION

When psychologists find evidence of impaired cerebral functions in a patient, frequently their first recommendation is to refer the patient for neurological (medical) examination. Curiously, however, many of these psychologists are not familiar with the neurological examination. They are not aware of the variability in procedures from one examiner (neurologist, neurological surgeon, internist, general medical practitioner) to another, and do not know the types of diagnostic conclusions which can validly be reached on the basis of this examination. And most important, perhaps, is that many psychologists do not realize that the information elicited by the neurological examination is largely subjective.

A detailed review of the examination a physician is likely to do will explain these comments. Both the neurological examination and the neuropsychological examination are concerned with behavioral manifestations of brain disorders. As a result, they have a number of things in common, such as evaluation of certain motor and sensory-perceptual functions. The neuropsychological examination, however, has been designed to expand the limits of the neurological examination by focusing more specifically on the higher-level aspects of brain functioning. Thus, one can view the neurological examination and the neuropsychological examination as complementary procedures.

The neurological examination is theoretically separated into two parts — the history and the physical examination — but most neurologists emphasize the advantage of integrating the two procedures. The neurologist can make important clinical observations while listening to the patient recount his medical history.

DeMyer (1980) suggests some questions the physician might ask him/herself while observing the patient. First, what is the *general behavior and appearance* of the patient? Is he hyperactive and agitated or quiet and immobile? Does he appear slovenly, or neat and appropriately dressed?

Second, is the *speech pattern* of the patient normal or deviant? Is his speech rapid, incessant, under great pressure, or slow and lacking in spontaneity? Is his *verbal communication* disorganized? Can he communicate points of information effectively?

Third, what is the patient's *mood or affect*? Is he euphoric, agitated, giggly, silent, weeping, or angry? Does his mood swing far in one direction or another during the course of the conversation?

Fourth, what is the *content* of the patient's verbal communication? Is there any evidence that the patient has illusions, hallucinations, or delusions? Are there any fears that may be classified as phobias, particularly concerning bodily complaints or illnesses?

Fifth, what is the patient's *intellectual capability*? Is he bright, average, dull, obviously demented or mentally retarded?

Sixth, is the patient's *sensorium* normal? Does the patient have an average *attention span*? Is he oriented to time, place, and person? What is his memory for recent and remote events? Is his general fund of information at an average level? Are his capabilities within a normal range? What is his ability in calculation?

Finally, is the patient's *speech* normal? Does he have difficulties in producing various sounds (dysphonia)? Problems articulating units of speech (dysarthria)? Does he demonstrate difficulty with the stress of syllables, inflections, pitch of voice, rhythm of words, or general tonal characteristics of verbal expression (dysprosody)? Is there any impairment of either expression or understanding of words as symbols of verbal communication (dysphasia)?

Although these capabilities may be evaluated by formal testing (including psychological evaluation) they are also judged by the neurologist as the patient presents a verbal description of his complaints and history. The reader can see that evaluation of all of these factors and abilities is quite a large undertaking, and one that is accomplished with varying degrees of success by different neurologists.

Talbert (1982) also emphasizes the importance of integrating the history with the physical examination. In his view, the neurological examination begins when the examiner first greets the patient. At that time the examiner begins to make observations of the patient's speech, movements, and mannerisms that may give clues leading to the localization and cause of the patient's disorder. If the patient has any evidence of intellectual impairment, Talbert recommends further questioning to obtain more definitive information. He says the patient might be questioned regarding ". . . the date, recent news events, and the like, which test orientation, memory, general fund of knowledge, and ability to calculate and think abstractly. . . . After sufficient questioning to elicit the information sought, proceed directly with tests of language function by presenting the patient with pencil and paper and a passage to read."

Although the neurological examination does not pretend to be a sophisticated psychological testing procedure, it can provide a basis for estimating an individual's general intellectual integrity and capability. Many neurologists and neurological surgeons use this part of the examination as a screening procedure to determine whether a patient needs a comprehensive neuropsychological examination.

Other physicians, however, feel that they can gain valid and detailed insights into the intellectual and personality factors as well as neurological inferences of the patient through the interview. Toole (1984) says that after listening to the patient's history, the experienced physician should, in 80%-90% of the cases, be able to answer the following questions: (1) What area of the brain is involved (location)? and (2) What is the cause of the problem (etiology)?

According to Toole, the clinical neurological interview should have three objectives: (1) to provide an accurate record of the events, in sequence, that relate to the patient's illness; (2) to gain the patient's trust so that all relevant information is divulged; and (3) to instill in the patient such confidence about the

physician's motivation, skills and judgement that he will heed his advice and act on it. This third element, according to Toole, is a culmination of the art of interviewing and a prerequisite for success in managing patients. Toole points out that, "Elicitation of a history is dynamic and often cannot be confined to one interview. Like an artist, the skillful physician often completes his history by sketching in the background on the first interview and adding details and color on subsequent occasions."

A patient with a neurological disorder may also have impaired brain function; he may not be appropriately aware of his condition, may neglect telling the physician significant points of information, or may be unable to communicate his concerns effectively. In order to overcome these problems, Toole recommends that a spouse (or other person with valid information regarding the patient's illness) corroborate information derived from the history.

Nonverbal behavior during the interview also contributes significant information: "The way the patient sits, his facial expression, and his eye movements can give important clues to the symbolic significance and emotional tone related to the symptoms." But it is not only the *patient* who demonstrates behavior that is important during the interview; Toole also points out that the *physician* must be cognizant of the effect of his own verbal and nonverbal communication on the information obtained from the patient. He believes that the interview establishes a relationship between the physician and patient that permits evaluation of any defensive behavior used by patients who are apprehensive, for one reason or another, concerning their illnesses.

As the reader can see by this discussion, neurologists and neurological surgeons feel obliged to gain a considerable amount of information about the patient and his illness from the history. However, competency in providing such information varies a great deal from patient to patient. The information obtained from the history is almost always incomplete, frequently inaccurate, and sometimes may actually be misleading. The situation may be especially compounded by the neurological patient, who may have some degree of intellectual or cognitive impairment. Thus, regardless of the expertise of the clinician, he/she should be cautious about accepting history information as a complete and valid expression of the patient's problems.

## Technique of the Neurological Examination

Talbert (1982) recommends several steps in administering the neurological examination.

The clinician should initially direct his attention to the patient's area of complaint. This will seem logical and reassuring to the patient. After examining the specific area of complaint (if any), the examiner should begin an orderly procedure of examination. The head and neck are evaluated next. First, examine coordinated movements and other reactions of the eyes: Standing about three feet in front of the patient, move your finger in various directions within the patient's visual field. Ask the patient to follow your finger closely, being careful not to move his head as he does so. The examiner should determine whether there is any incoordination, lag, or weakness in the eye movements. At the same time, note whether lid and brow movements and pupillary reactions are within normal limits.

The next examinations are done using an ophthalmoscope. Examine the eye grounds (fundi) for any abnormalities. Inspect particularly the optic disc and the macular area and test for the pupillary light reflex. Next, use the ophthalmoscope to examine the oropharynx. At the same time, test for the gag reflex and any deviations or abnormality in tongue protrusion. Finally, inspect the auditory canals. The next procedure is to examine for visual acuity. Following this, one should examine for losses in the visual fields, testing each eye separately, quadrant by quadrant. Then, using a pin, one should examine for pain sensation on both sides of the face.

The next examination concerns the sense of smell, testing each nostril separately using substances that smell of peppermint, clove, or tobacco.

The examiner should request the subject to whistle a common tune so that contraction of the orbicularis oris muscle may be observed. Spontaneous smiling should be observed to evaluate contraction of facial muscles on both sides under conditions of emotional response. The next procedure is to examine the masseter and temporalis muscles while the patient is deliberately clenching and relaxing his teeth.

Talbert recommends that hearing be tested by rubbing the thumb against the fingers near each of the patient's ears. If any abnormality in auditory acuity is noticed, recommendation should be made for more precise hearing tests.

The sternocleidomastoid muscles should be palpated while the patient turns his head toward the left and right. As the patient shrugs his shoulders, the trapezius muscle should be palpated. The patient should be asked to extend his head backward and then forward to touch his chin to his chest, with the examiner observing for possible range of limitation or pain.

The next examining procedures are intended to (1) elicit evidence of tremors and other abnormal involuntary movements; (2) afford an opportunity to inspect the musculature of the trunk and upper limbs for evidence of atrophy; (3) show any abnormal curvature of the spine and other aspects of the trunk; (4) demonstrate motor weakness that might occur on one side or the other; and (5) determine any loss in coordination or position sense.

To accomplish these aims the patient is asked to sit erect, close his eyes, extend his arms forward with the palms in a downward position and the fingers spread apart, and maintain this posture for 90 seconds. During this period of time the examiner observes the patient for any deviations from normality.

Next, the patient is requested to touch the tip of his nose with the index finger of each hand, first while his eyes are closed and then with his eyes open. Abnormalities in this response may indicate the presence of proprioceptive sensation difficulties and possible cerebellar dysfunction.

The patient is requested to sit with his arms in his lap and his legs extending freely. At this time the examiner moves each of the patient's arms passively, examining for any alteration of muscle tone. Following this, deep tendon reflexes are tested in all four of the limbs, comparing the two sides of the body.

The next step in the procedure is to have the patient lie supine on the examining table. First, the abdominal reflexes (plantar, cremasteric, and cutaneous) are examined. Examination of position sensibility, light touch, and discriminatory capabilities should then be performed. Testing the extremities, trunk and face for light touch discrimination should be done using a cotton wisp. Elicitation of corneal reflexes is also done at this time. Pinprick perception should be examined on both sides, with the detail of these various sensory examinations varying in accordance with any suspected problems of the patient.

Following these procedures, the patient is questioned regarding any disturbances of sphincter function; a rectal examination for sphincter tone should be done if there is any history of incontinence or if one suspects spinal cord disease.

The examination should be terminated by having the patient stand and walk. The examiner should observe gait, posture, swinging of the arms, instability or change in direction while walking. In addition, heel-to-toe walking should be observed and the subject should be evaluated for his ability to stand on a narrow base. These tests provide evidence of coordinated motor ability dependent upon the status of the cerebellum. The strength of the pelvic girdle and lower limbs, together with motility of the lower spine, can be assessed by having the patient sit in a low chair and then rise, rise from a squat, and flex the trunk beginning from an erect posture.

Talbert notes that sometimes a more "meticulous" evaluation is called for, but recommends that this be done at a later examination because of possible fatigue on the part of both patient and examiner. He also notes, however, that an examiner with some experience can complete the examination within a period of 15 or 20 minutes.

The above description obviously does not identify all of the specific abnormalities that may be elicited by the neurological examination. However, Talbert feels that the "keystone of consistently accurate diagnosis" depends on the history and the above examination. The next steps involve using the information elicited to localize the lesion or the disease process and to arrive at an etiological diagnosis or differential diagnosis. Additional diagnostic techniques and laboratory procedures are often necessary for this purpose as well as to plan management of the patient's illness.

DeMyer (1980) has written an entire book on the neurological examination, identifying normal and abnormal responses, including many illustrations, and discussing the significance of abnormal findings. This book is intended to instruct the examiner in the details of administration and interpretation of the neurological examination. The general format and content is similar to Talbert's (1983).

In examining the head and face, DeMyer first calls for careful inspection of the patient's appearance, including the general appearance of the face and motility under both voluntary and emotional conditions of expression; careful inspection of the eyes for ptosis, width of palpable fissures, the relation of the iris to the lids, pupillary size, and distance between the eyeballs; inspection of the contours of the features of the face and the hair of the scalp, eyebrows, and beard; and inspection of the head for abnormalities in shape and symmetry. The skull is palpated and the sinuses and mastoid processes are percussed for tenderness if the patient has complained of headaches. Auscultation is done for bruits over the eyes, temples, mastoid processes, and the great vessels. Finally, if the patient has complained of headaches, the sinuses should be transilluminated.

Although some variability may occur from one examiner to the next, DeMyer recommends that the formal examination follow an orderly sequence. He also suggests that the next step in the procedure be devoted to an examination of the cranial nerves, beginning with the optic group (optic, II; oculomotor, III; trochlear, IV; and abducens, VI). In addition to evaluating visual acuity and testing peripheral aspects of the visual fields by confrontation, the tests include evaluation of the size of the pupils and pupillary light reflexes as well as ocular motility.

The next tests are for the functional condition of the branchimotor group and the tongue (trigeminal, V; facial, VII; glossopharyngeal and vagus, IX and X; hypoglossal, XII; and spinal accessory, XI). These tests include evaluation of the motor functions of the masseter and temporalis muscle group (V); movement of muscles involving the forehead, eyelids, mouth, skin over the neck, and lips (VII); evaluation of phonation, nasality of articulation, swallowing, the gag reflex, and elevation of the palate (IX and X); articulation ability in speech and ability to protrude the tongue in the midline or to either side (XII), and evaluation of the sternocleidomastoid and trapezius muscles through testing strength of head movements and shoulder shrugging (XI). DeMyer also notes that fatigability of muscular function may have pathological significance and suggests that 100 repetitive movements (such as eye blinking) be requested if there is any concern in this regard.

Continuing with evaluation of the cranial nerves, the examination tests olfaction (I) using an aromatic substance for each nostril; taste (VII) using salt or sugar; hearing (VIII) using conversational speech as well as lesser stimuli such as a watch tick or light rubbing of the fingers followed by evaluation if deficits are detected; and vestibular function (VIII) testing for nystagmus induced by caloric irrigation or by rotary movement, especially if the history suggests any possible deficit.

The next set of tests involve sensory functions in the facial area, focusing particularly on the trigeminal (V) distribution. The corneal reflex (integrating the function of nerves V and VII) is elicited. Light touch is tested over the three divisions of the trigeminal (V) nerve followed by determination of pain and temperature perception in the same divisions.

The next phase of the neurological examination involves assessment of motor functions (exclusive of the cranial nerves) of both a voluntary and involuntary (reflex) nature. At the initial phase of the examination, before and during the history, the patient should

have been inspected for his posture, general activity level, tremors, and involuntary movements. In addition, the entire skin surface of the patient should be evaluated for surface lesions that might have neurological significance.

The size and contour of muscular configurations should be observed for atrophy, hypertrophy, asymmetry, improper alignment of bones at joints, fasciculations, tremor, and involuntary movements. Observations should be made of free walking, toe-to-heel walking, tandom walking, and deep-knee bends. Muscles should be palpated if they show evidence of atrophy, hypertrophy, or any tenderness or spasm activity. Muscles should also be tested for strength, including the muscles of the shoulder girdle, upper extremities, lower extremities, and abdominal muscles. Observation should be made of whether there is any particular pattern to muscular weakness, such as differential strength on the right or left sides, the upper or lower extremities, or a change in muscle strength in a proximal-distal dimension. Passive movements of the joints should be evaluated for spasticity, clonus, or rigidity. Muscle stretch (or deep tendon) reflexes should be tested and graded on both sides. These reflexes relate particularly to the functional status of levels of the spinal cord (cervical, lumbar, sacral).

Additional reflexes are elicited as skin-muscle interactions and are referred to as superficial reflexes. These relate particularly to various levels of spinal cord function and include abdominal skin-muscle reflexes (elicited by stimulating the skin of the abdomen), the cremasteric reflex (elicited by stimulating the skin of the medial portion of the thigh), and the extensor toe sign (Babinski sign), elicited by plantar stimulation. In addition to gait, which was tested previously, cerebellar signs may be evaluated by finger-to-nose tests, rebound tests, tests of alternating movements, and heel-to-knee tests. Nerve root stretching tests (straight-knee leg raising or bent-knee leg raising) may also be done if meningitis, nuchal rigidity, or disc or low back disease is suspected.

Evaluation of the somatic sensory system is next performed examining for temperature discrimination and light touch and pain perception over the hands, trunk, and feet. Deep sensory functions are tested by using a tuning fork to determine perception of vibration at the knuckles, fingernails, and malleoli of the ankles. Position sense of the fingers and toes is tested by moving the digits up or down. The Romberg test for swaying requires the patient to stand erect with heels together, first with the eyes open and then with the eyes closed. Finally, the patient's ability to recognize objects through the sense of touch (stereognosis) is tested.

The next phase of the examination relates to evaluation of cerebral functions. If the history or any of the previous findings implies the presence of a cerebral lesion, DeMyer suggests that the patient should be tested for two-point discrimination, ability in tactile finger localization, ability to recognize numbers or letters written on the skin, right-left confusion, and ability to perceive bilateral simultaneous tactile and visual stimuli (as compared with ability to perceive such stimuli when given unilaterally). The Reitan-Indiana Aphasia Screening Test is administered if additional information is needed with respect to adequacy of cerebral functioning.

The response to vestibular stimulation by caloric irrigation of the auditory canals includes subjective symptoms of vertigo, nausea, and sometimes a feeling of anxiety. The objective responses (or signs) which may be observed by the examiner include nystagmus, falling or postural deviation of the patient, sweating, pallor, vomiting and hypotension.

DeMyer (1980) lists various categories of neurological disease or disorder. In addition, he lists the general categories of neurosis, psychosis, and personality disorder because of the frequency with which they must be considered together with, or as an alternative to, neurological disease. In some respects, the general neurological categories are open to debate, and other authorities would deviate from the listings somewhat. DeMyer lists the following major categories to be considered in the neurological patient: allergy (demyelination); collagen disease; congenital malformation; genetic; inflammation; metabolic endocrine or electrolyte disorder; neoplastic disease; toxic diseases; trauma; and vascular diseases. It should be noted that a category for degenerative brain disorders, including Alzheimer's disease, was not included.

The above description of the neurological examination presents only an overview and is not complete in describing all of the tests and procedures that might be used. The major additional diagnostic procedures that may follow the neurological examination, such as EEG, computed tomography of the head, cerebral angiography, etc., will be described separately.

It should be clear that administration of the neurological examination requires close inspection of the patient throughout the testing. In fact, the results of the examination depend upon observation of abnormalities (as contrasted with manifestations of normal responses). Some of these abnormalities are deliberately elicited by specific examining procedures, but in some instances abnormalities are noted by observation of the patient's casual and spontaneous behavior. Since the results of the examination depend upon observing abnormalities in various aspects of behavior, it should be apparent that a heavy responsibility falls upon the examiner. Under examining circumstances of this type, a tremendous degree of variability occurs from one examiner to another in elicitation of the clinical data. In turn, interpretation of the observed abnormalities will show inter-examiner variability.

The physical neurological examination can be performed quite quickly in patients without neurological disease. Talbert suggests that the examination requires only about 15 minutes; DeMyer emphasizes that it is possible to complete the examination of an intelligent, cooperative patient in about six minutes. In fact, he recommends that a person learning to do the neurological examination use a criterion of six minutes for completion as a basis for knowing that he has practiced enough to be able to do the examination properly and efficiently. Of course, in patients with neurological disease, various types of abnormalities may be present and a much longer period of time may be required for elicitation and description of these abnormalities.

The reader will note that the neurological examination, although variable from one examiner to another (especially with respect to assessment of higher-level brain functions), relates to aspects of the neuropsychological examination in several respects. The history and general observations of the patient (which are usually not considered part of the formal examination) obviously may be similar. In addition, many neuropsychologists observe the types of functions that are included under the mental status examination, such as the general behavior and appearance of the subject, mood and affective responses, confusion in content of thought, disorders of speech, and obvious impairment of intellectual capability. In the neuropsychological examination, however, these areas of function are tested with standardized materials and procedures which permit a much more precise statement of the status of the patient.

Much of the formal neurological examination is oriented toward evaluation of sensory and motor functions, focusing upon the cranial nerves but also evaluating more general aspects of motor and sensory functions. Higher-level aspects of brain functions are relatively neglected in the neurological examination, although a growing number of neurologists now use many of the types of procedures that generally fall in the area of behavioral neurology (tests of aphasia and related disorders and the types of tests that Talbert [1983] refers to as measures of "discriminatory sensibilities"). The neuropsychological examination, in addition to being organized in such a way as to reduce the element of subjective interpretation by the examiner, concentrates on higher-level (central processing) aspects of brain functions.

# SKULL X-RAYS

Radiology of the skull may reveal many abnormalities, but, as with other x-ray evaluations, a considerable degree of experience is necessary to reach valid conclusions. X-rays of the skull have been used clinically for 75 years (Taveras & Wood, 1964). In prior times the clinical importance of plain skull films was much greater than at present because of the development of other diagnostic procedures. In fact, many of the radiological features of the skull that were once considered to have special diagnostic significance have been found to have little or no practical value in diagnosis or management of the patient. However, as will be noted below, plain skull films sometimes communicate exact and unequivocal diagnostic information, and such information should not be overlooked or neglected.

In evaluating skull x-rays it is first necessary to identify artifacts or normal variations so that these will not be confused with pathological findings. Schechter (1982b) has noted that sometimes even objects such as dense hair braids may resemble strange-looking lesions; gravel or sand in the hair may simulate intracranial calcifications; a glass eye appeared to be a calcified aneurysm in one instance; ulcerative lesions of the scalp may simulate skull lesions; and air in a gaping scalp wound may appear as a fracture on the x-ray.

Normal variations occur frequently and experience is necessary to be able to correctly identify these. Problems in interpretation relate to normal variations in calcification of various bony structures, variations in bony density and the configuration of structures, and the direction of the axis of a structure and its three-dimensional architecture with relation to the projection angle of the x-ray. Developmental variations in skull x-rays of infants and children constitute a special problem. A number of normal variations are confused with fractures, including bony sutures, suture lines along the inner surface of skull bones, and vascular grooves on the cranial bones.

Schechter (1982b) notes that certain questions present very frequent problems in differentiating normal variation from pathology. These include questions regarding the possibility of abnormally increased vascular markings (dural sinuses, dural veins, diploic veins, and arterial grooves), convolutional markings that may be associated with long-standing increased intracranial pressure, and skull lucencies that are sometimes associated with a number of pathological conditions.

If the conclusion is reached that the skull x-ray shows evidence of a pathological finding, an attempt must be made to determine if the problem is a primary skull condition, a manifestation of systemic disease, or an indication of intracranial disease. The sella turcica, which is well-visualized on plain skull films, must be studied closely because changes in the sella may be due to a number of intracranial conditions, including increased intracranial pressure, lesions in adjacent structures, or intrasellar lesions. Adjacent lesions include conditions such as pituitary adenoma, craniopharyngioma, carotid aneurysm, chordoma, metastatic lesions, and nasopharyngeal tumor. Pathological calcification of either a focal or diffuse nature may also be present. The principal lesions associated with focal calcification include arteriovenous malformation, aneurysm, tumor, Sturge-Weber syndrome, chronic subdural hematoma, and teratoma. Diffuse calcification occurs principally with tuberous sclerosis, either viral or parasitic encephalitis, endocrine disorders, turberculoma and tuberculous meningitis. Changes in plain skull films associated with lytic and hyperostotic lesions may also occur. Intracranial lesions which are associated with hyperostosis are usually meningiomas and fibrous dysplasia. Lytic and hyperostotic manifestations on skull x-ray are also associated with surgical defect, circumscribed osteoporosis, osteomyelitis, metastatic lesions, solitary myeloma, epidermoid, eosinophilic granuloma, and hemangioma. When multiple lesions of this type are present the associated conditions may be pacchionian granulations, Paget's disease, persistent parietal foramina, radiation necrosis, osteomyelitis, metastatic disease, or multiple myeloma.

Although findings of specific significance for intracranial disease are sometimes observed in x-rays of the skull, it should be noted again that unique contributions to understanding of the patient are rarely dependent upon skull radiology.

# ELECTROENCEPHALOGRAPHY

Electroencephalography (EEG) is a procedure in which fluctuations in the electrical activity of the brain are recorded by electrodes attached to the scalp. These electrical potentials are measured in microvolts; therefore, the original signal must be amplified about a million times before the difference in potential between two recording sites is large enough to drive a galvanometer. The galvanometer causes an ink-writing pen to produce a fluctuating trace on paper which is moving at a constant rate. The resulting fluctuating line provides a temporal recording of differences in potential between two input electrodes, attached to two different locations but connected to the single channel. In practice, 8, 16, or even more channels are used to record results from an individual subject. Recording from different locations is necessary because the rhythmic character of the recordings differs (at least to an extent) depending upon the region of the cerebral cortex that is represented. In addition, the level of alertness and age of the subject may also influence the recorded voltage fluctuations.

In general terms, the EEG is interpreted with respect to frequency of electrical fluctuations (in cycles per second), the contour or configuration of the waves recorded, and pathological alterations either in amplitude or frequency. Abnormalities are also described with respect to location (focal or diffuse) and comparisons of recordings over the two cerebral hemispheres (and locations within and between each cerebral hemisphere). Although formal and quantitative methods of EEG evaluation and interpretation have been a subject of study for many years, the customary procedure is for the clinician to observe, summarize, and evaluate the tracings.

As with any complex inferential procedure (including neuropsychological interpretation), evaluation of the EEG by visual observation is relatively complex. Three steps have been identified in this process (Sharbrough & Sundt, 1982).

The first step is to review the recordings from individual channels, following them from one page to another to assess short-and-long term variability of characteristics such as wave duration, frequency, amplitude, phase, and form. On the basis of these observations abnormalities may be identified and judged whether they are sustained or regularly intermittent in nature.

After identification of the characteristics of the tracings in single channels, the several channels being simultaneously recorded should be compared to identify similarities or differences in phase, latency, and amplitude of tracings from one channel to another. This procedure requires knowledge of the electrode placements of the channels being compared, and adds a dimension of spatial representation to the temporal dimension implicit in recording from a single channel. Thus, a very important aspect of clinical interpretation of EEG tracings refers to comparisons of recordings among various channels, especially emphasizing channels recording from homologous locations of the two cerebral hemispheres.

The third step in interpretation of EEG tracings relates to identification of variability caused by circumstances or events in the environment. It must be remembered that the recordings are not a reflection exclusively of electrical potentials of the cerebral cortex of the subject being examined; they may be influenced by the instrument (EEG machine) as well as environmental factors. Certain environmental influences are known to have an *activation* effect and others an *attenuation* effect. In fact, certain activation procedures, such as hyperventilation, photic stimulation, and sleep are regularly used in clinical recording in order to demonstrate abnormalities that may not be present during resting records. In addition, the cerebral potentials recorded with scalp electrodes may not represent only the dendritic potentials that arise from the large population of neurons in the cerebral cortex, but may be extracerebral in origin.

A common source of artifacts stems from the various sources of alternating current in the general environment of the patient and the EEG machine and electrical shielding is necessary to deal with this problem. Artifacts can also arise from inadequate contact of the electrodes with the skull. Technical errors of this particular type are often recognized when a high-amplitude potential is recorded from a single electrode with absolutely no corresponding deviation in nearby electrodes.

Extracerebral potentials may also arise from the internal environment of the patient. For example, the spontaneous ocular potential may have an influence on EEG recordings. This results basically from the potential difference between the more positive cornea and the more negative retina. However, because it is a direct-current potential, it usually does not influence the EEG amplifier unless there is a corresponding movement of the eye or eyelid. Eye movements may have an effect on the EEG but they are usually easily detected in clinical interpretation because the movement induces relative positivity on the electrodes toward which it moves and relative negativity on the electrodes away from which the eye moves. Nystagmus, for example, can sometimes be identified by the eye movement effect on EEG recordings. These influences make it quite clear that careful training of the EEG technician is imperative and that possible sources of influence on the EEG tracings be observed and noted.

Other sources of extracerebral influence on EEG tracings are stimulation of the retina by light, muscle contraction (including movements of the tongue and respiration as well as other movements) electrocardiographic potentials, and even pulsations of arteries that are located near an electrode site. Although these sources of influence on EEG tracings must be considered in evaluating the electrical activity of the brain, it should also be noted that in some instances they may provide the experienced electroencephalographer with ancillary diagnostic information.

### Placement of Electrodes

All generators of electrical potential must have two poles, one relatively negative and the other relatively positive with respect to each other. In record-

ing electrical potentials from the head (EEG), small metal discs (gold, tin, or chlorided silver) are used with a suitable electrolyte solution. In order to characterize the differential electrical activity of various areas of the cerebral cortex, it is necessary to use a sufficient number of electrodes. In fact, the International Federation has recommended that 19 scalp and 2 ear electrodes, as the minimal number, be used for clinical electroencephalography. The 19 scalp electrodes are distributed in standard positions. Eight electrodes represent the function of each cerebral hemisphere (three frontal; one anterior temporal and one posterior temporal; one centrally located; one in the parietal area; and one in the occipital area). In addition, three electrodes are positioned along the midline (frontal, central, and parietal). It is customary to number these various positions according to the area represented. Even numbers are routinely used for electrodes over the right cerebral hemisphere and odd numbers are used for electrodes over the left cerebral hemisphere. Additional scalp electrodes may be used for more refined localization and special electrodes, such as sphenoidal and nasopharyngeal, may be used to gain specific information under special circumstances.

It is apparent that the basic derivations from this array of electrodes can be organized in a montage that has a large number of different orders.

### Normal Patterns of Cerebral Electrical Potentials

Normal EEG patterns vary considerably with the age and general alertness of the patient, but in adults there are certain patterns that are customarily seen. The occipital leads usually reflect the *alpha* rhythm (8 to 12 cycles per second), which is symmetrically represented on both sides. The alpha rhythm is activated or accentuated when the eyes are closed and the subject is in a mentally relaxed waking state. Alpha is attenuated by such factors as eye opening and mental activity (such as doing arithmetic problems). Although alpha activity is principally recorded from posterior head regions, this same area may produce activity with the same distribution and reactivity pattern but in different frequency bands, such as beta or theta waves.

*Beta* activity (a fast alpha variant of 14 to 60 cycles per second) and *theta* frequency (a slow alpha variant of 4 to 6 cycles per second) are considered normal if they are harmonically related to activity which is in the alpha frequency band and if the alpha activity is in the same spatial distribution and has the same response reactivity. However, slow wave activity in the posterior part of the head is distinctly abnormal if there are no associated faster frequencies.

The central areas also sometimes generate a characteristic rhythm with a frequency in the alpha range. This is a spontaneous bilateral type of activity, often asymmetrical and asynchronous, that occurs in either sustained or short trains. This activity, referred to as the *mu* rhythm, is most apparent when the patient is relaxed, not moving any extremities, and not receiving somatosensory input. The mu rhythm may be attenuated by movement of the extremity or by somatosensory stimuli delivered to the extremities. Mu activity has a characteristic form in which the positive phase has a round contoured peak and the negative phase has a sharp peak.

The frontocentral regions may show activity of variable frequency but beta activity is frequently maximal and may even be confined to this area. Beta waves are usually continuous and may increase in amplitude during drowsiness but commonly disappear during deep sleep.

The temporal regions often show a wide variety of activity during the waking state. The posterior temporal regions usually show evidence of normal alpha activity but the temporal regions may generate asymmetrical single and serial transient waveforms that become increasingly prominent with advancing age as well as with states of drowsiness. EEG tracings of sleep patterns are also quite characteristic, with sequential alterations as the subject passes through stages of drowsiness, light sleep, and deeper sleep. With drowsiness the alpha rhythm often disappears and may be replaced by low-voltage, mixed-frequency activity or by rhythmic activity in the theta range. These particular changes represent patterns of drowsiness seen in the occipital area. The frontocentral area, however, usually persists in drowsiness with the characteristic beta rhythms and their amplitude may even increase. In the temporal lobes single and serial slow waves may occur independently and become more prominent during drowsiness. As sleep deepens, a characteristic type of single and serial slow-wave component may develop, as well as rhythmic faster components. In sleep, as in the waking state, different areas of the cerebral cortex show different patterns of electrical activity.

## Abnormal EEG Potentials

We shall not attempt to describe the various kinds of abnormal wave forms that characterize various conditions of brain disease or damage; excellent reference sources are available for this purpose (Kooi, 1971; Remond, 1974).

EEG abnormalities may be divided generally into two types: (1) distortion, alteration, and ultimate disappearance of both normal and abnormal wave forms; and (2) the appearance of abnormal rhythms with or without the disturbance of normal electrical activity. When abnormalities have been identified, they should be classified according to their degree of abnormality, their cerebral localization, and type of abnormality. There are several characteristics of neurological conditions that increase the likelihood of producing abnormal EEG tracings; however, the reader should be aware that abnormality on the tracing may not be clinically significant and may only represent a long-standing electrical disturbance not related to a disease process. Also, a normal EEG does not exclude significant underlying neurological disease. In many patients with significant brain lesions the EEG is normal. Finally, electroencephalographers point out the importance of integrating the clinical findings and results from other examinations, in order to gain the greatest clinical contribution from EEG.

Sharbrough and Sundt (1982) point out that if EEG is used only in the static phase of disease and after all other tests have been performed (and perhaps have identified the nature of the problem), and if EEG is done in the absence of any other clinical input, the procedure is rarely helpful. EEG is more useful when it is done (1) during the early course of the patient's evaluation; (2) after an acute, unexplained change in the patient's neurological status; and (3) sequentially for comparison of findings on different EEG examinations.

The EEG may provide valuable information when the lesion is near the surface of the brain and involves relatively extensive areas or if the pathological process produces epileptogenic activity. A lesion that is diffuse and infiltrating may produce distinct EEG abnormalities, together with evidence of clinical change in the patient's condition, before radiographic or contrast procedures demonstrate the lesion. However, if the lesion is far from the cortex, does not produce any change in consciousness and has a density different from normal brain tissue, it would be easily detected using procedures such as tomographic scanning but might be missed entirely by the EEG and clinical examination. Localized brain stem lesions which do not obstruct flow of cerebral spinal fluid frequently do not alter the EEG. Brain stem auditory evoked potentials (BAER), however, may detect such lesions even when the EEG is normal. These observations emphasize the necessity for integrating EEG with other findings as a basis for complete evaluation and diagnosis.

DeMyer (1980) summarizes the clinical conditions that would indicate an EEG. These include: (1) intermittent disorders of brain function, especially episodic disturbances of consciousness such as epileptic seizures; (2) episodes of unconsciousness of unexplained origin; (3) disturbances of the sleep-wake cycle; (4) clinical suspicion of a focal brain lesion or diffuse encephalopathy of unknown origin; and (5) suspected brain death. Criteria have been established for brain death protocols that combine clinical and EEG criteria. In terms of the EEG tracings themselves, sharp waves or spikes imply an epileptogenic lesion, usually of a static type (such as a brain scar) or a slowly advancing lesion. Slow waves, if focal, imply a focal destructive lesion. If slow waves are generalized, they imply

reduction of consciousness or a generalized brain disease. Flattening of the brain waves, if a phenomenon not immediately following an epileptic seizure, suggests the presence of a substance, such as a fluid, between the brain and skull or absence or complete destruction of the cerebral wall.

The clinical conditions for which EEG may be specifically helpful refer to identification of epilepsy. Nearly all epileptics have abnormal EEGs during a seizure and most have abnormalities even in the intervals between seizures. Probably no other diagnostic technique is as specifically helpful in the diagnosis of epilepsy. Patients with space-occupying lesions such as infarcts, neoplasms, abscesses, and some contusions show focal slow waves over the lesion site. In such instances the EEG does not identify the type of lesion but often provides information regarding the location.

Finally, diffuse slowing of brain waves is seen with coma of metabolic origin (e.g., uremic or diabetic) or infectious origin (encephalitic). Diffuse brain lesions may also cause diffuse EEG slowing. The EEG is usually of little help in differentiating the causes of coma although certain clues may be present in some instances.

After reviewing these indications for EEG, the reader may wonder about its popularity and frequency. DeMyer (1980) notes that EEG seems to have attracted its share of speculative physicians and psychologists, and cautions that it is not possible to read a person's thoughts from the EEG, match him or her with a proper marriage partner, etc. There have been certain correlations between learning and EEG but, as DeMyer notes, the general correlation of EEG with mental activity and behavior has been poor, and "in fact, downright disappointing." He observes that interpretation of EEGs is, at present, a visual art and hardly an objective science.

DeMyer notes that the EEG is generally worse than useless unless read by a physician who is trained in neurology; who personally diagnoses, treats, and is responsible for the care of a wide variety of neurological patients; who continually matches his diagnoses and interpretations against the clinical course and ultimate diagnosis of the patient; who regularly subjects his opinions and conclusions to the corrective influence of knowledgeable colleagues; and who is familiar with the structure of the brain, understands its pathologic reactions, and "regularly attends autopsy sessions to make rueful note of his errors."

# ECHOENCEPHALOGRAPHY

Echoencephalography is a diagnostic technique in which ultrasound is beamed from one side of the head to the other, from both the left and right sides, and a tracing representing reflection of the ultrasound beam as it encounters tissue of differing molecular density is obtained. The reflection of ultrasound, as shown on the oscilloscope screen, produces an "echo" at these points of differing molecular density. The procedure is performed with the patient lying supine with the head turned to one side. An experienced technician can perform an echo-encephalogram in one to three minutes. Tracings are obtained from both sides of the head; conventionally the upper tracing represents echos ranging from the right side of the head and the lower tracing is representative of the left side of the head. Echoencephalography, based upon demonstration of a shift of the diencephalic and midline structures (through a comparison of the two tracings), may produce useful information when an intracranial mass is suspected.

Dyck (1982) has briefly reviewed the history of the use of reflected ultrasound in neurological diagnosis. The original attempts were to use the procedure to outline the ventricular system, but the skull obscured any detectable variations within the brain. French, Wild, and Neal (1950) began experimentation with ultrasound reflection ("echos") and demonstrated that echos corresponding with tumors could be obtained (French, Wild, & Neal, 1951). Leksell (1956; 1958) demonstrated that midline structures of the brain reflected ultrasound and comparing echos from the right and left side of the head could show lateral displacement in craniocerebral trauma. Leksell coined the term "echoencephalography."

The position of diencephalic midline structures and the thickness of the cerebral mantle can be demonstrated by echoencephalography of the intact skull. This procedure is useful in management of infants with hydrocephalus. The technique has not turned out to be very useful in detection of intracranial neoplasms or hematomas associated with head injury. In fact, the availability of computed tomography has limited the use of echoencephalography and the procedure is relatively rarely used at present even though it has validity in the identification and evaluation of intracranial lesions. Dyck (1982) has pointed out that "assiduous attention to detail and anatomical correlation" and a considerable degree of expertise, gained only through experience and familiarity with the equipment, is necessary.

Echoencephalographic tracings customarily reflect five echos as they traverse through the head: (1) an initial echo from the scalp; (2) an echo from the skull; (3) midline or diencephalic echos (called "M-echos" because they tend to resemble the letter M); (4) echos from the inner and outer tables of the far side of the skull; and (5) echos from the far scalp-air interface. Tracings from the left and the right sides of the head must measure equal distances because interpretation requires "lining up" of the two tracings for purposes of comparison and interpretation.

Sonographic methods have proved useful in providing information regarding the dimensions of cerebral ventricles. The width of the third ventricle can usually be measured. The width of the cerebral mantle may be measured in young children, because their skulls are relatively thin and absorb less ultrasound, (Ford & McRae, 1966). Although computed tomography yields superior information, echoencephalography does not require that the infant be anesthetized, as is necessary to avoid movement of the infant when using computed tomography. Ultrasonic techniques are also useful in identifying cerebral tumors, especially when the skull has been removed and ultrasound can be delivered directly to the brain tissues. Although the difference between brain and cerebral neoplasms is slight in ultrasonic velocities, it is still sufficient to provide an interface from which ultrasound can be reflected. Tumor echos can be detected in almost all cerebral neoplasms when the skull does not interfere and can locate the regions of cystic degeneration and the area most severely involved. In addition,

the subcortical depth and medial extent of intracerebral hematomas may be determined, and this may
be of importance in the operative procedure. Nevertheless, the use of sonographic techniques has
diminished with the advent of procedures such as the
CT scan.

# ULTRASONOGRAPHY

Ultrasound uses acoustic pulse echo techniques derived from sonar to image biological structures. In this method signals are emitted from a piezoelectric crystal and the time required for echoes to return from interfaces between tissues is measured. This data is converted into points on an image plane, thereby outlining structures and organs. The resulting image is less detailed than the type obtained from CT scans because the sound pulse continually loses energy as it passes through tissue and, in addition, must return to the source in order to be detected. Strong boundaries between tissues, when they vary strikingly in density (such as bone and soft tissue or soft tissue and air) may reflect most of the acoustic energy in the form of echoes and prevent receiving echoes from more distant structures. Therefore, ultrasonography is most effective in producing images of soft-tissue structures that lie immediately below the skin surface.

Ultrasonography can also be used to visualize moving materials (such as blood) flowing within a vessel. This procedure is somewhat more complicated than imaging of a stationary object because echoes are shifted in accordance with the Doppler effect. However, in the neck area, the blood supply to the brain can be well visualized and show evidence of atherosclerotic plaque formation. At present, ultrasonography is not known to have any significant adverse biological effects and is the technique of choice when it is necessary to image the fetus. In addition, up to 60 images per second can be made, an important consideration in imaging of the heart. Since connective tissue contributes significantly to the detail obtained in ultrasonic images, disease processes that principally affect connective tissue can be evaluated with this method. However, the use of ultrasound has not proved to be of great value for visualization of either the lung or the brain. The acoustic waves are rapidly attenuated in air (lung) and, because they do not penetrate bone very well, brain structures are difficult to visualize. Ultrasound has proved useful in visualizing brain lesions, such as tumors, after a skull flap has been removed. However, by this time, diagnosis of the tumor has already been made, it probably has been visualized with other methods, and the surgical procedure has begun. In neonates, when the sutures of the skull have not fully closed, ultrasonography may provide useful imaging of the brain. Ultrasound techniques show some promise for differentiating particular tissues, and may have useful future applications in this respect.

Only ultrasonography and nuclear magnetic resonance (NMR) represent imaging procedures that are not dependent upon ionizing radiation. The adverse effects of ionizing radiation have been well publicized. There may be some eventual adverse effects identified even with the relatively low exposure required for imaging purposes. Considering the uses of these procedures for diagnosis, prevention, or treatment of serious illness, the benefits clearly outweigh the risks. Although no known adverse effects accompany the use of ultrasound imaging, prudent practice recommends restriction of use to situations in which medical indications are clear. Nuclear magnetic resonance imaging requires that the body be immersed in a high magnetic field, and possible tissue changes may occur at the molecular level; although there is no convincing evidence that magnetic energy has significant adverse biological effects, we cannot be certain that this procedure is entirely risk-free until further study is done.

# CEREBRAL ANGIOGRAPHY

**Cerebral angiography** is a technique in which x-rays of the brain and cerebral blood vessels are taken as an opaque substance (contrast medium), which has been injected intra-arterially, circulates through the brain. This permits visualization of blood vessels and identification of various abnormalities. These abnormalities often provide important information concerning the localization and type of underlying pathology.

Schechter (1982a) has given a brief summary of the historical factors in the development of cerebral angiography. Roentgen discovered x-rays in 1895. In 1913, Luckett published his observations of air in the ventricular system in a patient who had sustained a severe head injury. Noting the possibility of visualization of the ventricular system using x-rays, Dandy (1918) introduced air into the lumbar subarachnoid space and first described the procedure that has come to be known as *pneumoencephalography*.

Egas Moniz followed these examples with additional visualization attempts oriented toward delineation of the cerebral blood vessels (Moniz, 1927). Moniz's first attempts were not very successful. In a patient with severe general paresis he attempted to inject a solution of strontium bromide into the carotid artery but, since the patient reported no effect or sensations, presumed he had injected the jugular vein. In addition, the x-rays showed no filling of the vessels. He attempted the procedure a second and third time in patients with Parkinson's disease. These instances were also unsuccessful and in his fourth case he had technical problems with dislodging of the needle. Moniz therefore decided to expose the carotid artery surgically and made a direct injection of 4cc of 70% strontium bromide. The patient complained of pain, became agitated, and later had difficulty with speech, even though the injection was made on the right side. He recovered from these symptoms on the third day. However, timing between injection and taking the x-rays was not well coordinated and the exposures did not show any filling. In the sixth case, however, direct injection into the internal carotid artery was again made and the film showed contrast filling of the middle and posterior cerebral arteries. The patient died eight hours later from thrombophlebitis, possibly due to the use of strontium bromide as a contrast substance, and Moniz turned to using iodines as contrast substances.

Since that time, angiography has progressed from being a hazardous technique to one that is presently a simple and safe procedure. Both the technique itself and the contrast substances have been developed for safety, minimal complications, and technical excellence of the x-ray exposures. Many specific techniques are used to visualize the major vessels leading to the head and their cerebral distribution.

The two major approaches in cerebral angiography relate to carotid angiography and vertebral angiography. The reader will recall that the four major vessels supplying arterial blood to the brain are the two internal carotid arteries and the two vertebral arteries. Carotid angiography may be performed with direct puncture of the internal carotid artery, the external carotid artery, the common carotid artery, or through catheterization via the superficial temporal artery, the femoral artery, the brachial artery, or the axillary artery. Varying procedures are used when a catheter is introduced through one of these arteries. Carotid angiography may also be performed using an intravenous technique (Schechter, 1982a).

Vertebral angiography may also be performed by means of direct puncture of the vertebral artery or through catheterization via another vessel such as the brachial, femoral, radial, or subclavian artery. As with carotid angiography, a variety of specific procedures have been found to be effective. The patient usually lies in the supine position for the procedure. The three most useful x-ray projection views are the lateral view, the 20° anterio-posterior or frontal-occipital view and the half-axial or Towne's view. In this latter view, the central x-ray beam makes an angle of 30°–35°, coming through the forehead and emerging at the base of the skull. Additional projections are used for special purposes. Usually two films per second are obtained for a total of six seconds, but may vary according to the particular circumstances. The contrast medium usually used is 60% methylglucamine diatrizoate (Renografin) or 50% sodium diatrizoate (Hypaque).

The particular technique used depends upon many factors, including the clinical indications of the type and location of lesion. A greater degree of detail of the vessels of the brain is obtained with direct internal carotid puncture than with entry via the common carotid artery. When a comparison between the collateral supply of the extracranial and intracranial circulation is needed, the injection may be made directly into the external carotid artery. This technique is also useful in visualizing tumors that may be supplied principally by the external carotid artery (such as meningiomas).

Many additional details are important. For example, the type of lesion will influence the number of films and the time interval between them. When an aneurysm is suspected, the arterial phase will supply the vital information and a film in the intermediate or venous phase may demonstrate the pooling of contrast medium in the aneurysm. In occlusive disease, delayed films may show the collateral circulation. Arteriovenous malformations require a very short interval between films because of the rapid shunt of arterial blood through the anastomotic vessels to the venous system. The circulation time is faster in infants and children than in adults, and this factor will also affect the timing of the films.

# CEREBRAL ANGIOGRAPHY AS A DIAGNOSTIC PROCEDURE

## Extracranial Vascular Disease

It has long been recognized that symptoms of insufficient vascularization of the brain may be manifested even when examination fails to reveal evidence of an occlusion at the cerebral level. In many of these cases the explanation relates to lesions of the blood supply to the brain that are extracranial in location. As early as 1954, Fisher noted the high incidence of extracranial vascular disease as a localized entity. Fields, Crawford, and DeBakey (1958) found that more than one-fourth of their stroke patients had causative lesions that were located outside of the head. Recognition of involvement of the common and internal carotid arteries, and their diagnostic exploration, has prompted reports on their surgical correction over a number of years (DeBakey, Crawford, & Fields, 1961; Eastcott, Pickering, & Rob, 1954; Rob & Wheeler, 1957).

The clinical picture produced by common or internal carotid artery occlusion is somewhat variable. In most cases there is evidence of a rather sudden onset of complaints, but these lesions may mimic other conditions, such as cerebral neoplasms and strokes involving the cerebral vessels. Attempts have been made to identify specific clinically detectable manifestations that may characterize neck-vessel involvement. Conditions considered suggestive of such lesions were investigated (Silverstein, Lehrer, & Mones, 1960) and included diminished carotid pulsations, carotid or intracranial bruits, and response to manual compression of the carotid artery. These manifestations were of variable usefulness in identifying extracranial vascular disease, producing many false-positive responses. Opthalmodynanometric differences in retinal artery pressure provided a fairly accurate diagnostic test. However, by themselves, these clinical procedures were not very accurate and it is apparent that angiography plays a major role in the investigation and evaluation of neck-vessel disease.

The problem of differentiating these patients from those with strokes at the cerebral level continues to be formidable. Nevertheless, Schechter (1982a) indicates that it is still not at all uncommon to limit radiological examinations to the intracranial vasculature and to fail to include extracranial studies (which might produce evidence responsible for the patient's clinical condition). In studying patients with evidence of cerebral stroke, Schechter indicates that up to 80% of these patients may also have arterial disease in the cervical vessels. On the basis of his review of the literature, he strongly recommends a very careful investigation of the entire vascular tree, including selective vessel visualization. Many detailed studies have been published to support this position, including investigations based upon necropsy correlations (Hutchinson & Yates, 1956; 1957).

The sites of predilection for extracranial occlusive arterial disease have been published in a number of reports. Thus, there is no doubt that common and internal carotid artery involvement may be of great significance in explaining the clinical manifestations of cerebral vascular disease, including strokes involving the cerebral vessels.

Cerebral angiography may also be of advantage in defining additional lesions in extracranial locations. Dissecting aneurysms of the carotid artery may cause significant impairment of cerebral functions. These lesions are relatively rare and usually caused by trauma. Arteriovenous fistulae in the neck have also been reported, most often in association with traumatic injury. In these instances, the rapid shunting of blood from the arterial to the venous side may result in a poor filling of intracranial vessels. Congenital anomalies of the extracranial cerebral vessels may also occur and have been reported to be more common in the vertebral artery than the carotid artery. In either case, however, instances of complete absence of both carotid arteries (Fisher, 1913) as well as one vertebral artery with the other arising from the carotid artery (Morris, 1960; Sutton, 1950) have been reported. Hauge (1954) has also described instances in which the vertebral artery arose from sites other than the subclavian artery.

Carotid body tumors (usually benign and single) are also encountered and, despite having a distinct characteristic appearance angiographically, may clinically be mistaken for carotid aneurysms.

# Intracranial Vascular Disease

As indicated in the previous section, angiography has been shown to be a valuable diagnostic technique in revealing vascular occlusive disease in the extracranial circulation. Unfortunately, angiography has been less rewarding in the evaluation of an occlusion of a vessel directly involving the brain. In a patient with a clinical diagnosis of stroke, it is not uncommon to fail to find corresponding evidence in the cerebral angiogram. There can be a number of factors responsible for the negative angiogram in the presence of clinical evidence of a stroke. There are many vessels in the cerebral arterial tree, and it is possible that occlusive involvement of a small branch may not be noticeable in the angiogram. An occlusion of a vessel may go unrecognized because collateral vessels supply blood to the area that would have been supplied by the involved vessel. Technical aspects of angiography, including failure to obtain serial films, might also be a contributory factor.

Middle cerebral artery occlusions are more readily recognized in the lateral projections than in anterioposterior projections because the lateral films tend to superimpose branches of the middle cerebral artery. Occlusive involvement of the ascending fronto-parietal artery is more readily recognized than other branches. Diagnosis of occlusion of the anterior cerebral artery on the basis of angiograms must also be made cautiously, particularly because of anatomical variations of the circle of Willis and possible filling of the anterior cerebral artery after contralateral compression of injection of the other side. Finally, caution must be used in radiological diagnosis involving the posterior cerebral artery because of the possibility of anatomical variations in which the posterior cerebral artery arises from the carotid rather than the vertebral artery.

Neuroradiologists also point out other possible non-anatomical factors that may be involved in non-filling of vessels: the degree of pressure of injection on the two sides; factors influencing filling in one part of the cerebral vasculature as compared with another;

"streaming" spasm washout from the opposite vertebral artery; and temporary occlusion by the tip of the catheter or needle of the artery being visualized.

It is generally agreed that it is not possible to differentiate radiologically between thrombosis and embolism purely on the basis of the angiogram. Serial x-rays, however, may show migration of the point of obstruction; such movement would suggest an embolus rather than a thrombus.

## Aneurysms

Intracranial aneurysms represent an important pathological lesion because they are encountered fairly frequently and are the most common cause of spontaneous subarachnoid hemorrhage (Stubens, 1954). Wood (1964) believes that it is possible to identify ruptured aneurysms, even among multiple lesions, in more than 95% of the cases using several criteria (listed in order of decreasing value): angiographic evidence of a mass; the size of the aneurysm; and any indications of the presence of spasm of the vessel.

Several reports have appeared that have analyzed large series of cases with aneurysms and have attempted to identify their differential locations in the brain vasculature. Schobinger & Ruzika (1964) have provided evidence regarding the locations of aneurysms: vertebral tree–4%; posterior communicating artery–26%; bifurcation of the middle and anterior cerebral arteries–6%; middle cerebral artery–20%; anterior communicating artery–27%; anterior cerebral artery–3%. The remaining 14% of intracranial aneurysms were multiple in nature. Somewhat variable values have been offered in the analysis of intracranial aneurysms by other investigators. Thus, most aneurysms appear at the point of bifurcation of the branches of the circle of Willis and appear to be congenital in origin. However, other factors, such as high blood pressure and atheromatous lesions, may also cause the development of aneurysms in these vessels (Glynn, 1940).

Cerebral angiography is relatively effective in demonstrating subarachnoid hemorrhage associated with bleeding aneurysms. Sutton (1962) reported that 77% of 413 consecutive cases of subarachnoid hemorrhage demonstrated positive findings using bilateral carotid angiography. The group of 23% in which the findings were negative were further investigated by vertebral angiography and 40% of these cases showed positive findings. Additional positive findings were obtained in the remaining cases when a second vertebral angiogram on the contralateral side was performed.

## Arteriovenous Malformations

Because of the variability of arteriovenous malformations, both vertebral and carotid angiography are useful in their identification. These lesions vary in size and shape, may be superficial or deeply seated, may be found supratentorially or in the posterior fossa and in some instances are situated both above and below the tentorium. When bleeding has not occurred, these lesions are usually not space-occupying. They may, however, cause subarachnoid hemorrhage when bleeding has occurred.

## Tumors

Angiography is useful in determining both the presence and location of tumors. Two sources of information are used for this purpose: (1) the displacement of arteries and veins from their normal course; and (2) evidence of abnormal vascularity in the area occupied by the tumor. The displacement of vessels may be used to draw inferences regarding the size as well as the location of the tumor and whether the lesion is displacing or infiltrating other tissues. Displacement of structures may also reflect secondary changes, such as edema or swelling around the tumor and ventricular dilatation resulting from interference with flow of cerebrospinal fluid.

Some tumors are highly vascular while others have a poor blood supply. Vessels in a tumor differ from normal vessels in the regularity of their lumina and shape. Tumor vessels are more tortuous than normal vessels and connections may be present between arteries and veins. Malignant tumors, particularly, have numerous shunts between arteries and veins and may undergo necrosis, cystic changes, and focal hemorrhage that is demonstrated in the angiogram by areas of avascularity.

Inferences regarding the type of tumor may be made from the circulation rate of blood. Highly malignant tumors, which contain many arteriovenous shunts, may show filling of the tumor vessels only during the arterial phase of the angiogram with rapid disappearance of the contrast medium during the venous phase. Meningiomas, on the other hand, usually retain the contrast medium for a longer period (probably because of their numerous capillaries) and the contrast material will still be apparent during the venous phase. Metastatic tumors usually are intermediate to rapidly growing gliomas and meningiomas in this respect. Edema, or swelling of brain tissue, tends to delay circulation time and the contrast material may appear later in tumor tissue than in normal brain tissue. Large space-occupying masses (such as cysts and abscesses), which are relatively free of blood vessels, may crowd and displace blood vessels to the periphery of the mass and form a ring around the tumor. Displacement of vessel groups, and even of specific vessels, frequently indicates the general location of a tumor and sometimes serves as a specific sign of the probable type of lesion.

As mentioned above, the vascular architecture and the rate of blood flow through a tumor may be of assistance in inferring the type of tumor. Slowly growing gliomas are usually less vascular than normal brain tissue; rapidly growing gliomas and meningiomas usually have an enriched blood supply. Meningiomas often receive their blood supply from both external and internal carotid arteries, with the external carotid artery supply usually transported by the middle meningeal artery.

## Craniocerebral Trauma

The value of angiography in cases of head injury has been well established. In the past it was common to place multiple burr holes in the skull in an attempt to determine the presence of bleeding, but this procedure has been shown to miss collections of blood that can be recognized on angiograms. In addition, angiography may show the presence of lesions that were not suspected on the basis of clinical examination. Angiography is usually successful in demonstrating various lesions that may be present following trauma, including: (1) subdural hematomas, which are usually caused by tearing of the cortical veins as they enter the superior sagittal sinus; (2) epidural hematomas, which usually result from a tear of the meningeal arteries or veins, with the initial tear resulting in slow venous bleeding (although the bleeding may become both venous and arterial if small arteries are torn as the dura is stripped from the skull); (3) intracerebral mass lesions, including cerebral contusion and edema and intracerebral hematoma.

Cerebral contusion and edema are most frequently shown in the temporal, frontal, and occipital lobes. Sometimes the side opposite of direct injury shows the greater damage (contre-coup effect). A subdural or epidural hematoma may accompany the brain contusion and produce displacement of vessels that gives the appearance of a mass lesion. Intracerebral hematomas give the appearance angiographically of being avascular space-occupying lesions. Displacement of blood vessels may show improvement as the contusion subsides, but some degree of displacement often persists for a relatively long period. Traumatic occlusion of the middle cerebral artery occurs infrequently but may be demonstrated angiographically. Fistulae of the carotid artery have also been reported with penetrating wounds and fractures that involve the base of the skull.

# PNEUMOENCEPHALOGRAPHY and VENTRICULOGRAPHY

Pneumoencephalography and ventriculography are radiographic techniques used to demonstrate the ventricular system and cisterns. Pneumoencephalography involves the injection of air into the subarachnoid space at the lumbar level; ventriculography accomplishes a similar purpose through burr holes of the skull directly into the lateral ventricles. X-rays are taken at various intervals during the injections and the ventricular system and cisterns are visualized as the procedure progresses.

Pneumoencephalography is begun with the patient in a comfortably seated position. Proper positioning of the patient and correct placement of the needle are crucial. The needle should be placed in the subarachnoid (rather than the subdural) space. After about 10cc of air has been injected, a lateral film is made to show the posterior and craniocervical junction. This film gives information regarding placement of the needle, reveals any herniation of the cerebellar tonsils, and shows if there is any evidence of disease in the posterior fossa. After injection of another 10cc of air, a second film is taken to demonstrate the fourth ventricle and aqueduct of Sylvius. In this procedure the patient is seated with the forehead pressed against a headstand. The head is rocked from side to side and up and down in order to fill the ventricular spaces and cisterns with air. If disease in certain areas is suspected it may also be necessary to adjust the patient's head in special positions to visualize these areas. Next, a lateral film is obtained to demonstrate the roof of the lateral ventricle and verify that a sufficient amount of air has entered the ventricular system to permit additional studies.

For the next part of the examination the patient is shifted to a brow-up position. Several films are obtained, including frontal, anteroposterior and lateral views, which should identify the anterior horns and a portion of the bodies of the lateral ventricles together with the structures adjacent to these parts of the ventricular system (including the genu and rostrum of the corpus callosum, the heads of the caudate nuclei, anterior parts of the thalamus which make up the floor of the lateral ventricle, the lateral wall of the body of the lateral ventricle, and the septum pellucidum). Additional maneuvers are then carried out to demonstrate anterior portions of the ventricular system that may not previously have been visualized. The patient's head is rocked from side to side with the brow up and sometimes with the head hanging somewhat in order to cause air to pass from the lateral ventricles into the anterior portion of the third ventricle. The temporal tips of the ventricular anatomy may also be demonstrated with the patient in the brow-up position. The patient's head is extended as far posteriorly as possible, with the head off the edge of the table and a film beamed directly through the orbits is taken. Finally, the patient is turned to a brow-down position and additional films are taken to reveal the posterior portion of the bodies of the lateral ventricles, the occipital horns, and the posterior portions of the temporal horns. In addition, films are sometimes obtained 24 hours after injection of air because partial absorption is sometimes an aid in visualization of parts of the ventricular system and because certain types of lesions may be demonstrated that did not show up initially.

There have been recommendations that gas be employed rather than air for demonstration of the ventricular anatomy. Several gases have been studied, including carbon dioxide and nitrous oxide. There have been claims that the patient has less morbidity after the procedure using these gases because their absorption is more rapid. However, air is customarily used except in certain special circumstances.

It is not uncommon for the patient to experience headache, nausea, and vomiting for a short period of time following pneumoencephalography. In addition, morbidity and mortality may result from herniation of the cerebellar tonsils (usually associated with intracranial pressure as a result of a supratentorial mass lesion), air embolism, extracerebral hematoma formation, and meningitis.

Pneumography techniques (pneumoencephalography and ventriculography) have been largely supplanted by computed tomography for diagnosing intracranial disease. In addition, many aspects of ventricular and cisternal anatomy can be derived from angiographic studies. Nevertheless, the complete demonstration of all parts of the ventricular and cisternal systems is possible only with replacement of cerebrospinal fluid with contrast material. Pneumography has, in the past, been particularly important in demonstrating space-occupying lesions and structural changes, including cysts and tumors of various types, congenital anomalies, hydrocephaly, and cerebral atrophy.

Ventriculography is a procedure essentially similar to pneumoencephalography except that a hole is made through the skull and air is introduced directly into the lateral ventricle. The patient is in either a brow-up or brow-down position. The brow-up position permits study of all of the ventricular system; the brow-down position is useful especially for studies that involve only the posterior portions of the lateral ventricles, third ventricle, aqueduct, and fourth ventricle. Changes in the position of the patient's head, together with a series of films as air moves from one location to another, are used much as in the procedures described above. There are occasional instances in which ventriculography will be greatly facilitated in visualization of the ventricular anatomy if an opaque contrast agent is used instead of air. Sometimes an opaque material that is non-soluable and heavier than cerebrospinal fluid is used, and the x-rays visualize particular structures as the material moves from one position to another (Campbell, Campbell, Heimburger, et al., 1964; Zimgesser, & Schechter, 1982).

# COMPUTED TOMOGRAPHY

Computed tomography began in 1972 when Hounsfield developed the first computed tomography brain scanner. The name first used for these procedures was EMI scans (sometimes referred to as "Emmy" scans) because the scanner was developed at EMI Ltd. (Electronic Musical Industries, Ltd.). The CT scanner developed by Hounsfield was installed at Atkinson Morley's Hospital in Wimbledon, United Kingdom. CT scanners are now available in most hospitals and diagnostic centers around the world.

Since the beginning of clinical use of computed axial tomography (CAT) or computed tomography (CT), this type of scanning has had a great influence on diagnosis in clinical medicine, especially in identifying brain lesions. Wide experience with computed tomography has been gained across the full range of nervous system diseases and the diagnostic accuracy of the procedure in conditions that involve structural pathology or deviation of the brain has been accepted. The remarkable success and contribution of computed tomography is based on methodology that exploits the fact that the x-ray linear attenuation coefficients of many "soft" tissues in the body differ. In the past, it had been presumed that "soft" tissues were equally absorptive and therefore nondistinguishable. However, CT scanning permits visual separation of cerebrospinal fluid, blood, brain parenchyma and blood clots, and visual contrast of these various tissues. The CT technology uses multiple x-ray projections and brings out the differences in soft tissue better than standard radiography because the image produced is of a thin section, thereby permitting minimal x-ray scatter.

Computed tomography uses a scanner which rotates around the body part to be examined (e.g., the head). The procedure permits display of an image representing the tissue scan and initially reconstructs the images in the same plane as that in which they were taken. Thus, if the head is imaged in an axial plane, an axial slice is generated but coronal sections and sagittal planar images may also be obtained.

Computed tomography has advantages over conventional radiography because numerous x-ray slices are obtained and, through computer-assisted procedures, assembled into a single display image. The procedure uses equipment that emits x-rays which face radiation detectors during the scan. The detector signals are digitized and a computer-assisted display, composed of small picture points called pixels, is achieved. Each pixel has an assigned coefficient, or CT number, which corresponds with the appropriate anatomically accurate x-ray attenuation coefficient. This coefficient represents the brightness modulation of the pixel value and the overall display can be shown on a television monitor and photographed using Polaroid or standard x-ray film.

The CT number of zero is related to the absorption coefficient of water. In general, only fat and air are less absorptive than water and these substances, therefore, have negative CT numbers. Any material that is denser than water will be more absorptive and therefore have a higher CT numerical value. Cerebral spinal fluid values, for example, are slightly higher than those of water, and normal tissue ranges through considerably higher CT numbers. The higher the CT number the more dense the object or tissue and the "whiter" the image or object appears on the visual display. Bones generally appear to be quite white on the CT display, whereas cerebrospinal fluid is relatively dark. Other tissues, depending upon their density, appear as shades of gray.

The CT scan may be done either with or without contrast enhancement; contrast material improves visualization of the structure being examined. Contrast enhancement, which involves intravenous injection of iodinated contrast material prior to performance of the scan, is usually used if the patient shows signs or symptoms of focal brain involvement. In many instances, an unenhanced CT scan has been made initially and leads to a decision that greater detail or definition is needed through contrast enhancement.

CT scans are useful for detection of brain abnormalities as well as analysis of the nature of the abnormality. The remarkable success of CT scanning depends not only upon the differential density of "soft" tissues in the brain but also upon the striking symmetry of cerebral structures and the relative constancy of their locations. Thus, it is usually easy to distinguish normal anatomy from pathological involvement in the individual case. The reliability of CT scan interpretation, especially when contrast enhancement is used, has greatly decreased the frequency with which angiography and pneumoencephalography are performed.

Three general factors are of assistance in detecting brain lesions using computed tomography. First, when a space-occupying lesion is present within the brain, there is usually some deformity of the ventricular system. This information may assist in identifying the lesion and determining its location. Second, even when no ventricular deformity is present, brain edema may be indicated by an increased lucency of the brain tissues. Third, calcification within a lesion may be apparent on CT scans even when it is too faint to be identified by plain x-ray films.

In addition to a definitive localization of the lesion, CT scans have proved to be quite accurate in identifying certain general characteristics of many brain lesions. As an example, fairly accurate differentiation of slowly versus rapidly growing gliomas may be achieved (Davis & Kobrine, 1982).

## Glioma

Intrinsic primary brain tumors (gliomas) are usually discerned easily with computed tomography, even without contrast enhancement. Displacement or deformity of the ventricular system may provide a basis for estimating the mass of the tumor, its location, and its distance from the ventricular system. The actual location may also be identified by visualization of the mass itself or edema associated with the lesion. Gliomas with only slightly increased density and bulk, less edema, and less contrast enhancement are likely to be more slowly growing tumors. Malignant gliomas often show larger mass effects, a great deal of edema, extensive lucency, and pronounced enhancement. Studies of the accuracy of computed tomography in diagnosis of intrinsic brain tumors has been reported to be about 95% (Ambrose, Gooding, & Richardson, 1975).

Metastatic tumors are subject to identification based on essentially the same indicators as those used with primary intrinsic brain tumors. When single, metastatic tumors are usually impossible to differentiate from gliomas. However, because these lesions are often multiple, the presence of more than one tumor would suggest the possibility of metastatic brain disease.

## Abscess

Brain abscesses are usually identified by their edema and the mass effect of the lesion itself. On occasion, these indicators may be absent and the lesion invisible on non-enhanced computed tomography. With enhancement, a rim of the lesion may be identified with a cavity suggested in the central portion of the mass. It is often difficult to be certain of the spceific diagnosis of abscess based on the CT scan alone.

## Cerebral Infarction

Cerebral infarctions are usually identified correctly by their onset, signs, and symptoms. Computed tomography scans, however, are often quite variable in their manifestation of tissue damage. An acute stroke is usually demonstrated by an area of density in the region of brain tissue in which the stroke occurred (Kinkel & Jacobs, 1976).

Positive CT scans can usually be obtained within 4 to 7 days following the stroke, but more massive strokes can often be visualized immediately or within a few hours of onset. Midline shift or ventricular deformities may be apparent in some instances. Although

CT enhancement usually improves visualization, there are some conditions in which enhancement may reduce the appearance of abnormality, apparently through leakage of the contrast material. Serial CT scans, showing improvement over time, suggest the presence of a resolving infarct. CT scans are customarily normal after a transient ischemic attack. This is not surprising, considering the fact that damage in such instances is apparently insufficient to result in residual clinical manifestations. Among patients who suffer an acute stroke, 25%-30% show positive findings on the plain CT scans; contrast enhancement raises this percentage. Chronic infarcts are often difficult to detect. It is sometimes difficult to differentiate strokes from other lesions, such as an infiltrating glioma.

## Arteriovenous Malformations

Arteriovenous malformations are often difficult to diagnose using CT scans (Michaels, Bentson, & Winter, 1977) because they are variable in their characteristics and may be strongly or slightly hyperdense. Since blood is more dense than brain tissue, the CT scan may allow visualization of large blood pools in certain arteriovenous malformations. However, arteriovenous malformations are better diagnosed with contrast-enhanced CT scans than plain scans. If hemorrhage has occurred, it may be possible to identify a blood clot or find evidence of subarachnoid hemorrhage.

## Aneurysms

Aneurysms, like A-V malformations, may be hyperdense because of calcifications and this factor may permit identification. Although larger aneurysms are well demonstrated with CT scans because of the accumulated blood pool in the lesion, aneurysms smaller than 1.5 cm-2.0 cm usually cannot be visualized, even with contrast enhancement.

Computed tomography is especially helpful in evaluation of a ruptured aneurysm or arteriovenous malformation. Subarachnoid hemorrhage can be visualized approximately 90% of the time (Davis & Kobrine, 1982).

## Meningioma

Meningiomas show a considerable range of variation in density as a result of the degree of calcification of the lesion. Some meningiomas are diffusely calcified to a slight degree, and computed tomography will show these small amounts of calcifications even though they are too faint for visualization on plain skull films. In other cases, however, densely calcified meningiomas may resemble bone on the CT scan (Claveria, Sutton, & Tress, 1977). If the meningioma is located near the base of the skull, it is sometimes difficult to differentiate the positive result on CT scan from acoustic neuroma, aneurysm, or pituitary adenoma. Meningiomas along the cerebral convexity are more easily identified. Meningiomas regularly are more clearly visible with contrast enhancement than with plain CT scans.

## Acoustic Neuroma

Acoustic neuromas are rarely calcified and at least 50% of these lesions are invisible on plain CT scan (Davis & Kobrine, 1982). However, unless the lesion is quite small, contrast-enhanced CT scans show abnormalities with this type of tumor.

## Cranial Cerebral Trauma

CT scans vary greatly in instances of head trauma and tend to be correlated with the severity of structural damage to the brain (Dublin, French, & Rennick, 1977). Patients who have suffered only brain concussion frequently do not show any abnormality in the CT scan. However, in instances of brain contusion the findings may be quite distinct. Although skull fractures may be seen on CT scans, routine skull x-rays are more useful for this purpose. In instances of depressed skull fractures, the fracture may be correlated with evidence of tissue damage and possible bleeding underlying the fracture. Hemorrhage in the brain tissues associated with contusion appears on CT scans as a sharply defined increase in density similar to that of a hematoma.

Multiple areas of contusion may sometimes appear to be separate lesions on CT scans. In instances of severe contusion, the brain may be pulped, consisting of a variable mixture of edema, necrosis, and hemorrhage secondary to brain laceration. Although these indications of a pulped brain may occur in any location, they frequently are shown by CT scans as principally involving the frontal or temporal poles. The lateral ventricles may be in normal position but slit-like in appearance when bilateral masses are present or generalized edema has resulted from the head injury.

## Epidural and Subdural Hematomas

Epidural and subdural hematomas are clearly indicated in CT scans, with the classical appearance being a sharply defined radiodensity around the outer surface of the brain, adjacent to the inner table of the skull. It is usually possible to differentiate epidural and subdural hematomas on the basis of their shape. Epidural hematomas are usually represented by a lens-shaped configuration, with the layer adjacent to the internal table of the skull forming one curve and the opposite curve being formed by the inner part of the lesion adjacent to the dura mater. Subdural hematomas, in contrast, usually lead to a more extensive abnormality on the CT scan than epidural hematomas and are distributed along the surface of the brain. They may be quite large and extend from the frontal to the occipital poles or be more focal in nature. However, the inner margin of the hematoma parallels the outer margin and does not simulate the usual shape of the epidural hematoma in which the inner and outer margins are curved in opposite directions. Both epidural and subdural hematomas generally are dense and not distinguishable in this respect.

## Enlarged Ventricles

Enlargement of the ventricular system is clearly demonstrated by CT scan and is particularly important in evaluation of hydrocephalus and assessment of cerebral atrophy.

## Hydrocephalus

Computed tomography is useful in evaluation of the child with an enlarged or rapidly enlarging head. According to Davis and Kobrine (1982), patients who have a cranial measurement over the 98th percentile should have a CT scan. However, head size is not perfectly correlated with ventricular enlargement and often the CT scan serves to rule out the diagnosis of hydrocephalus. Enlargement of the ventricular system is also common in adults. Obstructive hydrocephalus is characterized by a relatively symmetrical and smooth enlargement of the ventricular system, often including the third (and possibly fourth) ventricle in addition to the lateral ventricles. Enlargement of the temporal horns is particularly prominent when an obstruction to flow of cerebrospinal fluid is present. Symmetrical bilateral temporal horn enlargement, compared with the amount of enlargement of the rest of the lateral ventricular system, serves as the criterion for diagnosis of obstructive hydrocephalus. A degree of enlargement of one or both temporal horns may, of course, be seen in persons who are otherwise normal or who have experienced some degree of temporal lobe atrophy. Judgments may be made regarding the location of the obstructing lesion, depending upon degree of involvement of various parts of the ventricular system.

## Cerebral Atrophy

Shrinkage of the brain tissue may be clearly demonstrated on CT scans by enlargement of the ventricular system and the sulci of the cerebral cortex. These changes are often described by neurologists and neurosurgeons as being clinically silent and do not imply any corresponding degree of clinical dementia. Detailed neuropsychological studies, however, have shown striking degrees of impairment of cortically related functions, even though the patient has not been subject to a clinical diagnosis of dementia. Thus, it would seem entirely possible that evidence of cerebral atrophy (brain shrinkage), in association with increasing age, may have definite neuropsychological (if not neurological) significance. It should also be noted, however, that many older persons have CT scans which show ventricular size that is essentially similar to that of younger persons.

On the basis of CT scans it is difficult to differentiate between cerebral atrophy and normal-pressure hydrocephalus. However, patients with normal-pressure hydrocephalus who have been subjected to a shunt procedure may have a series of CT scans to follow the effect of ventricular drainage procedures. Rapid reduction of ventricular size following shunting has been reported (Davis & Kobrine, 1982).

## Encephalitis

Patients with severe encephalitis may show a variety of changes on the CT scan. A focal mass effect is uncommon, but there may be focal or generalized areas of tissue lucency. Some degree of ventricular narrowing may be present due to generalized edema and it is not uncommon to see heterogenous and irregular areas of increased density. It is not possible to identify the viral cause of encephalitis by CT scanning, although supposedly characteristic types of lesions in some types of encephalitis (e.g., herpes simplex encephalitis) have been described (Dublin & Merten, 1977).

## Meningitis

Meningitis is not usually diagnosed by computed tomography, but, in instances of obstruction of cerebrospinal fluid circulation due to meningitis, hydrocephalus involving the entire ventricular system may be present.

## Lesions in the Region of the Sella Turcica

A number of lesions that occur in the region of the sella turcica may show abnormalities on the CT scan. These lesions include pituitary adenoma, meningioma, craniopharyngioma, aneurysm, optic glioma, teratoma, and hypothalamic intrinsic tumors. Characteristics of the CT scan may be of assistance in differential diagnosis of these various lesions, but some difficulty is encountered in this differentiation based on CT scans alone.

It is apparent from the above review that computed tomography is an invaluable technique for detection and, to some degree, analysis of structural abnormalities of brain tissue. Computed tomography has largely replaced pneumoencephalography and ventriculography as diagnostic procedures and, in many cases, provides information that previously was obtained with cerebral angiography and radionuclide imaging procedures. These latter procedures may complement computed tomography in some lesions, depending both upon their type and location.

# RADIONUCLIDE IMAGING STUDIES

In the late 1940s radioactive tracer studies were developed for diagnostic evaluation of brain lesions, representing a variation of the injection of dye compounds used in cerebral angiography. The procedure involves intra-arterial injection of a radiopharmaceutical tracer and detection with imaging devices. The image is displayed on an oscilloscope or television monitor and may be photographed for a permanent record. Computer or videotape may also be used for recording purposes. Current techniques permit serial recordings as the radiopharmaceutical tracer passes through the cerebral circulation following injection. In addition, some work has been done to permit quantification of the concentration of the tracer and comparison from region to region.

The first radionuclide tracer, diiodofluorescein labeled with $131^{130}$ iodine, was introduced in 1948 for brain tumor localization (Moore, 1948). Since that time a great deal of research has gone into development of radiopharmaceutical tracers, searching particularly for increased photon density in imaging, lower patient exposure dosage, and improved identification of various types of cerebral lesions.

The original technique for detection and localization of lesions involved point-counting using a Geiger-Muller tube positioned at symmetrically located points over the head. The scintillation camera, invented by Anger in 1957, led to increased sensitivity for gamma emissions and additional improvements in recording techniques have also been accomplished. Both stationary detector and moving detector imaging devices have been developed which produce images of the tracer distribution in the head and commercially available tomographic instruments may be obtained for this purpose.

In order to use radioisotopic brain scans for neurological diagnostic purposes, it is, of course, necessary to be aware of the normal appearance of the brain scan. Detailed descriptions of the normal scan are available involving anterior, posterior, and both lateral projections as well as certain special views (Overton, Haynie, Otte & Coe, 1965; Wagner, 1968; Webber, 1965).

Brain lesions are customarily manifested by retention (increased concentration) of the radionuclide tracer, showing a higher concentration of radioactivity in the diseased tissue than in the surrounding normal brain. There are some exceptions to this generalization. Cysts, for example, which have little or no vascularity, may show a decreased degree of tracer concentration compared with the homologous area of the other cerebral hemisphere. A number of variables have been related to the concentration of tracer activity, including tumor cell structure and location, size of the lesion, duration of symptoms, and other variables. Rapidly growing intrinsic tumors (astrocytoma grades III & IV) and meningiomas are seen as dense tracer concentrations. Metastatic lesions, when multiple, are quite distinctive in their representation; single metastases may range from concentrations that are minimal to quite dense. Vascular lesions of the brain are sometimes subject to specific identification because of the anatomical distribution of the tracer concentration in the region of the vessel system involved. Although differentiation of the type of lesion may not be possible using radionuclide imaging, this type of brain scanning may produce positive information in a wide range of neurological diseases, including brain tumors, arteriovenous malformations, intracranial hemorrhage, cerebral ischemia, cerebral infarction, hematoma (subdural, epidural, or intracerebral), venous sinus thrombosis, cerebral contusion, inflammatory cerebral disease, meningitis, abscess, and in conditions such as hydrocephalus, porencephaly, and cysts.

Wilkinson and Goodrich (1982) have presented summarical information regarding the accuracy of radioisotopic brain scans in various conditions, based upon an extensive review of reports in the literature. The percentage of positive brain scan results among brain neoplasms ranges from 53% (pituitary adenomas) to 95% (meningiomas). The total number of cases reported is variable and thus direct comparisons may not be entirely valid. However, the data may be summarized with respect to diagnostic accuracy as follows: 50%-59% range, pituitary adenoma; 60%-69%, craniopharyngioma; 70%-79%, the more rare types of gliomas as a group and astrocytomas grades I and II; 80%-89%, all gliomas considered as a group, ependymomas, oligodendrogliomas, acoustic neuromas and metastatic tumors; 90%-95%, astrocytomas grades III and IV, medulloblastomas, and meningiomas (Wilkinson & Goodrich, 1982). Excellent results have been reported in identifying cerebral abscesses (about 97%) and epidural and subdural hematomas (about 85%). Arteriovenous malformations also can frequently be identified as an area of abnormality (about 82%) but cerebral infarcts show positive findings much less frequently (about 47%). Some reports in the literature have indicated that positive scan results in patients with strokes tend to diminish in time following the onset of clinical symptoms. Transient ischemic attacks have also been studied but the identification of positive results varies with respect to the technique used and, in many instances, fails to show positive results.

The single static brain scan image, especially in cerebral vascular disease, has been shown in a number of studies to fail to reveal pathological involvement that is shown in scans which demonstrate rapid-sequence serial images of the tracer as it follows its progressive pattern. In fact, the combination of static brain imaging studies with the dynamic scan enhances the prospect of identifying cerebral vascular disease, even though the "dynamic" studies may frequently be positive when routine scans are negative. Traumatic injury of the head and brain often will yield a positive scan image, but, from the scan itself, it is difficult to differentiate between scalp contusion or laceration, skull fracture, and cerebral contusion. Thus, the interpretation of the brain scan must be made in conjunction with evaluation of skull x-rays and examination of the patient's scalp. In addition, positive results on the brain scan in cerebral contusion are most commonly seen early after trauma and, according to some reports, may be expected to resolve in 6 to 10 weeks.

Because of the rapid development of computed tomography (CT scan) as a diagnostic procedure in brain disease and damage, a comment should be offered with respect to the comparative performance of CT scans and radionuclide scans. Alderson, Gado, and Siegal (1977), in a compilation of published reports, found that CT scan had an accuracy rate of 93% in identification of lesions as compared with 85% for radionuclide scans. Evans and Jost (1977), in their comparative evaluation, conclude that consideration of both diagnostic accuracy and cost effectiveness indicate that in most cases CT scan is preferable to RN scan. Since both procedures are oriented toward the same aims, at least in a number of respects, it is apparent that the frequency with which RN scans are used will diminish because of the availability of CT scans. However, a number of investigators have emphasized certain complementary aspects of the two procedures (Fordham, 1977).

# POSITRON EMISSION TOMOGRAPHY (PET)

In 1895 Roentgen discovered x-rays. In this procedure a part of the body is irradiated with an x-ray emitting source and the x-ray photons pass through the body and fall on an x-ray-sensitive fluorescent screen. The light given off by this screen results in blackening of a light-sensitive film that is in close contact with the screen, showing darker images in the areas in which the x-rays pass through without obstruction and lighter images for more obstructive tissues such as bones. The combinations of fluorescent screen and film have been perfected to the point that they are able to register more than 60% of the radiation falling on them, thus reflecting quite accurately the three-dimensional structure (part of the body) in a two-dimensional image.

However, x-ray films are not very useful in differentiating organs composed of soft tissue because their x-ray attenuation values are very similar. This problem was overcome in visualization of blood vessels and certain other organs by injecting a contrast substance into the blood stream, thereby permitting visualization of blood vessels as well as the shape of organs that have a rich blood supply (angiography). In addition, certain elements can be introduced into organs which increase the absorption of radiation and enhance the contrast with neighboring tissues. For example, barium introduced into the digestive tract helps to outline its physical structure. X-ray films can be made quite quickly and, technically, up to 60 images per second can be obtained. Although this is an advantage for repeated visualization of a rapidly moving organ (such as the heart), x-ray photons are absorbed in the body and repeated images cannot be continued for very long without a harmful amount of radiation to the body.

Except for angiography, relatively little progress was made in film radiography and x-rays were used principally to provide images of bones and lungs, each of which have high contrast. In the late 1940s Moore (1947) discovered that he was able to identify tissues which contained tumor cells by injecting fluorescin into a brain tumor during surgery. As previously described, he later proceeded to inject radioactively-labeled substances into the blood stream and to locate the tumor through use of a detector that was placed over the cranium. Various improvements were made in the scanners that were used to detect radioactivity. Essentially this procedure located abnormalities in the blood-brain barrier which were represented by increased radioactivity.

Injection of positron-emitting radioisotopes was a logical next step and this procedure for detecting brain lesions was first described by Wrenn, Good, and Handler (1951). Technical developments in imaging systems followed and additional work was done to produce new radiopharmaceutical substances for brain imaging. However, the cameras (recording devices) still had poor spatial resolution and provided little anatomical detail. A major advance was made when a tomographic scanner was developed which performed linear scans at discrete angles around the human being or body part and permitted a transaxial reconstruction of the radionuclide distribution (Kuhl & Edwards, 1963). Technical developments continued into the 1970s, by which time it had become possible to quantitatively relate radionuclide concentration to a digital representation of an image. This technique was then pursued to quantify local cerebral blood volume in milliliters per 100 grams of tissue. The next step was to develop methods for measurement of regional blood volume in the brain and studies were performed in a variety of neurological disorders (including head trauma) that identified the extent of intracerebral bleeding as well as areas of decreased perfusion secondary to cerebral thrombosis. These developments made it clear that procedures of this type were of value in demonstrating regional cerebral changes that related to impaired function, even though they lacked precision in anatomic delineation.

Positron emitters (such as carbon, nitrogen, and oxygen) were studied and it was found that they could be tagged to a wide variety of natural substrates with the interaction between positrons and neighboring electrons giving rise to gamma radiation. Gamma-ray detectors, situated 180° apart, can then detect a signal from the X-axis and a signal from the Y-axis as well as a third signal reflecting pulse height or the measure of energy. However, the availability of positron emitters depended upon the availability of a medical cyclotron or accelerator within a short distance from the site at which the positron emitters were to be used. Phelps, Hoffman, Mullani, and Ter-Pogossian (1975) constructed the first clinically successful machine to map the regional distribution of positron emitters, and it was found to be valuable in outlining both anatomical and functional areas of damage in both the brain and heart. Additional developments have permitted determination of cerebral blood flow as well as metabolic rate for both oxygen and glucose. Although earlier procedures had been available for drawing certain inferences regarding such measurements, positron emission tomography promises to provide much more detailed information, particularly with regard to localized areas of deficient function.

Many studies of local glucose metabolism of the cerebral cortex in association with various conditions of sensory stimulation have been performed. In one study (Greenberg, Reivich, Hand, Rosenquist, Rintelmann, Stein, Tusa, Dann, Christman, Fowler, MacGregor, & Wolf, 1981) monaural stimulation was presented in the form of a factual story. In each subject investigated, this stimulation resulted in an increase in glucose consumption in the contralateral temporal cortex. Compared with the ipsilateral cortex, the increase in the contralateral primary auditory cortex was statistically significant. However, the evidence of glucose metabolism produced by PET scans appears to be somewhat more complicated than might be expected. Phelps, Mazziotta, Engel, and Kuhl (1981) used the Seashore Tonal Memory Test, which requires the subject to identify whether pairs of tone sequences are the same or different, with monaural presentation. Regardless of the ear stimulated, cerebral cortex glucose metabolism was increased in the right

frontal area, the contralateral transverse temporal area, and the contralateral posterior temporal area. When a verbal story was presented monaurally, an increase was noted in the right frontal and left associative visual cortex.

Greenberg et al. (1981) also found that the contralateral postcentral cortex increased in activity when the fingers and hand on one side were stimulated with a moderately stiff brush. Visual stimulation has generally shown an increased metabolic rate in the primary visual cortex contralateral to the hemifield stimulated. This effect was distinct in every subject examined and, even with small numbers, yielded a highly significant result. Several visual stimuli have been used: a bright white light at several levels of intensity, a two cycle per second alternating black and white checkerboard pattern, and a view of a park which was outside the window of the laboratory. The results were studied in conjunction with measurement of visual evoked responses. The white light resulted in an increase of glucose metabolism in both the primary and association visual cortex on the contralateral side. A somewhat larger increase occurred in both the primary and association visual cortex with the black and white checkerboard pattern. However, no reliable relationship was observed between the metabolic response and the visual evoked response. The largest PET response of glucose metabolism occurred when the subjects were asked to look at the park through the laboratory window. Compared to the PET activity when eyes were closed, an average increase of 45% occurred in the primary visual cortex and 59% in the association visual cortex. It would appear from these findings that complex scenes may bring about a degree of recruitment in metabolic activity of the association visual cortex.

Additional studies with individual patients have been done, particularly using persons with homonymous visual field defects. These patients show deficiencies of glucose metabolism contralateral to the side of the visual field defect. The metabolic activity is definitely lower than in normal subjects with their eyes closed. Thus, it would appear that interruption of the visual pathways results in a diminution of glucose metabolism in the occipital cortex beyond that found with mere reduction of visual input.

Kuhl, Phelps, Kowell, Metter, Selin, and Winter (1980) studied 10 patients with cerebral thromboses which probably involved the middle cerebral artery in most cases. In addition to determination of glucose metabolism from the PET scans, a measure of blood perfusion was also made. Glucose utilization was less impaired than the perfusion in the first two days following the stroke. In later stages, presumably when the infarcts had become more stable, glucose metabolism and perfusion tended to correspond. However, both measures demonstrated more brain involvement in these patients than was suggested by other radiological studies. Computed tomography, for example, identified areas of damage that were considerably more discrete than would be inferred from the PET studies. These investigators concluded that computed tomography might be misleading in estimating the functional state of tissue because it shows only the structural abnormality. The authors suggested that measures of local cerebral blood flow and cerebral metabolic rates for oxygen and glucose will improve understanding of the events that follow a stroke, response to therapeutic interventions, and possible identification of tissue with potential for recovery, particularly when used in conjunction with computed tomography.

Kuhl, Engel, Phelps, and Selin (1980) have studied patterns of local cerebral metabolism and perfusion among epileptic patients both during an active seizure and at intervals between seizures. CT scans usually appeared to be normal; however, in 12 of 15 patients PET scans showed broad areas of decreased metabolism and perfusion which correlated fairly well with EEG lateralization and localization findings. The results on PET did not correspond exactly, even when CT scans showed focal areas of atrophy. Thus, the findings suggest that these procedures may have complementary value in describing brain involvement among epileptic patients. As in previous studies of

cerebral blood flow, which have shown a marked increase during an active seizure, PET scans demonstrated about twice the normal metabolism and perfusion during the ictal period.

In another section of this book we have reviewed a number of findings of changes in brain functions with relation to age. As noted, most studies of cerebral blood flow have shown a decrease among normally functioning older persons, and an even greater decrease among older persons suffering from dementia. However, there is an argument, based principally on results reported by investigators from the National Institute of Aging, that the reduction in indicators of brain function among older subjects may be due to unrecognized atherosclerosis of cerebral vessels and other conditions that may be classified as a function of disease rather than aging. Alavi, Reivich, Greenberg, and Wolf (1982) refer to a study done by their group in which glucose consumption was evaluated with PET scans among 9 young normal volunteers, 4 elderly normal subjects who were carefully screened to exclude mental and physical disorders, and 8 elderly patients with dementia. The mean rates of glucose consumption for various areas of the brain showed a definite decrease from young normal to old normal subjects and an additional decrease among the old demented subjects. Only comparisons of the young subjects and the old demented subjects, however, were statistically significant considering the variability among subjects and the small numbers included in the groups. These very preliminary results suggest that glucose metabolism of the cerebral cortex decreases with age, but additional measures of oxygen metabolism and cerebral blood flow should be performed in the same subjects and group size obviously should be increased.

Some reports, based principally on individual schizophrenic subjects, have suggested that glucose metabolism as demonstrated by PET is decreased, particularly in the frontal cortex. Brain tumors have also been studied and results show a relationship between glucose consumption and the degree of anaplasia of the tumor. Highly anaplastic tumors appear to have a significantly higher rate of glucose metabolism than more slowly growing tumors, and, compared with the homologous cortex in the non-affected hemisphere, cortical glucose metabolism is reduced by as much as 50% in tissue adjacent to the tumor. It appears that PET scans may be helpful in early detection of intrinsic cerebral neoplasms and recognition of changes in growth rate as well as possible recurrence.

These various results suggest that computed emission tomography is a rapidly growing and exciting area of investigation of biological functions of the brain. It would appear that this imaging method will eventually provide much information regarding blood flow and metabolic activity of the brain in a great number of conditions of disease and deficit that have not previously been well understood in biological terms.

# NUCLEAR MAGNETIC RESONANCE (NMR) IMAGING

The theoretical basis and demonstration of nuclear magnetic resonance (NMR) dates back to the late 1940s and represents work for which Edward Purcell and Felix Block were awarded the Nobel prize for physics in 1952. Although the basic work for this procedure is not new, three somewhat diverse developments in science were necessary to produce the current imaging procedures using NMR. These were (1) an understanding of the nucleus (which contributed to the conception of NMR); (2) the discovery of superconductivity (which is an important component of the magnets used for NMR); and (3) the use of computers to combine multiple projections into a final image.

The first NMR images, using a computed tomography type of reconstruction, were published by Lauterbur (1973). As early as 1959 Singer had demonstrated the use of NMR in measuring blood flow. In 1971 Damadian used NMR to demonstrate differences between normal tissues and tumor tissues. It has been only in the last few years, though, that a strong general interest has developed in the use of NMR for imaging purposes. A review of these developments has been published by Kaufman, Crooks, and Margulis (1981).

NMR imaging requires that the subject be placed in a large chamber surrounded by a superconducting magnet that is capable of producing a magnetic field of up to 3,000 gauss. This magnet also contains radiofrequency coils which pick up signals emitted from hydrogen nuclei. The magnetic field causes alignment of hydrogen nuclei in the body as well as other nuclei with odd numbers of protons and neutrons which, in turn, results in a spinning of the nuclei. At a certain point of phase and radiofrequency of magnetic energy, the spin of the nuclei change direction and absorb energy in this process. The energy emitted from the nuclei is of a characteristic radiofrequency, depends upon the strength of the magnetic field and the density of nuclei in the plane of the body corresponding to that particular field and is picked up by receivers. Data obtained from different planes are fed into a computer, which plots the distribution of nuclei responsible for the emission and converts the data into a composite image. Although the spatial resolution of the image is not as fine as that of the CT image, in some respects differentiation of tissues (especially between gray and white matter of the brain) is better than in CT.

NMR images produced in coronal and sagittal views assist in visualizing brain lesions and determining their extent. NMR imaging responds to changes in water content, fat, and blood flow. Thus, these parameters determine the image obtained and diseases which have not changed these variables or grossly distorted the anatomy of the brain are not likely not be detected. Tumors are differentiated from normal tissues, but their characteristics overlap with abnormalities shown by lesions such as abscesses and hematomas. Vascular lesions (such as arteriovenous malformations) are clearly represented in NMR although they usually require use of contrast substances for clear definition using CT. A very sharp contrast between gray and white matter can be achieved with NMR, suggesting that NMR may be particularly useful in diseases that show a predilection for damage of the cerebral cortex as compared with underlying tissue. The differentiation probably depends upon the variation in water content of white versus gray matter. NMR produces excellent images in the region of the posterior fossa, with bone artifacts having little effect. Fast or slow blood flow in individual vessels can be judged by the degree of shading (dark to light) and tissue perfusion can also be estimated. However, blood flow measures are likely to be developed in much more detail in the future. NMR produces excellent visualization of the carotid arteries. Animal studies have indicated that induced infarcts as well as the eventual resulting atrophy of cerebral tissue are clearly shown by NMR.

Because of the sensitivity of NMR to fat, NMR has been studied in relation to in multiple sclerosis.

Using both NMR and CT, Young et al. (1981) evaluated 10 patients with multiple sclerosis. CT showed 19 lesions while NMR showed 131 lesions, including all of the 19 that were demonstrated by CT. Besson, et al. (1981) used NMR to investigate the effect of alcohol consumption. Their results indicated that changes in both the gray and white matter occurred during intoxication and increased during the period of withdrawal and abstinence. These effects may be due to a change in water content of the brain.

NMR has also been used to visualize the heart, breast, liver, spleen, kidney, abdominal muscles, blood vessels of the abdomen, and gall bladder. Preliminary studies indicate that abnormal structure and evidence of disease of these organs may be produced by NMR images, which provide sufficient anatomical detail to compete with results of CT scans.

It is apparent that NMR imaging represents a significant development and may be especially useful for evaluation of certain diseases of the brain and nervous system. Additional research will establish the full value of this procedure in comparison to other imaging methods.

# CEREBRAL SPINAL FLUID ANALYSIS

Under normal circumstances, cerebrospinal fluid (CSF) is a clear and colorless liquid. Detailed analyses have been performed to identify the chemical composition of cerebrospinal fluid, and most constituents of the cerebrospinal fluid are similar to those in blood plasma. All substances found in the CSF are found in the blood, but the reverse is not true and certain blood constituents found in the CSF are viewed as abnormal. The composition of CSF varies along the cerebrospinal axis, with distinctive differences occurring in the ventricular fluid, the cisternal fluid, and lumbar fluid, especially with respect to total protein and glucose. For purposes of analysis, cerebrospinal fluid is generally withdrawn at the lumbar level.

The major purpose of the cerebrospinal fluid is to lubricate and serve as a buffer between the brain and spinal cord on the one hand, and the more rigid framework of the dura mater, skull, and vertebral column on the other. In this manner, it appears that the cerebrospinal fluid, which bathes the entire central nervous system, may protect against injury. In fact, the weight of the adult brain has been calculated to be only 50 gm when it is suspended in fluid. In addition, the volume of the brain may be permitted a degree of change by decreases in the volume of the CSF (as in expanding intracranial lesions) or by increases in CSF volume (as in hydrocephalus ex vacuo).

The CSF must have unobstructed circulation for it to maintain its normal characteristics. The fluid is generated by the choroid plexus, a villous tuft enclosing a core of highly vascular connective tissue located within the lateral ventricles, the third ventricle, and the fourth ventricle. The path of circulation leads from the lateral ventricles through the foramina of Monro into the third ventricle, through the cerebral aqueduct (aqueduct of Sylvius) and then into the fourth ventricle. (*See* Fig. 3–1.) The path would ordinarily continue into the central canal of the spinal cord, but in human beings the central canal is usually obliterated by the twelfth year. Thus, from the fourth ventricle, the CSF communicates with the subarachnoid space through the two lateral foramina of Luschka and the medial aperture in the roof of the fourth ventricle, called the foramen of Magendie. The fluid enters the cisterna magna and from there circulates through the subarachnoid space of the cerebellar hemispheres, through the basilar cisterns, and caudally to the spinal subarachnoid space. Fluid arriving at the base of the cisterns progresses through the interpeduncular and prechiasmatic cisterns, the Sylvian fissures, and the cisterns of the corpus callosum to the lateral and frontal hemispheric subarachnoid space. The fluid continues its course to the medial and posterior cerebral hemispheric subarachnoid space. While the choroid plexus generates the cerebral spinal fluid, the arachnoid villi of the dural sinuses are responsible for absorption of the CSF. The CSF circulates through the ventricles and subarachnoid space at the rate of 500 ml per day. The composition of normal lumbar CSF has been determined in detail (Tourtellotte & Shorr, 1982).

For purposes of clinical evaluation, the cerebrospinal fluid is withdrawn from the lumbar level (the terminal ventricle — sometimes called the fifth ventricle). Under normal circumstances the CSF should be perfectly clear. It should always be inspected for turbidity, a condition that usually is due to the presence of cells in the fluid and becomes evident in the presence of 400 or more leukocytes or 200 or more erythrocytes per cubic ml. Normal CSF does not contain fibrinogen and, therefore, does not clot. Thus, the CSF is tested for clotting, a condition that relates to increased total protein content of the CSF. The CSF normally should never contain erythrocytes (red blood cells) and their presence indicates a distinct deviation from normality. The presence of erythrocytes may be due to faulty technique in entering the subarachnoid space at the time of lumbar puncture. The first few drops of cerebrospinal fluid, in this case, may show a bloody tinge, and various techniques are available

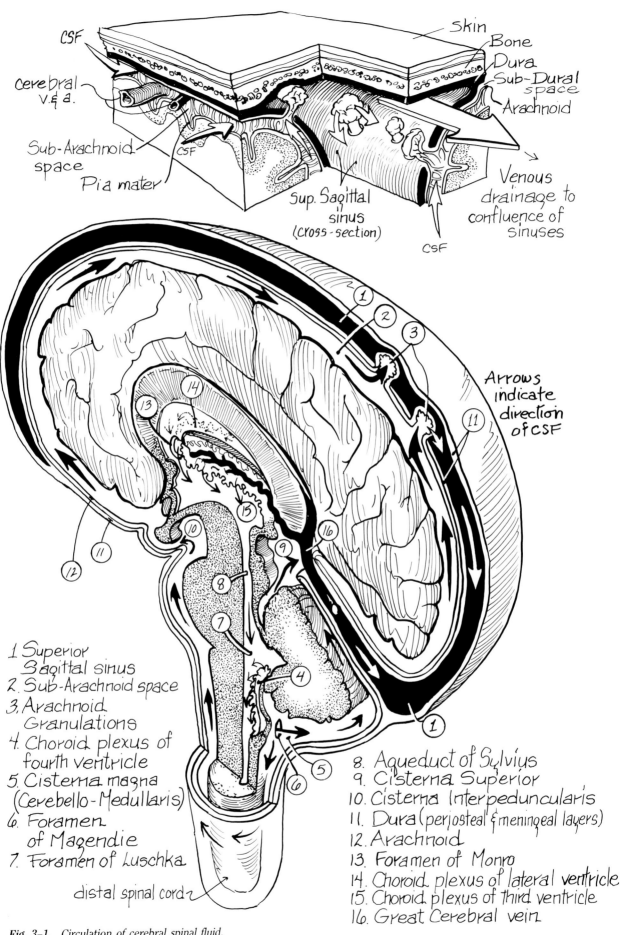

Skin
Bone
Dura
Sub-Dural space
Arachnoid

CSF

Cerebral v. & a.

Sub-Arachnoid space

Pia mater

Sup. Sagittal sinus (cross-section)

Venous drainage to confluence of sinuses

CSF

CSF

Arrows indicate direction of CSF

1 Superior
 Sagittal sinus
2. Sub-Arachnoid space
3. Arachnoid
 Granulations
4. Choroid plexus of
 fourth ventricle
5. Cisterna magna
 (Cerebello-Medullaris)
6. Foramen
 of Magendie
7. Foramen of Luschka

distal spinal cord

8. Aqueduct of Sylvius
9. Cisterna Superior
10. Cisterna Interpeduncularis
11. Dura (periosteal & meningeal layers)
12. Arachnoid
13. Foramen of Monro
14. Choroid plexus of lateral ventricle
15. Choroid plexus of third ventricle
16. Great Cerebral vein

*Fig. 3-1. Circulation of cerebral spinal fluid.*

to discern whether the needle entry has damaged a blood vessel, causing bleeding into the sample. The alternative possibility when blood is in the cerebrospinal fluid is that the patient has experienced a subarachnoid hemorrhage.

A related condition of abnormality of the cerebrospinal fluid concerns a yellow discoloration called *xanthochromia*. This term refers to any yellow discoloration of the fluid and such discoloration may be caused by bleeding as well as the presence of other pigments, such as carotene and melanin. The principal quantitative determination at the time of withdrawal of cerebrospinal fluid concerns the CSF pressure. The normal pressure is 150 ml of water but the standard deviation of 33 ml is relatively large. Thus, the normal range, in total, is fairly wide. In sitting position, when the effect of gravity is added, the normal adult has a CSF pressure of 400 mm of water. Variations in CSF pressure, over a relatively short period of time, have been related to various pathological conditions.

A second major concern in clinical evaluation of CSF concerns cellular analysis. No erythrocytes and few leukocytes are expected. Tourtellotte (1970) indicates that there should normally be 1.8 leukocytes per cubic ml with an upper limit of normal at 5. Monocytes may normally be present in the CSF, averaging 17 cells per cubic ml. Increases in the frequency of these cells suggest subacute abnormalities, including encephalitis due to virus or microbacterium, mycosis, resolving bacterial infections, tumor, response to foreign material, or a reaction to injury. The presence of other cells in the CSF, such as polymorphonuclear cells, eosinophils, basophils, plasma cells, macrophages, and tumor cells are always abnormal, even though the total leukocyte count may be within the normal range.

Because of the clinical importance in many cases of differentiating between bacterial and non-bacterial encephalomeningeal infections, the CSF is also evaluated for the presence of microbes. In addition, laboratory procedures have been developed for culturing viral agents that may be present in CSF.

In clinical practice, the CSF protein level is the most frequent abnormal component in laboratory evaluation. The total protein concentration in CSF is influenced by the site of sampling and patient's characteristics, including age, sex, and the degree of activity or recumbency of the patient. Males appear to have slightly more protein in CSF than females (although this difference is minimal) and prolonged recumbency increases the protein level. At the lumbar level, the normal range is considered to be 15-52 mg per 100 ml in normal younger subjects (Tourtellotte & Shorr, 1982) with an average value of about 38. Levels are lower in the ventricles with some increase in the cisterna magna. Adult levels remain relatively constant until about 40 years of age; at that time levels begin to gradually increase up to about 72 mg/100 ml in the elderly.

If the laboratory examination of CSF reveals protein fractions and combinations of proteins that differ from the normally expected relationships the results may have additional diagnostic value.

The CSF is also examined for glucose and normal values range from 50-80 mg/100 ml. Increases and decreases in the CSF glucose indicate the presence of hyperglycemia and hypoglycemia.

CSF has also been studied with respect to chloride concentration, acid-base characteristics, the presence of lipids, levels of neurotransmitters, and other constituents such as sodium, calcium, potassium, magnesium (among major cations) and chloride bicarbonate and phosphate (among major anions).

There are several contraindications to performing lumbar puncture. These include evidence of increased intracranial pressure due to a space-occupying lesion, the presence of a coagulation defect, acute trauma to the spinal column (especially in the lumbar area), skin or subcutaneous infections in the area of puncture, and other conditions. In addition, the *post-lumbar puncture syndrome* may occur several hours after the lumbar puncture. One of every three persons having lumbar puncture is said to experience mild to severe frontal and occipital headache (particularly on change of posture) and occasional nuchal pain. In severe cases, nausea, vomiting, and malaise may also accompany the headache when the person is in an erect posture. These symptoms are usually relieved when the patient lies down. This syndrome usually lasts for four days but may persist for two weeks or more. Experimentation has indicated that the size of the spinal needle used is relevant, and use of a small-gauge needle can decrease the syndrome to 10% of patients and also result in a milder and shorter course.

# Clinical Contributions

Analysis of CSF frequently proves to be abnormal in various infections of the nervous system, including both bacterial and viral infections. Various chronic infections causing meningoencephalitis show definite abnormalities, as does neurosyphilis and viral meningeal encephalitis. Vascular lesions do not usually cause significant abnormalities of CSF unless there has been intracerebral hemorrhage. In this case, abnormalities may be indicated by xanthochromia or the presence of erythrocytes. Intracranial tumors may cause elevation of CSF pressure, xanthochromia, and elevated cell counts and protein level. Abnormalities may be present following craniocerebral trauma, usually represented by the presence of blood in the CSF.

Abnormalities of the CSF have been found in a great number of other conditions, represented either by an increase in opening pressure, evidence of bleeding into the CSF, an increase in cells, or elevated protein levels. These abnormalities have been observed in various developmental defects, including congenital hydrocephalus, inherited diseases, metabolic systemic diseases, hepatic disease, renal disease, connective tissue disease, multiple sclerosis, degenerative diseases, paroxysmal disorders (including epilepsy), normal-pressure hydrocephalus, and benign intracranial hypertension. However, the abnormalities of CSF vary considerably among these conditions and usually do not have specific diagnostic significance.

# NEUROMUSCULAR ELECTRODIAGNOSIS

Neuromuscular electrodiagnosis is the recording of electrical activity from nerves and muscles. In general, electrodiagnostic testing is useful in the evaluation of disorders involving the motor unit, including the anterior horn cell, its axon, the neuromuscular junction, and all the muscle fibers supplied by the anterior horn cell. Usually, electrodiagnostic testing is of little or no value in evaluation of central nervous system disorders that involve the brain. In fact, these procedures are usually of limited value even in the evaluation of upper motor neuron spinal cord disorders. The greatest usefulness of these procedures is in evaluation of weakness, fatigue, decreased muscle tone, and muscular atrophy. We should note that these procedures are quite sensitive for these purposes and often allow detection of minimal dysfunction of the motor unit even when clinical signs may be absent or equivocal. In addition, muscular weakness resulting from hysteria or malingering can usually be differentiated from weakness having a neurological basis.

The majority of patients referred for neuromuscular electrodiagnosis have intervertebral disc disease, entrapment neuropathies, or traumatic neuropathies. In disc disease a motor nerve root may be compressed (leading to irritation) and this, in turn, may be followed by destructive changes within the root. Entrapment neuropathy refers to a localized area of nerve injury caused by impingement and continued irritation from a neighboring anatomical structure. The carpal tunnel syndrome is an example. Traumatic neuropathies result from physical damage to peripheral nerves. Electromyography and nerve conduction velocity testing permit accurate assessment of the degree and location of the damage. However, electrodiagnostic tests can evaluate only the lower motor neuron, neuromuscular junction, and muscle (on the motor side) and sensory nerve conduction velocity (on the sensory side), and indicate the functional status of these structures. These techniques do not provide evidence of etiology of the disorder and inferences concerning etiology must be derived from other sources of information such as the history, physical examination, and laboratory tests.

# BRAIN BIOPSY FOR NEUROLOGICAL DISEASE

There are instances when a definitive diagnosis of brain disease can be accomplished only by biopsy of the brain tissue. Brain biopsy is not usually considered unless the patient has a progressive brain disease, no cure is known on the basis of the patient's symptoms and other diagnostic procedures, and it is necessary to determine the diagnosis. A fairly large piece of tissue is needed for examination, usually taken from the right middle frontal gyrus, including the middle frontal gyrus and about ½ of the gyrus on either side. The specimen should be about 1.5 cm in length, about 1 cm deep, and about 1 cm wide.

General conditions in which brain biopsies are done with adult subjects include progressive dementia and central nervous system infections of unknown cause. In children, biopsies may be considered with progressive dementia, progressive loss of motor function, increasing dyskinesia or cerebellar dysfunction, obvious arrest of physical and psychological development, intractable seizures, or central nervous system infections of unknown cause. In the past, brain biopsy was used to diagnosis many diseases that may now be identified by enzymatic and serological techniques. Although most degenerative disorders still require brain biopsy for definitive diagnosis, a number of inborn metabolic disorders and demyelinating diseases may be diagnosed by other techniques. Previously, multiple sclerosis as well as viral encephalitis was diagnosed by brain biopsy. Laboratory examinations of serum and cerebrospinal fluid, or biopsy of non-neural tissues, has proved effective in diagnosis. Metabolic diseases that produce a diffuse storage of substances (such as lipids or glycogen) show changes in the tissue of liver, kidney, or adrenals. Other conditions, such as Reye's syndrome or Wilson's disease, may also be diagnosed by liver biopsy because of the association of primary liver disease with cerebral dysfunction. However, Alzheimer's disease, Pick's disease, Creutzfeldt-Jakob disease, and a number of less common conditions still require brain biopsy for definitive diagnosis. The purpose of brain biopsy, especially in adult dementia, may be related to additional information regarding prognosis, genetic counseling, and family reassurance.

Although the middle part of the right frontal gyrus is the site most frequently selected for biopsy, different sites may be used according to indications of maximal atrophy, as shown by computed tomography or pneumoencephalography and complemented by the patient's clinical manifestations. The frontal cortex is the usual site in Alzheimer's disease or in generalized conditions of brain involvement. In patients suspected of having Pick's disease, the maximal area of atrophy often involves the anterior two-thirds of the superior temporal gyrus, although in some instances the frontal area may be predominantly involved. In Creutzfeldt-Jakob disease, the occipital cortex may be involved initially and the biopsy is frequently taken from Brodmann's area 19. However, since this disease is rapidly progressive, by the time the biopsy is considered, the frontal cortex may also be involved. The anterior temporal and inferior frontal cortex are the usual sites of maximal involvement in herpes simplex encephalitis and the temporal lobe is the preferred site for biopsy in subacute sclerosing panencephalitis, although these latter diseases may be diagnosed by careful examination of the cerebrospinal fluid or serum. The cerebellum is the preferred biopsy site for identification of Lafora bodies in familial myoclonic epilepsy.

Experience has shown that the areas of maximal involvement should not be the selected site for biopsy in certain conditions. When the disease is long-standing and slowly progressive in nature, the area of maximal involvement may only show gliosis, necrosis, or calcification, whereas other areas of the cerebral cortex may provide more definitive histological changes.

Although complications of brain biopsy are generally reported to be low, the procedure is not without risk. Complications have included epilepsy, intracerebral hemorrhage, subdural hematoma or accumulation of fluid, mild and usually transient hemiparesis, porencephaly, post-operative fever of unknown cause, cerebrospinal fluid leak(s) and infection of the surgical site.

Biopsy of brain tumors is a common procedure during the course of surgical excision of a lesion. The resulting information derived from pathological evaluation, complemented by the observations of the neurosurgeon, provide important information regarding treatment and prognosis. The neurosurgeon is able to identify the general location of a tumor, the general tissue texture, and observations of tumor vascularity, necrosis, discreteness of tumor-brain interface, edema surrounding the tumor, and the presence of cysts and their contents. The pathological description includes many points of information concerned with identification of the basic tumor cell type, the degree of malignancy, and clinical correlates, including factors such as associated blood vessels, hemorrhage, evidence of calcification, edema, necrosis, etc. that may be useful in clinical management.

Needle biopsy may be used with deep-seated neoplasms such as thalamic or pontine astrocytomas, where attempted excision would be hazardous, or with lesions that are in highly characteristic locations. Computed tomography is sometimes used to assist in needle placement. The major disadvantages of needle biopsy are that small tissue samples are obtained and it is difficult to establish a histological diagnosis. In addition, the tissue extracted by needle biopsy may not be representative of the lesion. Depending upon the type of tumor tissue being examined, the common procedures used to analyze tumor tissue include light microscopy, electron microscopy, and immunohistochemical methods. We should also note that peripheral nerve biopsy is done in cases of peripheral neuropathy and skeletal muscle biopsy for conditions including neurogenic muscular atrophy, inflammatory myopathy, dystrophic myopathy, and metabolic myopathies, but these procedures have less direct relevance for the neuropsychologist (Ellis, Youmans, & Dreyfus, 1982).

# Section IV

# Neurological Diseases and Disorders

Tumors of the Brain

Cerebral Vascular Disease

Head Injury

Infections of the Brain

Demyelinating Diseases
    Including Multiple Sclerosis

Pick's Disease

Parkinson's Disease

Huntington's Chorea

Toxic and Metabolic Disorders

Effects of Alcohol

Aging

Epilepsy

# TUMORS OF THE BRAIN

## Overview

Tumors arise from tissues distributed throughout the body and about 10% of these lesions occur within the central nervous system, its meninges, and related bony structures. Eighty percent of these tumors are in the cranial cavity and 20% involve the area of the spinal cord. Tumors of the nervous system may be primary or metastatic. **Primary tumors** arise from tissue of the brain and spinal cord as well as their meninges and blood vessels, from the pituitary and pineal glands and residual embryonic tissue. Metastatic tumors account for about 20% of intracranial tumors. The most common primary sites of metastatic tumors are, in order, the lungs, the gastrointestinal tract, breasts, and kidneys. The lesions are multiple in 70% of metastatic tumors to the brain.

Little information is known about the etiology of most brain tumors. In general, hereditary factors seem to be significant for a limited category of tumors but the familial occurrence of brain tumors is rare. There have been occasional reports of tumors developing after brain trauma, but in general, trauma is not considered to be a significant etiological factor. Radiation may damage and impair tissues in the brain and lead to delayed degenerative changes, but there is no evidence that radiation produces intrinsic cerebral tumors. Some reports have suggested that long-delayed effects of radiation may be associated with development of meningiomas. Viral infections may have some relationship to development of certain rare brain tumors, such as lymphoma, but viruses appear to have little role in the development of most brain tumors. Chemical carcinogens have been used to produce experimental brain tumors in animals, and it has been suggested that carcinogens may play a role in the development of human brain tumors. However, there is little direct evidence or support of this hypothesis. Thus, while much is known of the types of cells from which tumors arise, little is known about factors that give rise to the development of brain tumors.

Brain tumors have been classified as intrinsic and extrinsic. **Intrinsic** brain tumors arise from tissues within the brain; **extrinsic** tumors arise from tissues outside of the brain, such as meninges. The principal categories of brain tumors, in order with respect to the frequency with which they occur, are the gliomas (arising from neuroglia and ependymal tissues); the meningiomas, arising from the meninges; pituitary adenomas, arising from the pituitary gland; neurilemmomas, including neurofibromas and acoustic neuromas; metastatic tumors from various primary sites throughout the body; and blood vessel tumors, which may also be classified under categories of cerebral vascular disease.

It is customary to classify tumors as benign or malignant. However, this division of tumors of the brain is nowhere nearly as clear as the classification of tumors involving other parts of the body. Gliomas customarily demonstrate characteristic features of malignancy, although some gliomas are slower growing than others. It must be recognized that any tumor of the brain, including one classified as benign, may gradually increase in size and produce damage that is eventually fatal. The particular location of the tumor may also influence the consequences. For example, a tumor near the aqueduct of Sylvius may obstruct cerebrospinal fluid circulation and result in a fatal rise in intracranial pressure. Figs. 4–1 and 4–2 illustrate some of the types of tumors.

Tumors may be classified according to their degree of malignancy. This applies particularly to gliomas because a number of other tumors do not show a significant degree of growth to be characterized as malignant. However, gliomas are classified according to the number of differentiated (as contrasted with embryonically immature) cells into Grades I, II, III, and IV. This grading of malignancy, from a practical and therapeutic point of view, is more important than the predominant cell-type of the tumor, although the type of cell from which the tumor arises is related to the degree of malignancy. Gliomas classified as Grade I have 75%-100% of differentiated cells; Grade II, 50%-75%; Grade III, 25%-50%; and in Grade IV

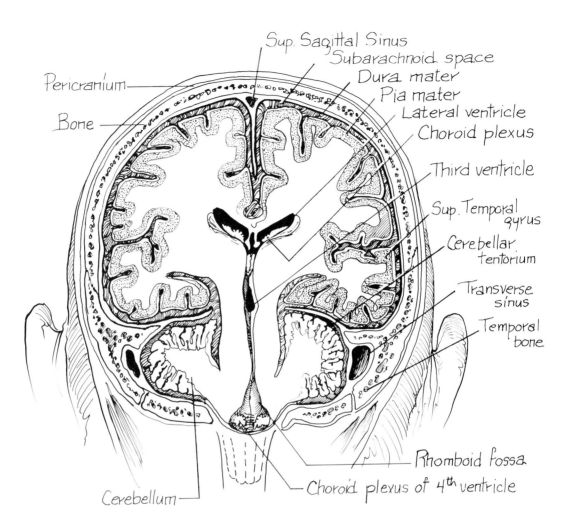

Sup. Sagittal Sinus
Subarachnoid space
Dura mater
Pia mater
Lateral ventricle
Choroid plexus

Pericranium

Bone

Third ventricle

Sup. Temporal gyrus

Cerebellar tentorium

Transverse sinus

Temporal bone

Rhomboid fossa

Choroid plexus of 4th ventricle

Cerebellum

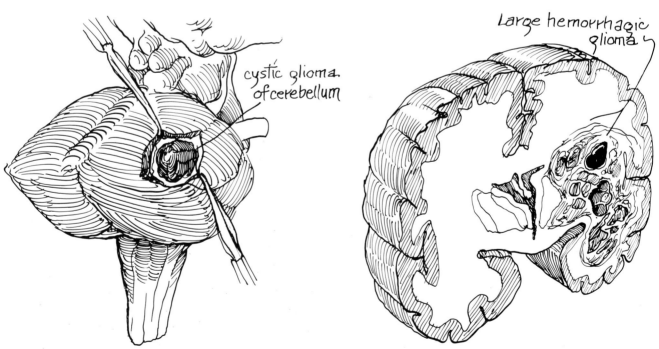

cystic glioma of cerebellum

Large hemorrhagic glioma

**Fig. 4–1.** Top: Normal relationship of intracranial structures. Lower left: Tissue of cerebellum has been exposed to reveal a cystic glioma, which typically contains xanthochromic or oily, dark brown fluid.

Lower right: Glioma of temporal lobe. Note shift of ventricles due to tumor mass.

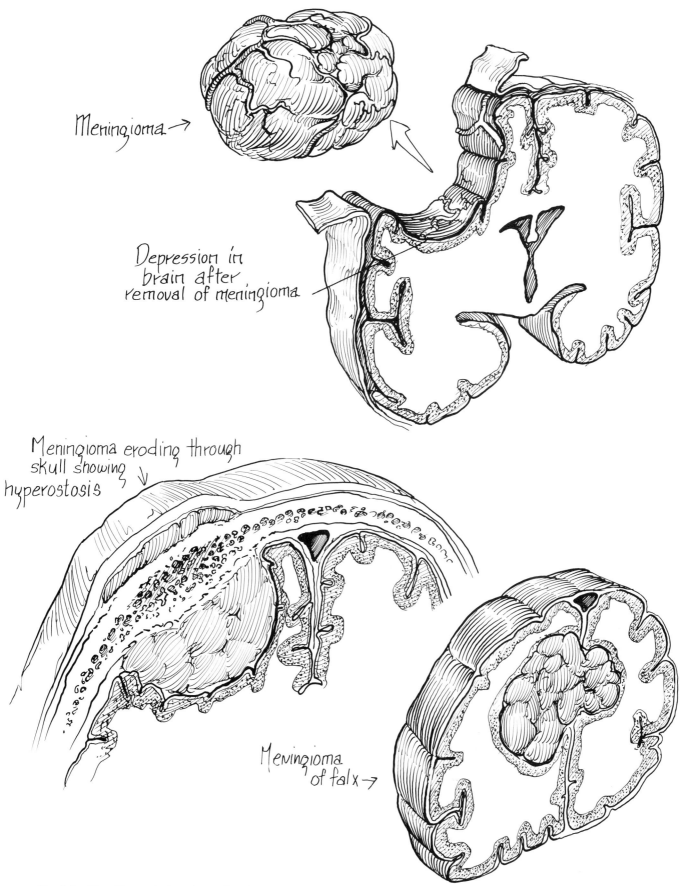

**Meningioma** →

**Depression in brain after removal of meningioma**

**Meningioma eroding through skull showing hyperostosis** ↓

**Meningioma of falx** →

**Fig. 4–2.** Top: The meningioma is usually a benign, well-encapsulated tumor. It is generally extracerebral (displacing but not infiltrating brain tissue).

Middle: Hyperostosis caused by meningioma is usually palpable through the scalp.

Bottom: Meningioma crossing the falx often produces bilateral spasticity.

(the most malignant), 0%-25% of the predominant glial cells are differentiated.

Intracranial tumors, due to the growth and resulting increase in the content of the skull, frequently cause increased intracranial pressure, compression of tissue, and edema or swelling. Intracranial pressure may increase not only due to the growth of the lesion, but because of infarction or hemorrhage within the tumor, swelling due to metabolic factors or an inflammatory response following infarction or venous obstruction caused by the tumor, or obstruction of the flow of cerebrospinal fluid by the tumor. Increased intracranial pressure may be particularly apparent in the eye grounds, a condition called *papilledema*, which may consist of congestion of veins, edema, elevation of the optic disc, and in later stages, the presence of venous hemorrhages around the optic disc.

An increase in pressure above the tentorium may also result in a range of symptoms due to herniation of brain tissue through the tentorium with resulting damage to the midbrain, pons, and medulla oblongata. In fact, chronic increases in intracranial pressure may actually cause damage of the skull, which is sometimes observable on plain skull films. In such instances there may be spontaneous repair of the bone damage, leading to new bone formation in the area overlying the tumor, referred to as *hyperostosis* (Fig. 4–2). Such changes are not exclusively due to intracranial hypertension, but instead are apparently associated with the proximity of the tumor to the bone and occur especially among meningiomas.

## Clinical Symptoms Associated with Intracranial Tumors

Headache is usually associated with brain tumors. It is usually worse upon arising in the morning, and is often made worse by coughing, sneezing, straining at the stool, lifting, or sudden exertion. It is frequently less severe when the patient is lying prone. Headache is thought to be the first symptom of brain tumor in about 20% of patients, although, of course, headaches occur with many other conditions as well.

Vomiting, also associated with increased intracranial pressure, is more prominent on awakening in the morning.

Epileptic seizures appear as the first symptom of a brain tumor in about 15% of patients. The onset of an epileptic seizure in adult subjects is cause for particular concern and most neurologists and neurological surgeons feel that unexplained epilepsy in an adult should be regarded as a possible symptom of brain tumor until proven otherwise. Seizures may be of a variety of types, depending particularly upon the area of the brain that is principally involved. Seizures occur with benign and slowly growing tumors as well as more malignant tumors.

Additional symptoms may include drowsiness (or even somnolence or stupor) and various clinical manifestations of dementia (impaired judgment, memory loss, etc.). Some patients also complain of abnormal or strange sensations in the head, which are usually vaguely described.

Brain tumors may give rise to a number of physical signs that are quite variable from one patient to another. These signs include evidence of papilledema, motor deficits, sensory abnormalities or losses, and other manifestations. However, the presence or absence of a brain tumor is best determined through use of contrast radiography or computed tomography.

## Treatment of Brain Tumors

Surgical removal of malignant brain tumors is the standard treatment. However, in most instances, it is not possible to effect a complete removal of the tumor and re-growth will occur. Surgery is frequently followed by radiation therapy, given in conjunction with high doses of corticosteroids. Adequate treatment may result in increased survival time, particularly in cases of more slowly growing intrinsic tumors. Although radiation therapy is also an important factor in survival time of patients with rapidly growing gliomas, the survival time is generally shorter.

Although much research has been done with chemotherapy of brain tumors, the results have not been particularly successful. The use of various drug combinations, together with chemotherapy and radiation therapy, is currently a topic of active investigation.

Nonmalignant tumors, such as meningiomas, can usually be removed surgically without difficulty. The recurrence rate is low, and the prognosis for recovery is good.

## Classification of Brain Tumors

Butler, Brooks, and Netsky (1982) note that as early as 1839 Bressler was one of many investigators who tried to classify brain tumors on the basis of their appearance and the tissues involved. It is interesting to note that this is about the same time that Johannes Muller first proposed the doctrine of "specific energies" of nerves — some nerves serve motor functions, some visual, some tactile, some auditory, etc. In addition, it was at this time that the French physician, Marc Dax, noted the association between the side of paralysis following strokes and involvement of the contralateral side of the brain. Thus, it is clear that interest and study of brain tumors dates back to some of the early physiological and clinical observations of nervous system functioning.

Tumors are presently classified largely according to the cell type from which they arise (but sometimes the location of the tumor) and have been correlated with outcome in great detail. The present-day classification of tumors stemmed from the work of Virchow (1863-1865), who recognized the supporting cells of the brain and called them neuroglia. Further, Virchow realized that many tumors arose from these cells and created the term "glioma," initiating an approach in which tumors were identified by the type of cell involved.

Tooth (1912) studied a large number of brain tumors at the National Hospital in London from 1902 to 1911 and published a description of 500 tumors, 258 of which were gliomas. This study represented one of the first instances in which extensive neurosurgical specimens were studied histologically and the morphological structure of the tumor was correlated with the patient's clinical course. Tooth differentiated between the benign and malignant gliomas and noted that different areas within the same glioma might show histological differences.

Bailey and Cushing (1926) began their extensive studies of brain tumors shortly afterwards and their classification of tumors has had a strong influence on current practices. These investigators tried to identify as many relevant considerations as possible with respect to developing an understanding of tumors basically organized around their cytology. For example, they considered the gross or macroscopic appearance of the tumor, the point at which it originated, aspects of growth and spread of the tumor, the life history of the tumor, the age of the patient, the clinical course of the patient, results of surgical procedure, results of radiation, and other variables and correlated all of these findings with the cellular architecture of the tumor. In 1926 they published a study of more than 400 verified gliomas, including 167 necropsy specimens.

Bailey and Cushing did not try explicitly to develop a theory of the origination of tumors (etiology) but, rather, based their study principally on resemblances among cells. A very significant aspect of their procedure related to the morphological stages through which each cell was believed to pass in embryogenesis. On the basis of these studies, Bailey and Cushing proposed that there were 11 categories of gliomas: (1) medulloblastoma; (2) glioblastoma multiforme; (3) spongioblastoma; (4) astroblastoma; (5) astrocytoma; (6) neuroepithelioma; (7) ependymoma; (8) pinealoma; (9) ganglioneuroma; (10) oligodendroglioma; and (11) papilloma choroideum (although Bailey had doubts whether papillomas of the choroid plexus should actually be included among gliomas).

While the above tumors were identified principally on the basis of the cells from which they originated, it has been general practice among pathologists to divide tumors into benign or malignant categories. As noted above, brain tumors can never be considered as "benign" in the true meaning of this word, although some are much less malignant than others. As early as 1912, Tooth observed that recovery from the more severely malignant tumors was practically impossible. However, it was quite clear that the degree of malignancy was of great clinical significance.

Broders (1920) suggested dividing tumors of the same cellular type into four grades of malignancy, essentially in accordance with microscopic evaluation of different degrees of cellular anaplasia (based on the number of mature cells that showed evidence of dedifferentiation). Kernohan and his colleagues have developed this idea into a specific system for grading gliomas in accordance with evidence of dedifferentiation (or growth) of cells and have correlated their findings with clinical development and prognosis. Kernohan and his colleagues proposed that gliomas be graded into four classes, and applied these gradings to astrocytomas, ependymomas, oligodendrogliomas, and another group of tumors that they called neuro-astrocytomas. Although medulloblastomas are considered to be among the glioma group, Kernohan et al. did not grade this type of tumor. They proposed a simplification of terminology, recommending that the terms "glioblastoma multiforme," "astroblastoma" and "polar spongioblastoma" be eliminated because these tumors were basically in the astrocytoma group. Their notion was that gliomas developed from existing adult cells that are still capable of proliferation (rather than retention of their adult cell status) by a process of dedifferentiation or anaplasia.

Using criteria related to these factors, Kernohan and his colleagues found a direct relation between the degree of anaplasia and the postoperative survival of the patient. They also noted that in individual patients well-differentiated astrocytomas (which at one point in time appeared to be relatively nonmalignant) might change in appearance to that of a glioblastoma multiforme. It has been observed by others (Butler, Brooks, & Netsky, 1982) that oligodendrogliomas and ependymomas, when recurrent, may finally appear microscopically to be essentially the same as glioblastomas.

The use of a grading system has been of definite value because the more malignant gliomas (Grades III and IV) develop more rapidly and are associated with a shorter survival time. This system, however, is not of great use with respect to certain tumors because their rate of anaplasia is not sufficiently great to require four grades (particularly oligodendrogliomas). The problem is even more significant with cerebral ependymomas because the histological findings are not closely correlated with prognosis (Cricheff, Becker, Schneck, & Taveras, 1964). The invasiveness of ependymomas does not depend on the histological characteristics of the tumor; the process is biological in nature. In addition, highly malignant ependymomas are rarely found, and (as pointed out by Butler, Brooks and Netsky, 1982) would probably be called glioblastomas if they were.

Nevertheless, grading of gliomas has been clinically advantageous. Usually, a patient with a well-differentiated tumor will live longer than a patient with a poorly differentiated tumor, although it must be recognized that it is far from possible to achieve a perfect correlation (prediction) in the individual case. The basic reason for this is that gliomas show many individualistic characteristics, regardless of the type. In many gliomas there is a mixture of mature oligodendrocytes, astrocytes, and ependymal cells; the pathologist usually names the tumor for the predominant type of cell. Many tumors contain both differentiated and anaplastic cells, and neuropathologists may then name the tumor for the most histologically malignant feature, rather than the proportion of cells of each type. Thus, the neuropathologist may identify the tumor as a glioblastoma multiforme if anaplastic cells and foci of necrosis are present (criteria for this type of lesion), even though the great majority of cells are represented by mature (differentiated) astrocytes.

Although general rules or criteria are used in each instance, interpretations among pathologists differ and it has been difficult to state rules or criteria capable of dealing with the great range of variability among individual tumors. Clinicians, particularly, point out that a histological classification of a tumor is not perfectly correlated with the clinical course and outcome; that factors such as intracranial pressure, position and size of the tumor, age, and general condition of the patient are important with respect to decisions regarding prognosis, possible repetitions of surgery, and radiotherapy; and that the consideration is not solely a function of the cells of origin (name given the tumor) nor judgments based on study of the tissue specimen.

These observations make it clear that there is still a problem concerning differential classification of tumors. The World Health Organization made an attempt to develop an internationally acceptable classification. This effort classifies tumors under the headings of neuroepithelial tissue, tumors of nerve sheath cells, meningeal and related tumors, primary malignant lymphomas, tumors of blood vessel origin, tumors originating from germ cells, vascular malformations, tumors of the anterior pituitary body, metastatic tumors, tumors that represent local extensions from tumors of specific regions, a broad range of malformations that are space-occupying and fall under the general tumor category and unclassified tumors. These various subdivisions, in turn, have a great number of more specific classifications and subclassifications. More detailed information regarding this classification system of the World Health Organization may be found in an article by Cobb and Youmans (1982). A system of classification quite popular in the United States also has been devised by Russell and Rubinstein (1977).

Finally, the basic classification system proposed by Bailey and Cushing as well as the grading system proposed by Kernohan and his associates is still frequently used. Thus, we should turn our attention briefly to a correlation of these systems of terminology. Bailey and Cushing referred to astrocytomas as relatively slowly growing gliomas arising from astrocytes. Kernohan et al. referred to these lesions as astrocytomas, Grades I and II. The glioblastoma multiforme of Bailey and Cushing is referred to by Kernohan et al. as astrocytoma, Grade III and IV. Oligodendrogliomas are included in both systems, but

Kernohan et al. grade them from I to IV, even though there are few that qualify in grades III and IV. Ependymomas are listed in each classification system without grading, as are medulloblastomas and pinealomas. Ganglioneuromas and neuroblastomas are classified by Kernohan et al. as neuroastrocytoma, grade I and neuroastrocytoma, grades II to IV. The principal difference in the two systems is that Kernohan et al. used a Roman numeral grading system whenever possible. This translates into grading principally of astrocytomas and oligodendrogliomas, with astrocytomas in the Bailey-Cushing system being astrocytomas Grade I and II in the Kernohan system and glioblastoma multiforme in the Bailey-Cushing system being astrocytomas Grade III and IV. Grading is not as relevant, as has already been mentioned, in the case of oligodendrogliomas because most of them do not fall in grades III and IV.

## Etiology of Brain Tumors

As was mentioned above, relatively little is known about the etiology of brain tumors. There is a genetic predisposition in certain tumors of the nervous system, including the neurofibromas of *von Recklinghausen's disease*, a disease characterized by multiple neurofibromatosis of the nervous system and particularly involving the auditory nerve; *tuberous sclerosis*, a disease usually afflicting children or adolescents in which there are firm hyperplastic nodules in the cerebral hemispheres that consist of malformed and often extremely large glial cells; and *von Hippel-Lindau disease*, a disorder that usually becomes evident in adults and consists of vascular tumors of the cerebellum and, less frequently, of the brain stem and spinal cord, together with vascular tumors of the retina. *Sturge-Weber disease* — angioma of the brain and meninges associated with an angioma on the same side of the face — is less securely identified as having a hereditary basis. Cytogenetic studies, as well as investigations of blood groups, have been done to investigate the possibility of genetic factors in the occurrence of tumors, but the results have been relatively unrevealing and unconvincing.

As noted previously, physical trauma has been associated with the development of some tumors, and the general belief is that it may be associated with a small number of meningiomas; it is more likely, though, that the trauma aggravates clinical symptoms of a tumor already within the cranial cavity. Radiation is well known as a factor inducing carcinoma of the skin as well as other tissues. Chemical carcinogens have been studied with respect to producing experimental brain tumors in animals in order to determine pathogenesis and growth rates and produce models for testing therapeutic agents. Although tumors can be induced through infection or placement of various chemicals, it is apparent that most tumors in human beings do not have this type of etiology. Finally, it is well-established that viruses, including many obtained from human tissues, are capable of inducing brain tumors when inoculated directly into the brain tissue. This has been demonstrated in species ranging from chickens to primates. Again, however, although tumors may be induced from viruses, there is little direct evidence that virus infection is responsible for the development of tumors in human beings. Much more investigation is needed to determine the role of viruses in the production of brain tumors in man.

## Growth of Brain Tumors

Tumors grow either by expansion, infiltration, or both. **Expansion** refers to enlargement of the tumor around a central core and tends to occur approximately equivalently in each direction. Tumors growing by this mechanism are usually spherical in shape. Growth by expansion depends upon proliferation (multiplication) rather than enlargement of cells. In addition, as a tumor develops, other factors may be present to increase the apparent size of the tumor, including fluid accumulation related to hemorrhage, increased permeability of blood vessels, or swelling and edema.

**Infiltration** or **invasion** by a tumor is the spread of tumor tissue into the interstices (small spaces or gaps) of the surrounding tissue. Infiltrations may extend for a considerable distance from the primary site of the tumor. Malignant tumors are more likely to show growth by infiltration, whereas benign tumors (such as meningiomas) seldom infiltrate but grow by expansion. Metastatic tumors grow principally by expansion, but may also infiltrate, especially around blood vessels. While gliomas of the brain may expand, the characteristic growth of a glioma is by infiltration. Growth by expansion or infiltration is not necessarily related to the rate of growth of the tumor. Some rapidly growing tumors simply expand and some slowly growing tumors, such as a diffuse astrocytoma, are highly infiltrative.

**Metastasis** refers to a tumor which has detached from the primary focus and is growing separately. The detachment of tumor cells from the primary tumor is usually transferred by way of systemic arterial circulation. Spread through lymphatic channels may also occur. Finally, metastasis may also refer to the spread of cells in the cerebrospinal fluid. Metastatic spread of primary intracranial tumors is quite rare, although a number of reports have been published that such metastases do occur. It is much more common for carcinoma in other locations of the body to metastasize to the brain than for primary brain tumors to metastasize either within the central nervous system or to other locations outside the central nervous system. Courville (1967) reported that multiple gliomas in a single individual was quite rare, occurring in about 1.5% based on a study of 1,000 autopsies. When limiting the sample to intracranial neoplasms, the figure rose to 4.3%, and with glial tumors, the figure was 8%. More specifically, Courville reported about 10% of glioblastomas multiforme and about 6% of astrocytomas were multiple. In Reitan's series of more than 500 brain tumors, only one brain was definitely identified as having more than one primary tumor.

## Incidence of Brain Tumors

The overall incidence of brain tumor is estimated to be within 4.2 and 5.4 per 100,000 population

(Kurland, Myrianthopoulos, & Leksell, 1962; Zuelch, 1965). Our concern in this volume is tumors in the brain that occur in adulthood rather than childhood. A number of tumors, however, occur most commonly in children, including cerebellar astrocytoma, medulloblastoma, craniopharyngioma, tumors of the choroid plexus, brain stem glioma, and optic glioma. Ependymomas occur among children, but also extend into the adult age range. Oligodendrogliomas occur in teenagers, but most commonly are seen in adult subjects.

A considerable number of tumors occur principally after the age of 20 years, although the peak incidence ranges from about 35 to 50 or even 55 years of age. These include, in ascending order of frequency of peak incidence with advancing age: slow growing astrocytoma, pituitary adenoma, hemangioblastoma, Schwann cell glioma, meningioma, glioblastoma multiforme, and metastatic carcinoma. With the exception of tumors dependent upon production of hormones, the incidence of most neoplasms in the body generally increases progressively with advancing age. In the case of brain tumors, however, there seems to be a decrease in number after about 60 to 65 years of age. This represents a fundamental difference between brain tumors and most other neoplasms in the body.

It should be noted that about two-thirds of tumors which occur in childhood and adolescence are located in the posterior fossa. Ependymoma is the most common tumor above the tentorium in children. The frequency of intracranial tumors decreases in adolescence and then gradually increases again in early adult life. Gliomas increase in frequency in the middle decades, especially glioblastoma multiforme. In old age, glioblastomas, meningiomas, acoustic neuromas, and metastatic tumors of the brain constitute 80% to 90% of all intracranial tumors (Netsky, 1960).

Tumors occur more frequently in men than in women. On an overall basis, the ratio is about 55% to 45%. It appears that the increased incidence of tumors in males is more striking in adults than in children. Pinealomas are about three times more common in males than females and a number of

tumors are about twice as frequently encountered in males including glioblastoma, angioblastoma, craniopharyngioma, epidermoid tumors, and medulloblastoma (Zuelch, 1965). Certain tumors have only a slight perponderence in males, including more slowly growing astrocytomas, ependymomas, and cerebral metastases. Meningiomas and acoustic neuromas occur about twice as frequently in women as in men.

Studies indicate that psychiatric patients have only a slightly greater incidence of brain tumors than the normal population. Nevertheless, popular opinion mistakenly often holds that bizarre or psychotic behavior may result from brain tumors. Anderson (1970) found a brain tumor incidence of only 3% in autopsies of 5862 hospitalized *psychiatric* patients.

## A Review of Specific Types of Tumors

The next section will briefly review a number of tumors of the brain and present information regarding their location, incidence, clinical symptomatology, diagnosis, treatment and outcome. The tumors to be reviewed will include glial tumors (astrocytomas, oligodendrogliomas, ependymomas, and glioblastomas multiforme), lymphomas, tumors in the region of the pineal gland, tumors resulting from abnormal nervous system development (craniopharyngiomas, epidermoid cysts, teratomas, colloid cysts, and lipomas), acoustic neuromas, meningiomas, sarcomas, and blood vessel tumors.

### Astrocytomas

Using the nomenclature of Bailey and Cushing, astrocytomas are the second most common primary tumors of the brain constituting, according to various estimates (Davis, Martin, Padberg, & Anderson, 1950; Fan, Kovi, & Earle, 1977; Zuelch, 1965) 17%-30% of all gliomas and 11%-13% of all brain tumors. Astrocytomas have varying degrees of malignancy. Less malignant astrocytomas, and those with cystic degeneration, firm consistency, and little cellularity, tend to have a more favorable prognosis (Finkemeyer, Pfingst & Zuelch, 1975). However, the majority of astrocytomas do not have these characteristics and do undergo anaplasia. In one study, 72 patients were identified who initially had astrocytoma Grade I and then suffered regrowth of the tumor after surgical removal. The second operation showed that in 55% of these persons the tumor had changed to astrocytoma Grade II and in 30% to glioblastoma multiforme. This study also included 65 patients who initially had astrocytoma Grade II. When these latter patients were reoperated, 45% had glioblastomas (Mueller, Afra, & Schroeder, 1977).

Headache is the most frequent symptom in patients with astrocytomas of the cerebrum, occurring in about 72% of patients. The headache is lateralized (or more pronounced on one side) in about 11% of the patients and the side involved corresponds with the side of the tumor in about 75%. Vomiting occurs in approximately 31%. Epilepsy is also a frequent initial symptom, being reported in 40%-75% of patients. Astrocytomas may produce either generalized or focal seizures. Seizures tend to be focal with tumors located in the middle part of the cerebral hemisphere, generalized with frontal tumors, and of a complex partial nature (temporal-lobe type) with temporal lobe tumors. Intracranial tumors are eventually found in 5%-10% of patients being treated for epilepsy in large general hospital clinics, as confirmed by CT scan (Gall, Becker, & Hacker, 1977; White, Liu, & Mixter, 1948).

Focal neurological deficits are common in patients with astrocytomas. Paresis of a limb occurs in 41% and of the face in 55%. About 15%-20% show evidence of homonymous visual field losses. Approximately 13% have unequal pupils and in these cases the smaller pupil is on the side of the lesion in 80% of cases (Gol, 1961). In addition, patients with astrocytoma frequently have evidence of impaired vision and other sensory losses, diplopia, vertigo, and dysphasia. Papilledema has been reported to be present in approximately 60% of patients (Gol, 1961).

Psychiatric disorders have been reported in patients with intracranial tumors, and occasionally (but rarely) patients who are initially diagnosed as having psychiatric disease are found to have gliomas. Malamud (1967) identified nine patients with temporal lobe masses who originally were diagnosed as having psychiatric disease (schizophrenia [4], depression [4], and anxiety state [1]).

Although astrocytomas may be suspected on the basis of the history and physical and neurological examination, definitive diagnosis usually requires other methods. Plain x-rays of the skull show abnormalities in about 50% of patients with astrocytomas, with the most common abnormality being erosion of the sella turcica (Gol, 1961; Twining, 1939). Visible evidence of calcification on plain x-rays occurs only in 8%-12% of astrocytomas (Martin & Lemmen, 1952). The EEG is normal in many patients with astrocytomas, showing the location of the lesion in approximately 45% of patients, and the hemisphere involved in an additional 30% (Gol, 1961; Rasmussen, 1975). However, a wide variety of abnormal EEG patterns may be present and the EEG is particularly helpful in making the diagnosis in only about one-third of the patients with astrocytoma (Gonzales & Elvidge, 1962). When the patient has demonstrated seizures due to the astrocytoma, the incidence of abnormal EEGs rises to approximately 85%.

Radionuclide scanning has been reported to have variable accuracy in identifying Grade I and II astrocytomas, ranging from below 50% to approximately 67%. This variability probably relates to differences in anaplastic features of the tumors included in various series. Grade II astrocytomas are more likely than Grade I astrocytomas to show a positive scan (Finkemeyer, Pfingst, & Zuelch, 1975; Moreno & DeLand, 1971). Pneumoencephalography and ventriculography were the definitive methods for diagnosis of brain tumors until cerebral angiography became widely used in the late 1950s. Air encephalography is quite accurate in showing the location of astrocytomas, being correct in about 90% of the patients (Gol, 1961). Cerebral angiography became the most widely used procedure and also showed an excellent accuracy rate, being within normal limits in only about 10% of astrocytomas, Grade I or II

(Finkemeyer, Pfingst, & Zuelch, 1975). At present, however, computed tomography is generally the procedure of choice and accuracy rates have become very high with the development of clinical experience and more sophisticated scanners. Accuracy rates approaching 95%-100% have been reported in both Grade I and II astrocytomas (Ambrose, Gooding, & Richardson, 1975; Steinhoff, Lanksch, Kazner, Grumme, Meese, Lange, Aulich, Schinder, & Winde, 1977).

## Oligodendroglioma

Oligodendroglioma, as the name implies, arises from neoplastic growth of oligodendroglial cells. The term "oligodendroglia" was devised by Hortega, who observed glial cells with a paucity of dendrites. Tumors arising from this type of cell were first described by Bailey and Cushing (1926) and Bailey and Hiller (1924). Bailey and Bucy (1929) presented a thorough clinical and pathological discussion of oligodendrogliomas.

Oligodendrogliomas make up only about 4% of all gliomas, but about 90% of oligodendrogliomas are in the cerebrum. When a person is first diagnosed as having an oligodendroglioma the average age is about 40 years and 60% of these persons are male.

The history and course of patients with oligodendrogliomas is quite variable. These tumors are usually slowly developing and the average patient has symptoms 7-8 years before definitive diagnosis. Seizures are the initial symptoms in approximately 50% of the cases, and, by the time diagnosis is established, about 70%-90% of the patients have seizures. Headache is also common as an early symptom. Papilledema and focal neurological deficits are each present in approximately one-third to one-half of the patients at the time of definitive diagnosis. Plain x-rays of the skull identify some degree of calcification in the tumors in about 40%-60% of the cases. EEG is usually abnormal, but the abnormality may not necessarily even be focal or suggest the presence of a neoplasm. Spinal fluid findings usually are not helpful in diagnosis. Radionuclide brain scans and cerebral angiography are frequently helpful in identifying oligodendrogliomas, and computed tomography has yielded excellent results (Vonofakos, Marcu, & Hacker, 1979).

The standard treatment for oligodendroglioma has been surgical removal. If a considerable portion of the tumor can be removed, the survival period is extended. Tumors located in the occipital lobe have a somewhat better prognosis following surgery than tumors at other sites because it is possible to remove a large part of a tumor in that location. Frontal and temporal oligodendrogliomas tend to grow enough to invade such structures as the basal ganglia or the corpus callosum before diagnosis and surgery and therefore have a poorer prognosis.

## Ependymoma

Ependymomas are glial neoplasms composed predominantly of ependymal cells and constitute approximately 5% of gliomas. The average age of patients who develop ependymomas is approximately 20 years, although there is a great deal of variation. These lesions are slightly more common in males than females. Approximately two-thirds of all ependymomas occur below the tentorium and ependymomas account for approximately 25% of tumors in and around the fourth ventricle. The infratentorial ependymomas occur principally in children; adults may develop either supratentorial or infratentorial ependymomas.

Ependymomas that arise within the ventricles customarily conform to the shape of the ventricle, but others burrow into the cerebral white matter. Approximately 50% of supratentorial ependymomas are primarily intraventricular or arise in the ventricle and grow into the cerebral white matter. The other 50% are separate from the ependymal surface of the ventricle and apparently arise from ependymal cells which are adjacent to, but not contiguous with, the ventricular surface. Of the intraventricular supratentorial ependymomas, approximately 25% are in the third ventricle and the other 75% either in or near the lateral ventricles. Most ependymomas are relatively slowly growing or well-differentiated neoplasms, but some are more rapidly growing.

The duration of symptoms before diagnosis is quite variable, but is estimated at about 16 months. Patients with infratentorial ependymomas have symptoms for longer than those with tumors of the lateral ventricles. Tumors that are relatively discrete cause symptoms for longer periods before diagnosis than those that are more invasive. Ependymomas within the ventricles are often clinically silent until they become quite large. Eighty percent of patients with ependymomas complain of headaches and 90% have papilledema. Nausea and vomiting are present in about 75% and about 60% have ataxia or vertigo. Seizures are present in only about one-third of patients having supratentorial lesions. The presenting symptoms of patients with fourth ventricle tumors are headache and vomiting; persons with tumors of the lateral ventricles are more likely to show focal neurological deficits.

Plain skull x-rays show evidence of calcification of supratentorial ependymomas approximately 20% of the time. Radionuclide scanning is abnormal in about 90%. Techniques of ventricular visualization and cerebral angiography had been the standard diagnostic procedures for identification of ependymomas, but these techniques have been largely replaced by computed tomography. Supratentorial ependymomas are treated with surgery and the approach is the same as with other tumors in the hemisphere. Because these lesions are not as rapidly growing or malignant as some others, the surgical procedure is sometimes more conservative in order to avoid producing unnecessary neurological deficits. In addition, ependymomas rank second only to medulloblastomas in their radiosensitivity. Radiotherapy followed by surgery has shown necrosis of the tumor and even patients treated by radiotherapy without surgery have had remission of symptoms. Operative decompression followed by radiotherapy can add months or years to a patient's life, but, as with most primary brain tumors, the prognosis for cure is slight. Estimates have been made that the chances of the patient living for five years following surgery and radiotherapy are about 80% with supratentorial tumors and about 90% with infratentorial ones. However, supratentorial ependymomas are more likely to be anaplastic and, therefore, likely to recur sooner than infratentorial ones.

### Glioblastoma multiforme

Bailey and Cushing (1926) originally called these tumors spongioblastoma multiforme but later (Bailey, 1927) recommended the term "glioblastoma multiorme." In practice, the term frequently is shortened to "glioblastoma."

These tumors represent about one-fourth of intracranial tumors and approximately one-half of all gliomas. They are reported to occur most frequently between the ages of 40 and 60 years, but a number of reports have indicated that they are comparatively more frequent than other tumors among older persons. They are rare in childhood. Males are affected more frequently than females, with estimates ranging from 55% to 65%.

Glioblastomas vary in gross appearance, depending upon the presence of necrosis, cystic degeneration, or hemorrhage. About one-fifth of these tumors are well circumscribed and approximately 60% are solid. Necrosis is present in about 50%, small areas of hemorrhage in about 40%, and massive hemorrhage in about 2%. Although certain areas are reported to be more commonly involved, no area containing glial tissue is exempt from the development of this tumor (MacCabe, 1975). Glioblastomas are extremely invasive and are characterized by a great deal of microscopic variability. Pathological changes include hypercellularity, pleomorphism of cells and nuclei, mitoses, capillary endothelial proliferation, and necrosis. The neoplastic cells may be so undifferentiated that it is impossible to identify their astrocytic origin.

Patients with glioblastoma multiforme customarily show such a rapid progression of symptoms that diagnosis is made fairly early in the course of the disease. The duration of symptoms before diagnosis is less than one month in about 30%, three months in 60%, six months in 70%, and longer than two years in only about 7% of patients. Onset of symptomatology is sudden only in about 4%.

Patients with glioblastoma multiforme have a wide variety of symptoms. The most common initial symptom is headache, (40% of patients), and eventually occurs in over 70%. Headache is unilateral only in about 25%, but in those patients the tumor is on the same side in over 90%. Motor disorders are rarely present initially (only about 3%) but have been noted by the patients themselves in about 43% of the cases by the time of diagnosis. Mental changes of various types are noted in about 45% of the cases and are the initial symptom in approximately 7%. Seizures are the initial symptom in about 15% and occur, in total, in about 33%.

The neurological examination frequently shows obvious abnormalities in these patients. Jelsma and Bucy (1967) have estimated the frequencies as follows: abnormal reflexes, 83%; confusion or disorientations, 50%; papilledema, 45%; drowsiness or lethargy, 28%; visual field abnormalities, 25%; "parietal lobe" signs, 26%; hypesthesia or hypalgesia, 19%; stupor or coma, 19%; and third or sixth cranial nerve palsy, 5%.

The symptoms of glioblastoma multiforme may be caused by a number of factors, including generalized increase of intracranial pressure (either from the tumor mass or obstruction of cerebrospinal fluid pathways), focal neurological deficits due to displacement and distortion of fiber tracts, replacement of brain tissue by tumor, or edema interfering with brain function. Considering these factors, it is clear that glioblastoma multiforme may have "distance effects." Cysts can develop, especially in lesions that have been previously treated surgically. Involvement of vessels by neoplasms can also occur, although this appears to be a less common cause of symptoms. Vascular involvement, however, may be due to ischemia or hemorrhage.

In past years, encephalography (pneumoencephalography and ventriculography) were the diagnostic procedures that identified the presence of these tumors. In the late 1950s cerebral angiography was developed with sufficient precision to be very helpful diagnostically. By about this time, published reports indicated that angiograms were abnormal in about 90% of patients with glioblastoma multiforme.

Improvement in cerebral angiography has continued and Grunert, Jellinger, Sunder-Plassmann, and Wober (1973) reported that every one of 335 patients with glioblastoma multiforme had abnormal angiograms.

Plain x-rays of the skull are abnormal in 60%; EEG is reported to be abnormal in about 92% with localizing indicators in 75%; radionuclide scanning is abnormal in 90%. However, the current diagnostic procedure of choice for glioblastoma multiforme is computed tomography with a water-soluable iodinated contrast material (Ambrose, Gooding, & Richardson, 1975).

In the presence of a glioblastoma, spinal fluid pressure is usually elevated, protein level is increased, the number of white cells is often high, and polyamine content in cerebrospinal fluid is often elevated. However, these findings are not definitive in diagnosis nor of any particular help in the management of such tumors. In addition, lumbar puncture should *not* be performed on patients who are suspected of having glioblastoma multiforme because of the significant risk involved in possible downward shifting of the brain through the foramen magnum, other shifts in position of brain tissue, and resulting stress and tear. Thus, the information that might be gained from lumbar puncture and examination of cerebrospinal fluid does not justify the significant risk that accompanies the procedure.

The traditional treatment for glioblastoma multiforme is surgical. Neurosurgeons have learned to adopt an aggressive approach in treating these lesions. The general recommendation is that it is advisable to remove as much tumor as possible. Tumor may either displace or infiltrate brain tissue. If displacement occurs, Cobb and Youmans (1982) point out that excision of the tumor may be done, even in areas that are probably important in a functional sense, without increasing neurological deficit. It is possible to identify tumor tissue that is displacing brain tissue because it is usually necrotic or hemorrhagic and, therefore, of a different color than normal brain. However, tumor tissue that infiltrates brain tends to be more similar in appearance and color to normal brain tissue.

Removal of infiltrating tumor in areas of neurological significance is generally not recommended. Cobb and Youmans (1982) believe that brain tissue may still be functional in areas of tumor infiltration and that excision of this tissue could produce additional significant deficit.

Aggressive resection of these rapidly growing tumors is associated with longer survival time than limited resection. Three-year survival rates as high as 20% and five-year survival rates as high as 12% have been reported after extensive resection followed by radiotherapy (Bloom, 1975; Onoymama, Abe, Sakamato, Nishidai, & Suyama, 1976). Jelsma and Bucy (1967) performed extensive resection in a series of patients with glioblastoma multiforme and found that the six-month survival rate was twice as high as in patients who had been subjected to only partial resection. Many factors appear to be correlated with survival time in patients having glioblastoma multiforme. Young adults survive longer than older adults, but this factor may be related to a lesser degree of anaplasia in the younger group. Jelsma and Bucy (1967) found that only 10 of 162 patients survived two years or longer and Russell and Rubinstein (1977) reported that only two of 74 patients survived three years or longer.

## Lymphomas of the Brain

Tumors may arise from any of the cellular elements of the brain, including the lymphoreticular system (represented by lymphocytes), plasma cells, macrophages, and reticulum cells. When tumors arising from this system are clinically diagnosed, they are already malignant and have been referred to as "malignant lymphoma." The cell of origin of lymphoma of the brain has not been determined. Lymphomas usually contain a mixture of microglial and reticulum cell elements as well as additional small, undifferentiated cells. Lymphomas of the brain may occur as a discrete mass or may consist of widespread infiltration. If a discrete mass is present it usually has a gray-pink color, may be soft or firm, and generally is homogeneous without significant necrosis or hemorrhage. If the neoplasm occurs as a diffuse, unlocalized process, the brain usually looks relatively normal grossly. Microscopic examination, however, reveals widespread proliferation of microglia. Diffuse infiltrative growth and the occurrence of multiple foci are characteristic of lymphoma, even in patients with discrete tumor masses.

Lymphomas can occur in any part of the central nervous system with approximately half of the primary tumors of the central nervous system occurring in the cerebral hemispheres and 10%-30% in the posterior fossa. The two sides of the brain are affected with about equal frequency and the distribution of discrete masses involving the cerebral hemispheres is not systematic. However, a lymphoma is particularly likely to involve the choroid plexus and the septum pellucidum. This disposition may be related to spread of the tumor through the ventricular system. Lymphomas also frequently involve the corpus callosum and may have a "butterfly" distribution involving areas of the cerebral hemisphere on each side of the corpus callosum. Lymphomas of the central nervous system are not a very common type of tumor, accounting for 1%-3% of the central nervous system tumors in general.

The presenting signs and symptoms of lymphomas of the brain are essentially similar to those of glioblastoma multiforme and the latter condition usually is the clinical diagnosis. In some instances, lymphoma is suggestive of encephalitis; the patient may have developed malaise, lethargy, anorexia, headache, and fever, sometimes with clinical signs of cerebellar involvement. The more common form of presentation, as mentioned, mimics a glioblastoma multiforme or other highly malignant tumor. Increased intracranial pressure, producing headache, is frequently present early in the clinical course. Reported symptoms frequently include personality changes, confusion, irritability, drowsiness, and inability to focus attention. Focal neurological signs and symptoms may or may not be present, depending largely upon the location of the tumor. Localized motor deficits are present in fewer than half of the cases, and seizures are uncommon.

Lymphoma is a rapidly developing condition and, without surgical treatment or radiotherapy, the average length of survival after diagnosis is only three weeks. If the patient is not too ill for surgery, and operative treatment is given, the survival time increases to approximately two months. Lymphoma is very radio-sensitive and radiotherapy often produces a dramatic decrease in symptoms. When radiotherapy, together with surgery, has been used, the average survival varies from 17 months to four years.

Skull x-rays are abnormal in approximately one-half of the patients with lymphoma, showing signs of increased intracranial pressure and usually a shift of the pineal gland. EEG shows either diffuse or focal abnormality in approximately 80% of these patients. In patients with focal lymphomas, EEG shows abnormalities in nearly all patients. Radioisotopic brain scans are highly accurate in identifying lymphomas, with certain tracers (e.g., technetium) being particularly accurate. However, isotopic scan may be interpreted as showing evidence of multiple lesions and is sometimes confused with metastatic carcinoma. Angiograms are abnormal in more than 80% of the cases, usually pointing toward a localized intracerebral mass. Pneumonencephalography also is quite accurate in showing these tumors. Computed tomography usually shows evidence of the tumors in the brain tissue but often does not identify tumors that principally involve the meninges.

Because of the therapeutic value of radiotherapy, the role of surgery frequently is delimited to tissue biopsy in order to establish a definite diagnosis. Sometimes analysis of the cerebrospinal fluid is significant for diagnosis, in which case treatment often begins immediately with radiotherapy.

Because of the relative infrequency of lymphomas of the brain and the rapid clinical course, patients with these lesions are not often seen for neuropsychological evaluation.

## Tumors in the Region of the Pineal Gland

Another group of tumors is often considered together because they arise from the same general loca-tion — the pineal gland and surrounding regions, including the posterior third ventricle and the quadrigeminal area. This group represents a relatively small percentage of brain tumors in general and they are quite varied in terms of histological types. In neurosurgery, a particular interest centers on these tumors because they are difficult to reach surgically and have a rich venous system which adds to the hazards of operation. Thus, there have been a number of reports concerning surgical approaches and techniques for excision of these tumors.

Increased intracranial pressure appears early with these lesions because of their location. Total obstruction of the aqueduct of Sylvius, even in the presence of large tumors, is not invariable. However, in the majority of cases, a blockage of the aqueduct has been reported (Jennett, Johnson, & Reid, 1963). Cerebellar signs of limb ataxia and abnormalities of gait are often present. These patients also frequently show limitation of upward gaze, impaired eye convergence, inequality of pupils, and impaired reaction to light and accommodation.

X-rays of the skull frequently show evidence of calcification of the pineal gland; a large or dense area of calcification would be considered suggestive of the presence of such a tumor in children less than 10 years of age. Radioisotopic brain scans may also identify tumors in this region and cerebral angiography may be useful in ruling out vascular abnormalities. Ventriculography has been the means by which a definitive diagnosis was made, but computed tomography more recently has proved to be of great value in identification of these tumors. CT scans may precisely define the limits of the tumor and its relation to the third ventricle, midbrain, and quadrigeminal cisterns and may also show whether there are cysts within the tumor.

Because of the deep-seated location and invasive character of most of the tumors in the region of the pineal gland, surgical intervention has been difficult. Shunting procedures have been used to relieve intracranial hypertension, together with radiotherapy. These lesions constitute a difficult problem with respect to proper treatment, but some neurosurgeons feel that they have developed a reasonably safe operation which may be of therapeutic benefit (Stein, 1982). These tumors are quite variable in their histological characteristics and there is no way to be sure, in advance of surgical biopsy, of the nature of the tumor. Histological identification of pineal tumors is of paramount importance in selection of therapy, and, in addition, direct operation may in some instances permit total removal.

## Tumors Resulting From Abnormal Nervous System Development

A number of tumors of the brain develop as a result of disorders of embryogenesis and may not produce symptoms leading to diagnosis until adulthood. These tumors represent a group of mass lesions that are quite heterogeneous. Some are classified according to the structure involved (e.g., pituitary masses), but the lesions show variability in their location, histological characteristics, and degree of anaplasia. A group of these lesions has been described by Kernohan as congenital tumors of the central nervous system (Kernohan, 1971) and these include craniopharyngiomas, teratomas, epidermoid cysts, dermoid cysts, other cysts, and lipomas.

### Craniopharyngiomas

Craniopharyngiomas are suprasellar tumors and usually contain both solid and cystic portions. These tumors are usually located in the subarachnoid space just above the sella turcica. The infundibulum of the pituitary gland usually is just posterior to these tumors. The tumors are in the vicinity of the optic chiasm, lying posterior to the chiasm in approximately one-third of the cases, with the additional two-thirds lying either beneath the chiasm or anterior to the chiasm. Visual pathways are not infiltrated by the tumor, but visual field defects are common.

Craniopharyngiomas make up approximately 2.5% of brain tumors in general. Because of their congenital nature, they are more frequently identified in children than in adults. In children they make up about 7% of brain tumors, are the most common non-glial tumor, and constitute approximately half of the tumors in the region of the optic chiasm. In adults they make up approximately 20% of tumors in this area. Approximately 50% of craniopharyngiomas are identified in persons less than 20 years of age, but they are not uncommon even in old age.

The duration of symptoms prior to diagnosis is quite variable. The mean is about one year, but it is not uncommon to find the onset of symptoms being as little as one month before diagnosis. The rate at which symptoms develop is related to the eventual outcome. For patients whose symptoms gradually develop for more than two years before diagnosis is made (compared with persons having symptoms for less than two years), the longer duration of symptoms correlates with a longer survival after treatment (Bartlett, 1971). The most common initial symptom is headache. By the time diagnosis is made, 75%-90% of patients have headache, 30%-38% have vomiting, and approximately 67% have visual disturbances. A variety of other symptoms occur in 10%-20% of patients at the time of diagnosis.

In adults it is likely that visual symptoms will be particularly prominent at the time the patient seeks medical help. In children early complaints of visual difficulties are less than half as frequent. Visual difficulties in adults are represented by visual field defects in 90%-95% of the cases. In two-thirds of these patients, a bitemporal hemianopia is found, homonymous hemianopia is present in about 15% of the patients, and paracentral scotomas are seen occasionally. Visual acuity is impaired in about 75%. Papilledema is frequently present in children (30%-50%) but in only 10%-15% of adults. The presence of papilledema suggests that the lesion has developed in such a way as to cause some obstruction of cerebrospinal fluid spaces and circulation. Sixty percent of patients with craniopharyngioma show neurological abnormalities other than visual manifestations, including cranial nerve palsies and pyramidal and cerebellar motor signs.

Psychiatric difficulties of a variety of types may occur, including hypersomnia, apathy, spatial disorientation, memory disturbances, and depression. Severe mental disorders, described as Korsakoff's syndrome, have been reported in as many as 25% of adults (Kahn, Gosch, Seeger, & Hicks, 1973). The presence of mental symptoms of this type are associated with an adverse prognosis (Bartlett, 1971).

Plain skull x-rays often show abnormal characteristics that are sufficiently specific to identify the lesion as a craniopharyngioma. These radiographic abnormalities represent fairly characteristic changes in the sella turcica and often include calcification of the tumor. The EEG is abnormal in most patients with craniopharyngioma, being more common in children than adults, and is most frequently represented by diffuse abnormalities of the tracings. Because of the likelihood of increased intracranial pressure, lumbar puncture is rarely done in these patients to avoid the risk of herniation of the cerebellar tonsils. Up until the 1960s, the diagnostic procedure of choice usually was air ventriculography. Angiography has also been useful in demonstrating ventricular enlargement, which usually is apparent in about 75% of the patients. However, CT scan is abnormal in almost all patients with craniopharyngiomas and currently is the standard diagnostic technique.

Cobb and Youmans (1982) note that there are difficulties in assessing the results of treatment in patients with craniopharyngiomas. They point out that the natural history varies greatly from one patient to another, different investigators have reported very different results, relatively few clinicians have gained sufficient experience to be able to reproduce the results of clinicians in other centers, and treatment techniques are improving rapidly. However, in children, craniopharyngiomas are more rapidly progressive than in adults. As noted, mental or psychiatric symptoms are associated with diminished survival time and the presence of motor signs is also ominous.

The standard treatment for craniopharyngioma is surgical excision. Total excision seems to be possible in about three-fourths of all patients and there is general agreement that surgical intervention is the treatment of choice. Even if only most of the tumor can be removed, survival, even without radiotherapy, may continue for a number of years. In one study, 87% of children were alive at a follow-up averaging 6.4 years after operation (Hoffman, Hendrick, Humphreys, Buncic, Armstrong, & Jenkin, 1977). Partial excision is more successful in adults than in children. Nevertheless, many patients who survive the operation may die from recurrent tumor, which may eventually be fatal more than 20 years after the initial surgery. A combination of surgical excision, followed by radiotherapy, has shown evidence of prolonging survival and delaying recurrence of the tumor.

## Additional Congenital Tumors

There has been a lack of uniformity in the histological analysis and evaluation of tumors at the base of the brain and the findings range from invasive and often highly malignant tumors to ones that are essentially of a benign dermoid character. Some of these tumors have a rather simple degree of histological organization (epidermoid cyst) but the entire spectrum ranges to tumors that include tissues that are quite diverse embryologically (teratoma).

Epidermal cysts contain only epidermal elements. Many are quite benign in neoplastic potential but they may range to epidermoid carcinoma. If hair and dermal glands are included in the cyst, it is called a dermoid cyst. If the mass lesion contains histological elements that are not found in the dermis or epidermis, including multiple tissues of kinds foreign to the part in which it arises, the term "teratoma" has been used. A variety of tumors could be classified as teratomas according to this general criterion, indicating the problem in deriving a basis for discrete classification of these masses.

Several embryological theories have been advanced to establish the relationship between the epidermoid cyst, dermoid cyst, and normal skin, as well as to explain the difference between epidermoid and dermoid cysts. Both are inclusion tumors that represent congenital malformations. Apparently the epithelium included in the nervous system during neural tube closure differentiates into dermal as well as epidermal elements and the depth of included epithelium might be the basis for differentiation of epidermoid as compared with dermoid cysts.

Cerebrospinal fluid studies are usually within normal limits with these lesions, but approximately 15% of patients may show elevation of protein levels. Routine skull x-rays and radioisotopic scanning studies often show abnormalities. Pneumoencephalography usually discloses not only the tumor mass but also shows characteristic markings. Computed tomography reveals these lesions as a dense rim around a low density center, the latter representing the cystic area.

Epidermoid cysts constitute about 0.5%-1.5% of brain tumors; dermoid cysts are less common and represent only about 0.3%. Teratomas are more common than dermoid cysts and account for about 0.5% of brain tumors. Epidermoid cysts can occur at any age and about one-half of the patients are between 20 and 40 years. Dermoid cysts tend to be more symptomatic and are diagnosed at a younger age; about half the patients with dermoid cysts are children. Teratomas are more likely to occur in children and the average age at diagnosis is 12 years. Epidermoid and dermoid cysts appear to occur about equally among males and females, but teratomas are probably somewhat more common in males.

Epidermoid cysts contain concentric layers of desquamated epithelium surrounded by a capsule of stratified squamous epithelium. The surface of the lesion is smooth, often nodular, and resembles mother-of-pearl. Dermoid cysts may closely resemble epidermoid cysts if the dermal elements occur in only a small area of the capsule. These dermal elements, such as hair and sebaceous glands, may be in only a small area or pervade the entire capsule. Teratomas are variable in their appearance. They may be solid and consist of a large cyst or multiple cysts. A variety of tissues may be included and solid portions may contain all elements of primitive tissue, including teeth.

Epidermoid cysts occur in a variety of locations in the nervous system, with approximately half being intracranial. Other areas in which epidermoid cysts arise include the cerebellopontine angle, the posterior fossa basal cisterns, and the suprasellar region. The Sylvian fissure is not an uncommon location for epidermoid cysts that involve the cerebrum. Dermoid cysts tend to occur in the midline. Approximately one-third are in the area of the fourth ventricle and another one-third lie in the subarachnoid space at the base of the brain. The remainder are in other locations.

It should be noted that epidermoid cysts are not usually anaplastic but the epithelial cells can become anaplastic. The diagnosis of the tumor, in this case, would change to squamous cell carcinoma.

Microscopic examination reveals that dermoid cysts may be thought of as variants of epidermoid cysts, with the difference relating to inclusion in the dermoid cyst of dermoid structures (e.g., hair follicles and sebaceous glands). Dermoid cysts cover a gradual transition to teratomas. Technically, the lesion would be classified as a teratoma if it included even a single nondermal structure, though the teratoma would appear grossly to be very similar to a dermoid cyst. Customarily, teratomas may include muscle, respiratory epithelium, gastrointestinal epithelium, cartilage, bone, fat, and even neuroepithelial plaques.

Patients with epidermoid cysts and other inclusion tumors may have a great variety of symptoms, which usually have been present from many years before diagnosis. Generally, it is not possible to make a diagnosis on the basis of history and clinical examination. Symptoms may include abnormal cranial nerve activity (particularly trigeminal neuralgia), hemifacial spasm, or deficits involving the optic nerve. Approximately half of all patients with intracranial epidermoid cysts have seizures. Seizures are relatively uncommon with dermoid cysts, probably because of differential location of the lesions. The clinical symptomatology of patients with teratomas is even more diversified than that of patients with epidermoid and dermoid cysts.

The treatment for these lesions requires surgical excision. The ease and success of excision depends in large part upon the location of the cysts. Epidermoid cysts can often be totally removed; dermoid cysts represent an intermediate area with respect to the prospect of total excision; teratomas are usually the most difficult to treat. Some authorities have emphasized the importance of total excision whenever possible in order to prevent clinical recurrence, but others have found that recurrence, even with partially excised inclusion cysts, is relatively rare. In a recent series of 29 patients with intracranial epidermoid and dermoid cysts (Guidetti & Gagliardi, 1977), 21 patients were able to return to work or school; 2 were able to work but were incapacitated by seizures; 4 were unable to work because of continuing neurological deficits; and 2 had recurrence of the tumor that lead to death.

## Colloid Cyst

Colloid cysts constitute about 2% of all gliomas. They may occur in any age range, but usually appear between 20 and 50 years of age. The tumor is a spherical mass with a wall that encapsulates a thick gelatinous material. They usually originate from the roof of the third ventricle, just posterior to the foramen of Monro, although, on rare occasions, they have been found to occur between the leaves of the septum pellucidum.

Clinical diagnosis of colloid cysts cannot be made reliably because there are no characteristic signs and symptoms. Headache is the presenting complaint in 85% of patients and, as the condition progresses, increases to include a total of 96%. A variety of signs may be present in individual cases, but probably about 25% present only with headache and papilledema without any other signs or symptoms. In one series of 54 cases, 15% of the patients had an initial attack that was acute and fatal; 63% had repeated attacks with only short intermissions, and the remaining 22% had repeated attacks with long intermissions (Yenerman, Bowerman, & Haymaker, 1958). A classic picture has emerged, characterized by repeated episodes of headache (sometimes accompanied by neurological deficit) usually manifested by paroxysms of headache with vomiting and sometimes amblyopia. Perhaps 20% of patients with colloid cysts have sudden attacks of leg weakness, possibly related to intermittent ventricular obstruction with sudden ventricular enlargement or episodes of sudden increase in intracranial pressure. Attacks of sudden leg weakness rarely occur in patients with other tumors. Intermittent episodes of dementia may be present and sometimes progressive dementia occurs. About 20% of these patients have epilepsy, with the seizures being of a major motor type.

Angiography has been useful for demonstrating hydrocephalus in these lesions, often suggesting an anterior third ventricle obstruction. However, the definitive diagnostic procedure has been ventriculography, used to identify the outline of the lateral and third ventricles. Computed tomography has simplified the diagnosis of colloid cysts and is quite reliable in showing the presence of a mass in the anterior portion of the third ventricle. If non-enhanced CT scans are used, it may be helpful to inject an iodinated contrast agent directly into the intraventricular area. This enhancement makes it relatively simple to demonstrate anterior third ventricle tumors.

Surgical evacuation of the cyst is required as nonoperative treatment is not effective. A number of surgical approaches have been studied and current surgical methods, including micro-operative techniques, generally result in rapid and uncomplicated recovery.

## Intracranial lipoma

Intracranial lipomas are masses of fat consisting of mature adipose tissue with variable amounts of collagen. Ganglion cells and areas of neuroglia may be included in these tumors. These tumors usually produce little in the way of clinical manifestations and have been observed principally in routine autopsies. They probably constitute about 0.1% of brain tumors in general, and occur in patients of all ages, but the average age is probably about 50 years.

# Acoustic Neuromas

Acoustic neuromas are tumors of the VIIIth (auditory-vestibular) cranial nerve. These tumors have been observed at autopsy for more than 200 years and the first clinical report of an acoustic nerve tumor was given in 1830 by Charles Bell. The first attempt at surgical removal was done by Cushing in 1906 (reported in Cushing, 1917). In the early operations for these tumors, preservation of the VIIIth nerve to the extent that hearing was preserved was essentially impossible. Usually the facial (VIIth) nerve was also involved and a permanent facial palsy followed the operation. There has been an excellent development in surgical techniques and it also has become apparent that complete removal of the acoustic tumor is a great advantage. Partial removal almost invariably leads to recurrence and death of the patient. At the present time hearing can occasionally be preserved and the facial nerve can usually be saved.

Hearing loss on one side, often associated with tinnitus, is one of the earliest signs of an acoustic neuroma. The patient also experiences episodes of vertigo that are often difficult to distinguish from Meniere's disease. In addition to having periods of unsteadiness in the early stages of the disease, impairment of word discrimination ability is a characteristic finding. These early symptoms are a manifestation of involvement of the cochlear and vestibular divisions of the VIIIth nerve. Compression of the facial nerve also occurs early in the course, but a clinically apparent motor deficit is rarely obvious. An electromyogram of the facial muscles may show abnormalities before clinical findings become apparent. Loss of the corneal response, on the same side as the tumor, suggests that the tumor has reached a moderate to large size with upward and medial growth against the pontine trigeminal nuclei. Occasionally a patient will notice paresthesias and numbness of the face and when this symptom occurs the tumor is usually quite large.

Nystagmus is a frequent neurological manifestation of acoustic tumors, and when such a tumor is suspected, electronystagmography should be done. This technique records the electrical activity of the eye as it moves and can detect clinical nystagmus as a response to caloric (both heat and cold should be used) stimulation of the vestibular nerves. Cerebellar dysfunction occurs rather late in the course of symptom development. The patient usually complains of a staggering gait and incoordination of the *ipsilateral* upper extremity.

Audiologists have developed a number of routine as well as specialized tests that provide additional information. First, auditory acuity should be evaluated by pure tone air and bone-conduction audiometry. This procedure will identify the impairment of auditory acuity and may be useful in differentiating between a conductive and neural hearing loss, but does not yield information regarding the location of the lesion. Additional tests may determine whether the lesion is located in the cochlea or involves the VIIIth nerve. These procedures include impedance studies and measurement of brainstem auditory evoked responses (BAER). Tumors that affect the VIIIth nerve or involve the brainstem disrupt the latency and overall shape of the evoked response and the differential influence on successive waveforms (Selters & Brackmann, 1977). In addition, a threshold tone delay test described by Jerger (1961) measures the rate of adaptation of the auditory system and a loudness recruitment test originally described by Fowler (1936), in which there is an abnormally rapid increase in the sensation of loudness, have also been found useful.

A number of neuroradiological techniques have been used in diagnosis of acoustic neuroma, including plain skull films, laminagraphy, positive contrast encephalography, cisternography, vertebroangiography, and pneumoencephalography. The current use of computed tomography, however, has greatly reduced the use of other neuroradiological procedures. CT scan has a high degree of accuracy for medium and large-sized acoustic neuromas, especially when contrast enhancement is used. Even some small acoustic neuromas can be identified. Vertebral and carotid angiograms are often helpful in differentiating between tumors and aneurysms. Posterior fossa pneumoencephalography may aid in identification of tumors of the cerebellopontine angle. In clinical practice, a combination of these procedures is frequently used in order to gain as much information as possible before surgical intervention.

The results of surgery are related to a number of factors but a significant variable is the size of the tumor. It is possible to completely resect smaller tumors and nearly 95% of medium-sized and large neuromas. When complete resection is not possible, the residual tumor tissue is destroyed by using cryosurgical techniques to repeatedly freeze and destroy the remaining tumor fragments.

Involvement of the facial nerve has in the past been a frequent complication of surgical removal of acoustic neuromas, but recent results have indicated that facial nerve function is preserved in essentially all cases with small tumors, in about 80% of persons with medium-sized tumors, and in about 32% with large tumors. Many additional patients have only mild paresis of facial muscles following surgery (Rand, Dirks, Morgan, & Bentson, 1982).

## Meningiomas

Meningiomas are tumors that arise from the meninges of the brain and, more specifically, from the dura mater. Various estimates of the proportion of intracranial tumors represented by meningiomas have been made, ranging from about 13%-38%. In most medical centers, gliomas outnumber meningiomas by about 2 to 1 or 3 to 1. About 10% of meningiomas occur in persons below the age of 45 years and the greatest frequency is beyond 65 years. Females have meningiomas about twice as frequently as males.

Meningiomas of the brain are most frequently located in the parasagittal region, followed by the regions of the sphenoidal ridge, the convexity, and the posterior fossa. However, meningiomas may arise wherever meningeal tissue occurs.

Although some meningiomas are malignant, most are benign and do not show anaplastic characteristics. Jellinger (1975) reviewed more than 1200 meningiomas and found that 1.2% were malignant. Cushing and Eisenhardt (1938) found a frequency of 1.9%. However, Zuelch and Mennel (1975) reported that 9% of 1400 meningiomas were not histologically benign. The differences in results of these studies may relate, at least in part, to different criteria with respect to number of mitoses, indications of cellular pleomorphism, and evaluation of invasion of adjacent tissue. In any case, in the great majority of instances, meningiomas are classified as benign tumors.

Meningiomas are extra-axial (extrinsic) intracranial tumors and produce neurological symptoms primarily due to compression of adjacent brain tissue and cranial nerves. Thus, there is no specificity in the presenting clinical pattern to identify this tumor type with any degree of certainty. The fact that meningiomas tend to arise in certain locations and grow slowly sometimes causes hyperostosis in adjacent bone and this may be a definite clue to the presence and location of the tumor. Meningiomas of the sphenoidal ridge, for example, cause hyperostosis of the sphenoid wing, reduction of the volume of the orbit, and vascular compression which produces, in total, a non-pulsating, painless, unilateral exophthalmos. This lesion occurs most commonly in middle-aged women. Parasagittal meningiomas and those in the region of the falx show nearly classical symptoms when they arise in the central area near the Rolandic fissure. These tumors frequently cause epilepsy of a relatively focal onset. Typically, the seizure involves the lower extremity, spreads to the upper extremity, and then may become generalized. Hemiparesis involving the contralateral side may also develop in a progressive fashion, frequently affecting the lower extremity to a greater degree than the upper. Large bilateral parasagittal meningiomas in the central region may cause severe spastic paraparesis, which sometimes is incorrectly thought to be caused by a spinal cord lesion. Lesions that are rather far anterior or posterior in the midline are associated with a higher incidence of headache. Posterior meningiomas may cause compression of the occipital lobe, and resulting homonymous hemianopia, but such visual defects rarely occur.

Meningiomas of the cerebral convexity usually do not present localizing symptoms and the diagnosis may not be possible on the basis of clinical findings alone.

Radiographic changes on plain x-rays of the head may show characteristic changes.

Intraventricular meningiomas, estimated to represent about 1% of these tumors, show symptoms of headaches, vague and general complaints possibly reflecting obstruction of the flow of cerebrospinal fluid, and homonymous hemianopia.

About 5% of meningiomas develop in the olfactory groove underlying the frontal lobe. These lesions frequently cause central scotoma and primary optic atrophy of the eye on the side of the lesion and papilledema in the opposite eye. Loss of smell, involving the nostril on the same side as the lesion, is frequently present and motor deficits on the contralateral side are sometimes seen. Meningiomas in the region of the tuberculum sella, which are estimated to include about 9%-10% of meningiomas, usually occur in middle-aged persons and show progressive loss of vision, either papilledema or optic atrophy, bitemporal hemianopia, and a normal-appearing sella turcica on skull x-rays. Early diagnosis of meningiomas that cause loss of vision is desirable because the impairment may be irreversible. Meningiomas also may swell during pregnancy and produce visual impairment that will show improvement after delivery.

Meningiomas arise from many additional locations, including the tentorium, the lateral sinus, the dura of the posterior fossa and the region of the foramen magnum. Because of the wide and varied range of symptoms, misdiagnosis is frequent. It is not uncommon for these lesions to simulate carpal tunnel syndrome, syringomyelia, cervical spondylosis, myelopathy, or even multiple sclerosis.

X-rays of the skull are frequently helpful in diagnosis of intracranial meningioma, showing evidence of hyperostosis, increased vascularity and tumor calcification, but rarely bone destruction. Approximately 75% of patients with intracranial meningiomas show at least suggestive evidence on skull x-rays and the specific diagnosis reportedly can be made in 30%-60% of cases. Diagnostic techniques including radionuclide scanning, echoencephalography, and air encephalography have all been used in the past to effect a diagnosis. However, at the present time, computed tomography has essentially replaced these procedures. Not only does the CT scan detect the tumors, but it often permits a specific diagnosis of meningioma to be made. Despite the validity of the CT scan, cerebral angiography remains the definitive test for complete evaluation of the tumor and planning of the operation. Although meningiomas can usually be dealt with quite successfully by surgery, surgeons generally recognize that these tumors continue to challenge their skill and experience.

The prognosis for patients with meningiomas of the brain is influenced by many factors, including the age of the patient, the site of the tumor, the completeness of the removal of the tumor, and the presence or absence of malignancy. Recent studies (MacCarty & Taylor, 1979) found that among patients surviving for at least one month after the operation, 96% survived the first year and 63% survived for 15 years. As would be expected, the 15-year survival rate of older patients was much less, but in many cases their deaths were due to other causes.

Meningiomas do recur and a great deal depends upon the extent to which the initial lesion is fully removed. Simpson (1957) found that for patients in whom the surgeon felt that he had accomplished a total removal, including the site of dural attachment, the recurrence rate was 9%. For patients with total removal except for the site of dural attachment, the recurrence rate was 19%. When the meningioma was only partially removed, recurrence rates were 40%. Recurrences are usually manifested within five years following surgery and tend to decrease after five years.

## Sarcomas and Blood Vessel Neoplasms

There is a group of intracranial neoplasms involving connective tissue and blood vessels that includes sarcomas (composed of anaplastic connective tissue), meningiomas (generally composed of benign connective tissue) and tumors called hemangioblastomas and hemangiopericytomas (vascular tumors). These tumors would probably be organized as a group except for the fact that Cushing described meningiomas as if they were primary tumors of the leptomeninges rather than in terms of a common cell of origin. Thus, in practice, meningiomas have tended to be treated separately from other tumors that derive from connective tissue.

Intracranial sarcomas are composed of anaplastic connective tissue and, since most intracranial connective tissue is located either in the meninges or in vascular structures, most intracranial sarcomas derive from the meninges or vascular tissues. Vascular tumors, composed of hemangioblastomas and hemangiopericytomas, tend to resemble angioblastic meningiomas. Thus, in terms of classification, there appears to be an overlap of a small percentage of highly vascular meningiomas with blood vessel tumors. The distinction, however, may be quite important. Angioblastic meningiomas that resemble hemangioblastomas have a rather favorable prognosis; those that resemble hemangiopericytomas have a poor prognosis.

Hemangioblastomas arise from proliferation of endothelial cells that are not markedly anaplastic. They constitute approximately 1.5%-2% of all brain tumors. Hemangioblastomas of the cerebral hemispheres are rare and occur more frequently in the posterior fossa. Only about 10% of hemangioblastomas are supratentorial. These tumors also occur in the retina and other locations. This type of tumor is slightly more frequent in males than in females and the average age of initial diagnosis is usually between 30 and 40 years.

Headache is often the first symptom experienced with this type of tumor. Vomiting occurs in approximately 60% of the patients; vertigo and diplopia are also common. Skull x-rays show evidence of increased intracranial pressure in about one-third of patients with this tumor, but calcification rarely occurs. Diagnosis and localization customarily is made with computed tomography or angiography.

The approach to treatment involves surgical resection. If the entire tumor can be removed, morbidity usually is minimal and regrowth is unusual. In fact, this tumor is one of the most favorable for operative treatment.

Hemangiopericytomas are rare lesions, making up only about 1% of meningiomas. They present as firm vascular tumors attached to the meninges and tend to compress and displace brain tissue rather than to invade it. Approximately 80% of these tumors are supratentorial, but they can also occur in the cerebellopontine angle, the foramen magnum, or the spine. These tumors are composed of a proliferation of capillary blood vessels with normal endothelial cells surrounded by neoplastic perivascular cells. As noted above, there is an apparent overlap of these tumors with tumors earlier identified as angioblastic meningiomas. These tumors cause clinical manifestations that are essentially similar to meningiomas, with the most common symptom being headache. Computed tomography, particularly with enhancement, is effective in identifying the tumor.

Surgical intervention may be complicated by hemorrhage during the operation. Symptoms of tumor regrowth occur in approximately 75% of cases and the mean survival time is 7.3 years following the initial operation.

As noted above, the practice of identifying tumors that arise from the leptomeninges, regardless of histogenesis, causes confusion with respect to differentiation of meningiomas and sarcomas. Confusion of sarcomas with other types of tumors is a problem in determining the frequency, but this tumor is estimated to represent 1%-3% of brain tumors.

Fibrosarcoma, arising from the meninges, may develop in any part of the brain. Approximately 20% of these lesions are in the posterior fossa. When these tumors arise from the meninges, they usually appear to be firm and white; when they arise from perivascular connective tissue and occur in the brain tissue, they appear to be soft and gray. The interface between the neoplasm and brain is usually poorly defined and surrounding edema may be quite marked.

Many patients with fibrosarcomas present with headache and evidence of increased intracranial pressure, but there are no specific clinical manifestations. Seizures occur in approximately 25% of these patients. They are about equally divided among males and females, but the more anaplastic forms of these tumors tend to occur in younger patients and especially in children. Enhanced CT scans are usually accurate in identifying these lesions.

The standard treatment is surgical removal. Few patients with markedly anaplastic fibrosarcomas live more than six months. Patients with non-anaplastic lesions usually survive more than two years. Although the number of patients studied is small, some reports have indicated that patients with relatively non-malignant lesions average a survival time of 74 months following surgery.

## Neuropsychology of Brain Tumors

One purpose of the present volume is to provide a brief description of the neurological and neuropathological abnormalities of various brain lesions. Because the brain is the organ of behavior, biological damage to the brain tissues may cause profound changes in the most fundamental aspects of the individual, involving intelligence, behavior, and personality. Such concomitants of the brain have been referred to as the *higher-level aspects of brain functions*. Within the last 50 years methods for measuring and evaluating higher-level brain functions have been developed and the consequences of cerebral lesions can now be assessed clinically. Because the companion volume of this book, *The Halstead-Reitan Neuropsychological Test Battery — Theory and Clinical Interpretation* (Reitan & Wolfson, 1985) describes in detail how this is done, in the present book we shall give only a brief insight into the nature of higher-level brain functions and the deficits that may be experienced by individuals who sustain the brain lesions that have been described.

The behavioral correlates of brain functions can be subdivided into three categories: (1) *receptive or input mechanisms* concerned with delivery of information through the senses to the brain; (2) *central processing mechanisms*, in which the brain registers, analyzes, integrates, and prepares an appropriate response; and (3) *effector or response mechanisms*, in which the brain guides the muscular contractions

representing the response of the individual. Each of these subdivisions is immensely complex. The human being has an exquisite capability in sensing and perceiving the environment as well as fascinating competence in muscular and motor responses (consider, for example, the highly refined movements necessary for production of speech). However, the input and output mechanisms are far less complex than central processing and represent only interfaces with the principal aspects of brain functions.

Information learned about the mechanisms of central processing by the brain has been derived largely through careful study of persons with brain lesions and detailed comparisons of such persons with individuals who have normal brain functions. This research has indicated that central processing may be subdivided into three areas: (1) *language functions*, enjoining the entire area of use of verbal symbols for communicational purposes; (2) *temporal and spatial organization of the environment*, both in terms of receptive and expressive functions; and (3) the *complex analytical processes* involved in problem-solving, including abstraction, reasoning, and logical analysis. It is apparent from this brief presentation that brain functions underlie not only one's contact with the external as well as internal environment and one's ability to modify the environment, but also a person's entire ability to comprehend and interact with that environment. In brief, the essence of human individuality is represented by brain functions.

Rapidly developing intrinsic brain tumors constitute a severe biological insult and may have extremely adverse effects on all three of the major areas of brain functions and any of the sub-areas included. Depending upon the part of the brain involved, a brain tumor might, for example, severely restrict primary aspects of vision. A brain tumor might cause paralysis of large muscle groups, especially on one side of the body or the other, and greatly limit response potential. However, each of the higher-level aspects of brain function may be equally compromised. Ability to use language for communication, either receptively or expressively, may be grossly impaired with lesions of the left cerebral hemisphere. Ability to appreciate and understand temporal and spatial relationships may also be affected, a circumstance that frequently leads to grossly inappropriate and inefficient behavior. Probably the most serious loss that may occur is in the area of abstraction, reasoning, and logical analysis, because such deficits undercut the essential quality of intellectual and cognitive functioning.

We shall attempt to communicate some insight into the higher-level impairment experienced by persons with brain tumors by giving a brief description of the types of changes and problems experienced by individual patients.

The first patient to be described had been getting along very well in his life until he was 44 years of age. He and his wife had three healthy and normal children. Since graduating from high school the patient had made excellent progress working for a large firm. He had progressed through successful employment as a draftsman and currently was emerging as a middle-level management executive.

His first indication of neurological difficulty came as quite a surprise and he completely failed to understand its significance. He began having spells during which he stared straight ahead, his pupils became somewhat dilated, and he smacked his lips. However, these spells were very brief and, even though noticed by others, rarely attracted any specific comment. At the same time the patient began to notice that he had a mild degree of incoordination of his movements, tended to be somewhat clumsy, and dropped things more frequently than he had before. He went to his family physician and reported his symptoms, but physical examination revealed no abnormalities. A decision was made to wait and see if the problems would resolve themselves spontaneously. Instead, however, the patient's difficulties became progressively worse. Within three years of the initial manifestations the patient had become forgetful, inefficient in his behavior, and was encountering increasing difficulty in carrying out his occupational duties. He sought medical examination again and a more detailed assessment was performed. Cerebral angiography indicated

a lesion principally in the right temporal lobe; a craniotomy was performed and an astrocytoma Grade II was partially removed.

The patient recovered well from the operation, was given a course of x-ray therapy over a period of four weeks, and was placed on anti-epileptic medication. He returned to work and got along fairly well, although he did not show his former degree of ability and efficiency. Six months after the operation he had a series of four epileptic seizures which began with contractions of muscles in the left hand and face and progressed to become generalized tonic-clonic seizures. Following this series of seizures the patient had transient paralysis involving the left extremities. Neurological examination done at this time revealed no obvious deficits but EEG showed focal slow wave activity in the right frontal-temporal area. The patient's anti-epileptic medication was adjusted and he returned to work. He interacted fairly well with his associates and they wanted to help in every way possible, but it became apparent that they were only "carrying" him in his work.

Two years later the patient began having additional convulsive episodes and was given another series of x-ray treatments. The irradiation of his brain probably contributed to the lethargy and vomiting which followed this series of treatments, and the patient continued to have severe headaches. However, in a general sense he appeared to be somewhat improved and again returned to work. Finally, at the age of 50 years (about six years after the initial onset of symptoms), he gradually began to become increasingly lethargic and non-responsive and was admitted to the hospital. He could obey only simple commands and his responses to questions were very brief and sometimes inappropriate. Neurological examination indicated some reduction in responses to painful stimulation on the left side of the body, but he did not show any distinct or definite reflex changes. Cerebral angiography showed definite displacement of branches of the right middle cerebral artery, suggesting a re-growth of the tumor in the right parietal area. A craniotomy with fairly extensive removal of tumor tissue was again performed. Pathological examination of the tissue indicated that it had become increasingly anaplastic in comparison with the sample originally removed about three years earlier. However, the patient was much more alert after surgery than he had been before and, in verbal communication, seemed essentially to be quite normal.

This man's surgeon felt that the operation had been very successful. When the patient was first seen by his wife and children, as well as co-workers, they were impressed with his verbal communicational skills and believed that he was scarcely, if at all, impaired. However, he was not able to get anything done effectively, easily became confused, and could not integrate elements of complex situations. It finally became clear that he had little, if any, higher-level brain functions remaining except for his verbal communicational skills. Verbal and language skills were intact, but his spatial and temporal abilities were severely affected and he was not able to analyze or understand problems of any degree of complexity. He became confused very easily and did not understand cause-and-effect relationships among events in his environment. In effect, it was necessary to lead him by the hand when it came to dealing with practical problems in everyday life. He had mild motor deficits on the left side of his body and only minor tactile-receptive losses. However, because of his spatial confusion, he could scarcely find his way from one location to another, even in familiar surroundings. This area of deficit, together with profound losses in abstraction and reasoning processes, made it quite clear that remaining verbal skills (he still had a Verbal I.Q. that was in the superior range) were entirely inadequate to subserve the requirements of normal living.

A glioma may change in its degree of malignancy over time; in this instance it progressed from an astrocytoma Grade II to a rapidly growing and highly anaplastic glioblastoma multiforme. Gliomas produce neuropsychological deficits in accordance with a number of characteristics of the lesion, not only including its degree of anaplasia but also its location. Less rapidly growing gliomas usually do not produce

such devastating impairment, though the deficits fall within the same framework as described above. At the other extreme of the continuum, in terms of neuropsychological deficits, are patients with tumors described as "benign." Meningiomas fall in this category. Depending upon location within the brain, meningiomas may cause serious generalized impairment; frequently, though, they have a very slowly developing progression with respect to symptomatology and the neuropsychological deficits are not as profound. For example, one particular patient who had a right parietal meningioma suffered from headaches and a variety of other vague complaints for a period of six years. His complaints were frequently attributed to a psychiatric cause before he finally had a major motor seizure that lead to diagnosis of the tumor. Even at the time of diagnosis, though, his general intelligence was essentially unimpaired, he was able to perform reasonably well in most practical situations, and only sophisticated neuropsychological testing showed the presence of certain selective deficits in cognitive abilities.

# CEREBRAL VASCULAR DISEASE

## OVERVIEW

Cerebral vascular insufficiency and cerebral infarction, major factors in the incidence of cerebral vascular disease, are both usually the result of cerebral vascular atherosclerosis. Thus, in a major sense, understanding as well as preventing cerebral vascular disease concerns understanding and preventing the development of atherosclerotic changes in the arteries that supply blood to the brain. **Atherosclerosis** is a form of arteriosclerosis in which deposits of yellowish plaques (atheromas) containing cholesterol, lipoid material and lipophages are formed within the intima and inner media of large and medium-sized arteries (*see* Fig. 4–3). It is a chronic degenerative process which usually begins at an early age and progresses through several decades of life.

Three factors are commonly associated with cerebral atherosclerosis: hypertension, heart disease, and diabetes mellitus. More than 80% of patients with cerebral vascular disease have, or have had, chronically elevated blood pressure. Cerebral vascular insufficiency and cerebral infarction occur two to four times more frequently in hypertensive patients than normal tensive individuals. The risk of cerebral infarction seems to be directly related in a systematic fashion to elevation of both systolic and diastolic blood pressure. In fact, the Veterans Administration Cooperative Study of antihypertensive agents (1970) has shown that effective treatment of hypertension significantly reduces the incidence of cerebral vascular disease.

Heart disease is also common in persons with cerebral vascular disease; some type of cardiac disease is present in about 60% of these patients. About 10% of patients with acute strokes have associated myocardial infarction. Of course, both of these conditions are principally the result of atherosclerosis. Study of patients with myocardial infarction shows that they have a high prevalence of severe atheroma in the carotid arteries (McAllen & Marshall, 1977). In addition, at least 30% (and perhaps more) of patients with diabetes mellitus also show evidence of cerebral atherosclerosis.

These findings make it clear that lipid metabolism is a significant factor in the development of cerebral atherosclerosis and patients with hyperlipidemia have an increased incidence of occlusive cerebral vascular disease. Elevated serum cholesterol and triglyceride values are associated with development of atherosclerosis as well as an increased risk of cerebral infarction occurring before the age of 50 (Fogelholm & Allo, 1973). Reitan and Shipley (1963) have shown that persons who have reduced their serum cholesterol levels for a period of one year, as compared with a similar group who had not reduced their levels, showed significant improvement on neuropsychological tests of brain functions.

Three major clinical conditions are associated with the development of cerebral vascular atherosclerosis: (1) transient ischemic attacks which appear to result from the early stages of cerebral vascular insufficiency; (2) infarction in specific areas of the brain causing focal neurological deficits; and (3) multiple areas of small infarcts with resulting dementia and associated arteriosclerosis (multi-infarct dementia).

## TRANSIENT ISCHEMIC ATTACKS

**Transient ischemic attacks** are by definition neurological deficits of sudden onset that last between a few minutes and 24 hours. When focal neurological deficits persist for more than 24 hours they are customarily referred to as *vascular infarcts*. As noted previously, the cerebral vasculature provides the opportunity for collateral circulation and many compensatory mechanisms. Symptoms of TIAs are the result of temporary failure of these compensatory mechanisms. The symptoms of TIAs are referred to either the carotid or vertebral-basilar systems, although it is well-recognized that blood flow is altered in both systems and one is unable to compensate for the other. In addition, temporary focal vascular insufficiency may involve small cerebral vessels and cause TIAs.

TIAs due to insufficiency in the carotid system may produce recurring attacks of symptoms involving

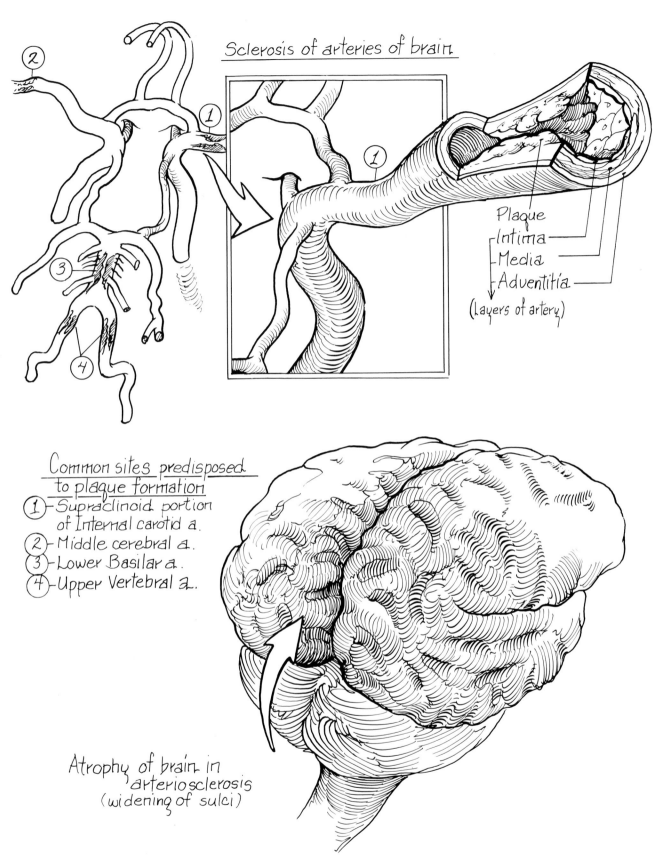

Sclerosis of arteries of brain

Plaque
⌐Intima⌐
⌐Media
⌐Adventitia⌐
(Layers of artery)

Common sites predisposed
to plaque formation
(1)-Supraclinoid portion
of Internal carotid a.
(2)-Middle cerebral a.
(3)-Lower Basilar a.
(4)-Upper Vertebral a.

Atrophy of brain in
arteriosclerosis
(widening of sulci)

**Fig. 4–3.** *Top: Detail of plaque formation in an artery and sites in the cerebral arterial system commonly affected by plaque deposits.*
*Bottom: The brain affected by arteriosclerosis shows irregularly prominent convolutions because of the widening of the deep sulci.*

only one eye, such as dimness of vision or complete blindness (*amaurosis fugax*). This is due to diminution of blood flow in the ophthalmic artery on the same side as the involved eye. The patient may show variable degrees of homonymous hemianopia, hemiparesis, and hemihypesthesia on the side opposite the diseased carotid artery. These episodes may be variable in their intensity and last from a few minutes up to 24 hours. The patient may also show evidence of transient dysphasia or losses in ability to deal with spatial configurations. Some patients develop a headache after a TIA but there appears to be a complete clinical recovery between attacks. We suspect that neuropsychological deficits of a general nature might be shown at any time these patients are examined, but there have been few studies testing this hypothesis. Some patients who suffer TIAs may show some mild positive signs on neurological examination for 24 hours or more after an attack and a considerable number have a bruit (murmur) at the origin of the internal carotid, presumably where a plaque in the vessel has caused turbulence of blood flow (Gilroy & Meyer, 1962).

TIAs involving the vertebral-basilar system usually occur for the first time in persons who are elderly. The attacks may continue for many years, and vary greatly in frequency from one individual to another. Some persons have these attacks several times a day and others experience them only once every several months. The symptoms are occipital headaches, dimness of vision or transient blindness, the experience of "flashing lights" and sometimes homonymous visual field defects. These manifestations are associated with involvement of the posterior cerebral vessels. Brain stem symptoms, including diplopia, ptosis, facial weakness, tinnitus, vertigo, nausea and vomiting, dysphagia (difficulty in swallowing) and slurring of speech may also occur. Feelings of numbness, especially around the mouth, are not uncommon. Patients may also demonstrate signs of cerebellar dysfunction, including ataxia. When the vertebral arteries are involved, it is not uncommon

for the patient to suddenly collapse without loss of consciousness.

Gilroy and Meyer (1979) have suggested that a number of factors may cause TIAs, including an intermittent release of emboli from ulcerated plaques in cervical vessels, sudden episodes of transient hypotension, sudden compression and temporary occlusion of vessels (particularly of the vertebral arteries) with turning of the head, a sudden and transient reduction in cardiac output, or atherosclerosis and occlusion of small arteries within the brain tissue in patients with chronic hypertension.

TIAs are a warning symptom and patients who experience these episodes must be considered as potential candidates for a major stroke. Estimates vary widely, but TIAs precede cerebral infarction in a substantial proportion of patients. One investigation has suggested that the majority of patients with TIAs resulting from carotid insufficiency and about half of the patients with vertebral-basilar insufficiency develop infarcts after only one or two TIAs (Marshall, 1964). It must also be noted, however, that some patients have TIAs over a period of many years and never develop cerebral infarcts (Ziegler & Hassanein, 1973). Finally, many patients with TIAs eventually develop myocardial infarcts and it would appear that the occurrence of TIAs is a warning for cardiac as well as cerebral vascular disease (Toole, Yuson, Janeway, Johnston, Davis, Cordell, & Howard, 1978).

Treatment of patients with TIAs is principally directed toward treatment of hypertension, and a number of medications have been found useful in this respect. In addition, associated medical conditions such as heart disease, diabetes mellitus, hyperlipidemia, obesity, and other conditions must also be treated. A great deal of disagreement exists concerning the value of anticoagulants. However, aspirin therapy has been shown to be effective, particularly in combination with other drugs. When a significant degree of narrowing of the internal carotid or veterbral arteries is present, the patient may be considered for surgical reconstruction of the involved vessel(s). In some instances patients with complete occlusion of one or both carotid arteries have been helped by a bypass from the superficial temporal artery to the middle cerebral artery.

## BRAIN INFARCTION

Cerebral infarction represents the most common type of stroke and is caused by a lack of oxygen or nutrients, possibly complicated by impaired removal of the metabolic products of these substances. There are three causes of infarction, but occlusion of an artery by thrombosis or embolism is by far the most common. This type of infarct is referred to as *ischemic infarction* and causes secondary hypoxia, impaired nutrition of brain cells, and cell death. *Anoxic infarction* occurs when there is a lack of oxygen despite normal circulation. *Hypoglycemic infarction* is the result of blood glucose levels being seriously reduced for a prolonged period of time.

Blood flow to the brain (or any other organ) depends upon the condition of the blood vessels, the composition of the blood, and perfusion pressure. The four major causes of ischemic infarction are (1) the formation of atheromatous plaques and resulting thrombosis in vessels which serve the blood supply of the brain; (2) severe hypotension over prolonged periods of time; (3) emboli which arise from pulmonary veins, the heart, the aortic arch, or arteries in the neck, and lodge in vessels of the brain; and (4) spasmodic contraction of blood vessels (vasospasm) which can be caused by migraine, hypertensive encephalopathy, or ruptured vessels resulting from vascular anomalies. Of course, additional factors may also be contributory, including compression of arteries by tumors, kinking of vessels on head turning, involvement of intracranial vessels by arteritis particularly associated with syphilis, etc.

The majority of infarcts involving vessels supplying the brain occur in patients who are atherosclerotic. The arteries may show generalized and diffuse narrowing or a number of areas of focal stenosis. The most common sites appear to be the origin of the internal carotid and vertebral arteries. On the basis of the clinical picture or the neurological examination

it is often difficult to differentiate between strokes due to thrombosis and embolism. However, it is our impression that strokes due to thrombosis give a more generalized picture of neuropsychological dysfunction in addition to evidence of the focal area of involvement. This could possibly be due to the greater degree of atherosclerotic involvement of the cerebral vessels in cases of thrombosis.

The composition of the blood may well be different in persons who are susceptible to developing a stroke as well as in those who have actually suffered a stroke. Low arterial oxygen tensions are frequently found in stroke patients, probably due to impaired pulmonary function. A variety of other conditions associated with cardiac disease may also be contributory. Changes in blood composition also include an increase in the adhesiveness of platelets and elevation of fibrinogen levels, both leading to an increased tendency for the blood to clot.

Reductions in cerebral blood flow due to a diminution of perfusion pressure may cause special problems for the patient with cerebral atherosclerosis. A sudden episode of hypotension may produce a critical decrease in cerebral blood flow in such patients because the autoregulatory mechanisms that work toward maintenance of cerebral blood flow may be unable to compensate during such reductions in perfusion pressure. A considerable degree of variation occurs among individuals and depends upon the degree of impairment of collateral circulation and the atherosclerotic involvement in smaller cerebral arteries.

Infarcts vary greatly in size but they have certain common pathological characteristics. Every infarct has a central area of tissue necrosis (coagulation necrosis), a surrounding edematous area with disintegration of nerve cells, axons, myelin sheaths, and some damage to astrocytes. The blood vessels are also necrotic in the center of the infarct but may be preserved toward the periphery of the infarct even though damage to the endothelial lining may be present. A sudden increase in blood pressure at this time may lead to rupture of necrotic blood vessels and produce hemorrhage in the necrotic area. Episodes of hypotension may also have an adverse effect by producing a decrease in regional cerebral blood flow.

The repair process begins within several days after the infarct has occurred. Active proliferation of glial cells and removal of degenerative products resulting from cellular disintegration and breakdown of myelin continues for a period of months, and a cystic space surrounded by glial tissue is gradually formed. Eventually a cyst containing clear or yellowish fluid may form. Infarction of the white matter follows a similar recovery process with removal by disintegrative axons, myelin sheaths, and oligodendroglial cells by microglial cells with eventual formation of a glial scar or cyst in the infarcted area.

### Clinical Aspects of Strokes

Strokes are often identified by the vessels or areas of the brain involved and occur more frequently in certain locations. This section will be organized to briefly describe the characteristics and clinical correlates of strokes involving the internal carotid arteries, the middle cerebral artery, the anterior cerebral artery, the anterior choroidal artery, the posterior cerebral artery, the midbrain, the pons, the cerebellum, and the medulla oblongata. Figs. 4–4 and 4–5 illustrate some of the more common sites of plaque formation.

In a patient with cerebral arteriosclerosis, thrombosis of an internal carotid artery is usually followed by an infarct in the distribution of the middle cerebral artery. The consequences in the individual patient, however, depend primarily upon the adequacy of collateral circulation. As noted earlier, the anatomy of the vascular system supplying the brain provides alternate routes when any particular system is occluded. Thus, clinical observations of patients with thromboses of the internal carotid artery range from manifestations of no clinical symptomatology to serious involvement of the entire hemisphere. In many patients occlusion of the internal carotid artery does not have to be complete to produce symptoms; these will be largely determined by the adequacy of collateral circulation. In the majority of cases, the thrombotic lesions that occur in the internal carotid artery form

at the origin of the vessel as it arises from the common carotid artery in the neck.

In addition to the degree of reduction of patency of the vessel, the length of the stenosed segment of the artery is significant in determining the reduction of blood flow. If the stenosed area is 1 cm or more in length, a substantial reduction in blood flow will occur. As mentioned earlier, a reduction in perfusion pressure will also be significant in this regard. Considering the biological differences between individuals, the clinical picture is quite variable.

In many cases episodes of TIAs will precede symptoms of an acute stroke. Some patients may slowly develop a pattern of neurological deterioration, suggesting that the condition is of a progressive nature rather than of acute onset. Thus, at least 50% of patients having carotid occlusions which lead to acute stroke had significant symptoms before the stroke occurred. A substantial proportion of patients have a catastrophic sudden onset. When the stroke (infarct) occurs, the onset of symptomatology is sudden and abrupt. The patient frequently becomes stuporous or comatose and develops a flaccid hemiplegia with decreased deep tendon reflexes on the affected side. In addition to impaired consciousness and hemiplegia, a variety of neurological signs may be elicited. The conscious patient may demonstrate dysphasia, homonymous visual field defects, facial weakness, hemihypesthesia, depressed deep tendon reflexes, and a unilateral extensor plantar response. With massive infarctions that involve most of the lateral portion of the hemisphere a considerable degree of cerebral edema occurs and intracranial pressure is increased. This often produces pressure on the lower centers of the brain and death from respiratory failure may result. In the less severely affected patient, however, the usual course is one of slow and partial recovery.

The clinical neurological manifestations of middle cerebral artery occlusion are difficult to differentiate from internal carotid artery occlusion on the same side. In cases of internal carotid artery disease there may have been symptoms such as amaurosis fugax (transient dimness of vision or blindness in one eye)

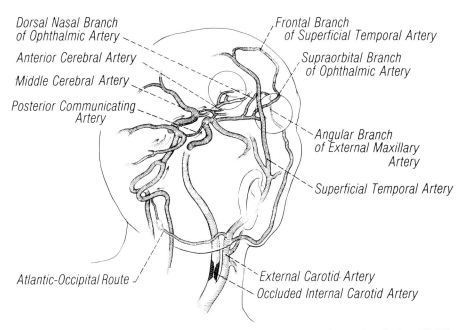

**Fig. 4–4.** *Major external carotid and vertebral collateral pathways associated with internal carotid occlusion. (© Edward B. Diethrich. Reproduced with permission.)*

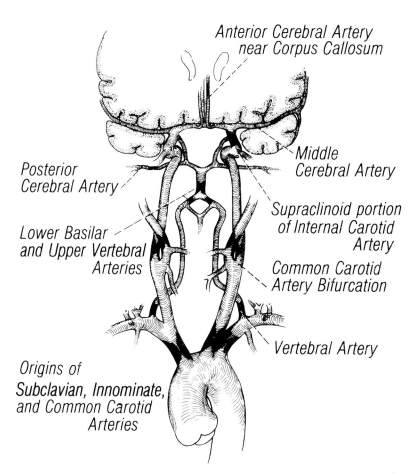

**Fig. 4–5.** *Extracranial cerebrovascular anatomy showing the areas predisposed to atherosclerotic plaque formation. (© Edward B. Diethrich. Reproduced with permission.)*

resulting from diminished blood flow in the ophthalmic artery. However, indications of internal carotid artery involvement do not exclude the possibility of concurrent middle cerebral artery occlusion. In fact, emboli arising from plaques in the internal carotid artery frequently lodge in the middle cerebral artery. If the stroke is associated with hemiplegia and a relative absence of other neurological signs, the area of involvement may be in the motor area or the internal capsule, both supplied by branches of the middle cerebral artery. In addition to motor dysfunction, middle cerebral artery occlusions may cause dysphasia, hemisensory losses and homonymous visual field defects. Such lesions may vary in severity; occlusion of the main trunk of the vessel and massive deprivation of blood supply will lead to death and small occlusions may be accompanied by only mild cerebral deficits.

Neuropsychological results show a considerable overlap between internal carotid artery occlusions and middle cerebral artery lesions, but the evidence of specific, focal involvement is often more pronounced in cases of middle cerebral artery thromboses. Internal carotid artery occlusions may produce a number of signs of involvement, especially of the middle part of the cerebral hemisphere; frequently though, at least one of the expected deficits is relatively absent (such as the relative absence of aphasia even though a pronounced contralateral motor deficit has occurred). However, severe hemiplegia in the relative absence of aphasia may also occur in some patients with discrete vascular lesions involving the internal capsule.

Occlusions of the anterior cerebral artery also vary, of course, with respect to severity. Unilateral lesions of the proximal portion of the artery, a relatively rare occurrence, may result in contralateral hemiplegia and sensory loss affecting the lower limb. The recurrent artery of Huebner, which supplies mainly the anterior limb of the internal capsule, may cause motor impairment of the upper limb when it is occluded. Thromboses of the distal portion of the anterior cerebral artery (which supplies the medial aspect of the frontal lobe and the paracentral lobules) may result in paralysis and sensory loss of the lower

limb without significant involvement of the upper limb. Occlusion of the left anterior cerebral artery may produce dysphasia characterized by motor or expressive deficits.

Occlusion of the anterior choroidal artery, which supplies the optic tract, part of the cerebral peduncle, the lateral geniculate body, part of the internal capsule, and the choroid plexus in the temporal horn of the lateral ventricle, may produce symptoms resembling middle cerebral artery occlusion. These include homonymous hemianopia, hemiplegia or hemiparesis, and hemisensory loss. With lesions at this level, however, cerebral cortical functions are relatively spared and aphasia is not usually present, even with lesions of the left cerebral hemisphere. However, patients with occlusions of this artery may show varying degrees of generalized neuropsychological impairment, depending upon the degree of generalized cerebral atherosclerosis.

The principal sign of posterior cerebral artery occlusion is the sudden and permanent onset of homonymous visual field losses without corresponding evidence of unilateral motor dysfunction. However, since the posterior cerebral arteries supply the upper end of the midbrain, the cerebral peduncles, portions of the thalamus, the subthalamic area, and parts of the hypothalamus in addition to the occipital lobes, a number of other symptoms suggesting midbrain involvement may also be present. Aphasic manifestations may be associated with occlusion of the posterior cerebral artery in the left cerebral hemisphere. Impairment in dealing with simple spatial configurations, of both an expressive and receptive nature, may be present when the right cerebral hemisphere is involved.

Occlusive lesions may also occur in the midbrain, the pons, the medulla oblongata, and the cerebellum.

Occlusions of the midbrain are relatively rare and are characterized by palsy of the third (oculomotor) cranial nerve and contralateral hemiparesis. Thrombosis of the superior cerebellar artery involves the junction of the midbrain and pons and frequently produces homolateral cerebellar signs. Nystagmus and facial paresis are fairly common and pain and temperature sensation on the opposite side of the body may also be impaired.

Infarcts of the pons produce many brain stem signs, including multiple cranial nerve palsies, dysphagia, vertigo, nystagmus, facial paralysis, diplopia, and gaze palsies. Damage of this area and higher levels of the brain stem may result in a state of akinetic mutism. Cerebellar signs including dyssynergia, dysmetria and dysdiadochokinesia of the same side as the lesion are common with infarction of the lateral and tegmental parts of the pons.

Isolated cerebellar infarctions, which are also rare, may cause abnormalities of ocular movements and other cranial nerve signs. Cerebellar signs, including vertigo, nausea, vomiting, nystagums and severe ataxia are prominent.

Medullary infarcts are associated with a number of signs, including motor deficits (not necessarily unilateral), disturbances of respiratory and vasomotor control centers, disruption of other aspects of vital functions, changes or deficits in pain and temperature sensitivity, vertigo, vomiting, and varying degress of paralysis of the palate, pharynx, and vocal cords.

## MULTI-INFARCT DEMENTIA

Autopsy studies in the late 1960s revealed the existence of a strong tendency to misdiagnose primary neuronal degenerative disease as cerebral arteriosclerosis. This was one fact that led to interest in presenile and senile dementia and primary neuronal degenerative diseases, with a special emphasis on Alzheimer's disease. Now there appears to be some tendency to limit diagnoses of cerebral arteriosclerosis or multi-infarct dementia. On the basis of clinical examination there is certainly a problem in differentiating multi-infarct dementia from Alzheimer's disease, or correctly diagnosing Alzheimer's disease in patients with cerebral arteriosclerosis. Thus, the comments below, which are intended to characterize multi-infarct dementia, will point out some of the differences in this condition as compared with primary neuronal degenerative diseases of the brain. Hachinski, Lassen and Marshall (1974) have provided a concise review of multi-infarct dementia for the reader interested in this area.

**Multi-infarct dementia** is the clinical diagnostic term applied to progressive dementia in a cardiovascular patient. The condition is associated with atherosclerotic changes in the arteries of the brain leading to cerebral arteriosclerosis. The dementia is due to the cumulative effect of repetitive infarcts widely scattered throughout the CNS (Sourander & Walinder, 1977). This condition, like primary neuronal degenerative disease of the brain, afflicts older people. Unlike TIAs, these small strokes produce permanent damage.

Patients with multi-infarct dementia frequently show (1) evidence of episodic intellectual deterioration and a somewhat fluctuating course (contrasted with the more steady deterioration observed in persons with Alzheimer's disease); (2) a history of at least one ictus (sudden attack of symptoms) or a history of prior transient ischemic attacks; (3) episodes of dysphasia, dyspraxia or ataxia followed by rapid recovery; (4) focal neurological signs and lateralized neurological deficits, such as hemiparesis or monoparesis (in primary neuronal degenerative disease more generalized deficits are present and there are fewer indications of specific motor and sensory losses); (5) a patchy reduction of cerebral blood flow generally distributed over the cerebral hemispheres (compared with the reduction principally in the frontal and temporal areas in primary neuronal degenerative disease); (6) angiograms demonstrating delayed blood flow as well as atherosclerotic deposits at various typical sites of vascular branches of the extracranial arteries and the circle of Willis together with evidence of narrowing of smaller cerebral vessels; (7) evidence of atherosclerosis in other parts of the body and signs of vascular disease, including systolic hypertension, wide fluctuations in pulse and blood pressure (including episodes of hypotension), cardiac enlargement and arrhythmias, and possibly diabetes mellitus; and (8) autopsy findings of reduced brain weight, widening of sulci, dilatation of the ventricles, and scattered infarcts in many parts of the brain with necrosis of tissue in the areas of infarct, and resulting gliosis.

Multi-infarct dementia demonstrates an overall course of progressive deterioration that includes not only the above manifestations but eventually is characterized by emotional lability, slurring of speech, dysphagia, generalized rigidity, and multiple, asymetric, hyperactive deep tendon reflexes and bilateral extensor plantar responses.

## SUBARACHNOID HEMORRHAGE

**Subarachnoid hemorrhage** refers to bleeding into the subarachnoid space. It may occur alone or in conjunction with bleeding elsewhere in the cranial cavity. Subarachnoid hemorrhage may be caused by a wide range of factors, the most common being trauma. Nontraumatic causes include ruptured cerebral aneurysms, vascular malformations, and intracerebral hemorrhages resulting from hypertension. Gilroy and Meyer (1979) use "traumatic" to identify a traumatic etiology and "spontaneous" to identify nontraumatic causes. Thus, "primary" subarachnoid hemorrhages are spontaneous and refer principally to bleeding into the subarachnoid space due to rupture of aneurysms or arteriovenous malformations. Primary subarachnoid hemorrhage may also be caused by bleeding from developmental defects, infectious diseases, neoplastic lesions, blood dyscrasias, other vascular disorders and degenerative conditions.

## ANEURYSMS

An **aneurysm** is a sac formed by the dilation of the wall of a blood vessel (*see* Fig. 4–6). A **berry (or subarachnoid) aneurysm** is a small saccular aneurysm of a cerebral artery. Berry aneurysms occur principally (about 90%) in the vicinity of the anterior part of the circle of Willis but may arise from the vertebral, basilar, and posterior cerebral arteries. They usually arise at the bifurcation of a cerebral vessel and the most common sites are the terminal portion of the internal carotid artery, the junction of the anterior cerebral and anterior communicating arteries, and the middle cerebral artery where it divides at the lateral sulcus. The most frequent sites in the vertebral-basilar system occur at the point the posterior inferior cerebral artery arises from the vertebral artery and at the division of the basilar artery into the posterior cerebral arteries.

A number of factors are believed to be significant in the production, development, and rupture of berry aneurysms, including continuous pressure of the blood as it divides at the bifurcation of arteries (together with possible absence of the usual development of hyperplasia of the intima of the arteries, which appears to form "cushions" at these points); direct effects of hypertension (in more than half of the patients); weakening of the internal elastic lamina of arteries due to inflammatory factors; and changes associated with atherosclerosis.

Ruptured berry aneurysms is a disease of middle age; 70% of these patients are aged 40 to 70 years. Until age 50, men predominate slightly; after age 50 women increasingly predominate. This may be because of the increasing porportion of women in the aging population. Most subarachnoid hemorrhages arise from berry aneurysms greater than 1 cm. The rupture of a berry aneurysm produces a sudden discharge of blood under high pressure into the surrounding brain structures. This may occur alone or be associated with intracerebral hematoma, hydrocephalus, or spasm of cerebral vessels caused by surrounding blood. Rupture of a berry aneurysm may result in cerebral infarction, cerebral edema, bleeding directly into the tissue of the brain without subarachnoid hemorrhage, and bleeding into specific structures with resulting symptoms related to the function of the structures involved. Berry aneurysms may vary greatly in size before rupturing.

About one-half of the men and perhaps two-thirds of the women have warning signs before the sudden and usually severe onset of subarachnoid hemorrhage due to a ruptured berry aneurysm. These consist of episodes of headache and stiff neck. Some patients develop focal or generalized seizures and others have episodes of facial pain.

Regardless of these warning signs, the onset of subarachnoid hemorrhage is sudden in 90% of cases. About 60% of the victims experience a sudden, severe headache; 20% rapidly go into a comatose state; the remaining 20% have various symptoms, including epileptic seizures, vomiting, pain in the neck or back, pain in the limbs, and focal paralyses. Although 20% of these patients develop unconsciousness almost immediately, an additional 50% have a delay of 6 to 12 hours before increased intracranial pressure is sufficient to produce stupor or coma. If the patient is not in a deep coma it is possible to elicit evidence of a stiff neck in almost all cases. About one-half of these patients show at least some degree of impaired alertness and consciousness at the time of admission; the others frequently show excitement, restlessness, irritability, disorientation, impaired retention and

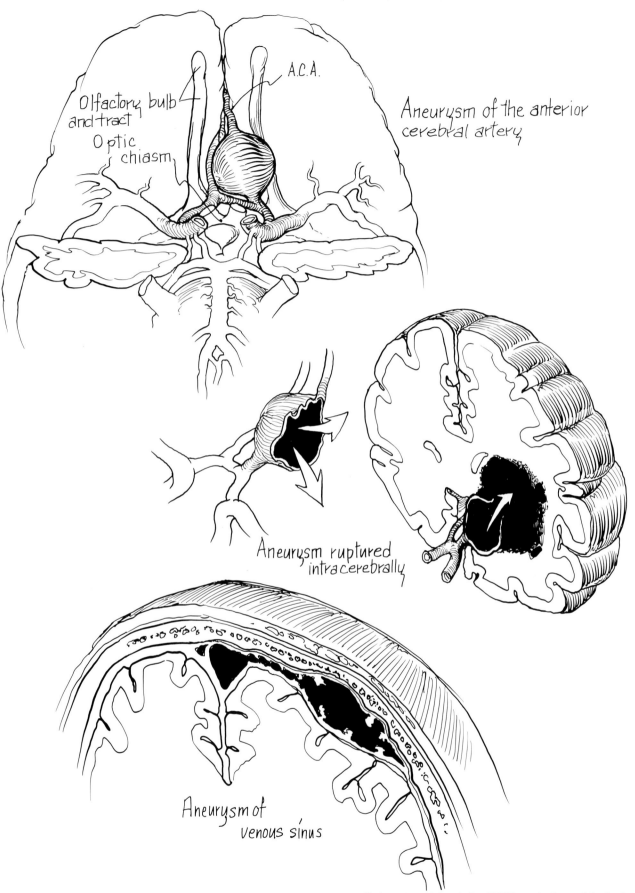

**Fig. 4-6.** *Top: Intracranial aneurysms are frequently located at the point of bifurcation of the circle of Willis at the base of the brain.*
*Middle: Rupture of an intracranial aneurysm is often due to an increase in intravascular tension (caused by extreme exertion).*
*Bottom: An aneurysm of the venous sinus will often compress the brain tissue. Frequently it will involve the dura and cause erosion of the skull bone.*

recall, deficient judgment, and dysphasia. Examination of the eye grounds may show *subhyaloid hemorrhages*, which are areas of bleeding between the retina and the hyaloid membrane having the appearance of large purple blots. Hemorrhages of this type are pathognomonic of ruptured aneurysms and usually imply bleeding of the anterior communicating or internal carotid arteries. Visual acuity may be reduced or visual field deficits may be produced due to damage in the vicinity of the optic chiasm, the optic nerve, or the retina. A careful examination and consideration of signs and symptoms often permits accurate clinical localization of the aneurysm.

Lumbar puncture frequently shows increased cerebrospinal fluid pressure and the CSF is grossly bloody in appearance. EEG is usually normal prior to subarachnoid hemorrhage but may show diffuse slowing after severe bleeding or focal slow-wave activity in the area of an intracerebral hematoma. Computed tomography usually does not show the presence of intracranial aneurysms unless contrast material is used and the lesion is quite large. However, CT scanning may demonstrate intracerebral or subdural hematomas, edema, and acute hydrocephalus resulting from the bleeding. Cerebral angiography, which detects about 80% of berry aneurysms, is also useful in identifying intracerebral or subdural hematoma as well as acute hydrocephalus.

There is general agreement that intracranial surgery should not be performed for at least seven days to three weeks after the onset of subarachnoid hemorrhage. During this period the patient should be on strict bedrest because excessive movement increases the possibility of further hemorrhage. Headaches should be controlled and blood pressure should be reduced in hypertensive patients. Besides the usual medical care of comatose or severly impaired patients, special circumstances (such as hydrocephalus or brain edema) may warrant specific treatment. There are a number of basic surgical procedures used in the treatment of berry aneurysms. The patient is usually considered to be ready for surgery if the immediate indications of acute illness have been overcome, the patient has only minimal neurological deficits or perhaps none at all, and severe spasm of the cere-

bral vessels and resulting ischemia is no longer present.

Many patients with subarachnoid hemorrhage due to ruptured berry aneurysms are not seen for neuropsychological examination because the onset is sudden and the mortality rate high. Thirty percent die within 24 hours of the hemorrhage and an additional 20% expire during the first week after the hemorrhage. About 50% of the patients who survive the first week have a recurrence of bleeding, usually occurring within two weeks of the initial episode. This second incident of bleeding carries an even higher mortality rate than the first. Total mortality is estimated at about 60% within six months following the initial insult. One-third of the surviving patients show residual paralysis, epilepsy, headache or mental symptoms (Leech & Shuman, 1982).

## ARTERIOVENOUS MALFORMATIONS

An **arteriovenous malformation (AVM)** consists of a tangle of abnormal blood vessels of various sizes. There is usually one or more large feeding arteries and a number of abnormal draining veins. The brain tissue in the area of the arteriovenous malformation may show evidence of old hemorrhage and the overlying leptomeninges are frequently thickened and stained. Microscopic examination may show evidence of hemorrhage, gliosis, and astroglial proliferation.

Arteriovenous malformations are the second leading cause (following berry aneurysms) of primary subarachnoid hemorrhage. They represent about 2%-4% of intracranial masses and are particularly common in young adults. Although they may be found in any part of the brain or spinal cord and may occasionally be multiple, the most common site is in the parietal lobe. They may be quite small or large enough to cover the greater part of a cerebral hemisphere.

Even prior to having a subarachnoid hemorrhage patients with arteriovenous malformations demonstrate a high incidence of abnormal symptoms and signs, including various types of epilepsy sometimes represented initially by focal motor manifestations of the Jacksonian type. Considering the frequent location in the parietal-temporal-occipital areas, seizures not uncommonly begin with auditory or visual phenomena. Before bleeding occurs, some patients with this condition have migraine-like headaches which are often unilateral although not necessarily on the same side as the arteriovenous malformation. Patients with large arteriovenous malformations may show a degree of chronic progressive dementia, possibly caused by chronic hypoxic deficiency affecting the cerebral tissue, progressive gliosis (secondary to repeated small hemorrhages) and hydrocephalus due to arachnoiditis resulting from recurrent subarachnoid hemorrhages.

The bleeding from arteriovenous malformations is often venous rather than arterial and the symptoms are less severe than customarily seen with arterial bleeding from ruptured berry aneurysms. Since the mortality from hemorrhage of an AVM is less than that of ruptured aneurysms, a history of recurrent episodes of subarachnoid hemorrhage is more common in persons with an AVM. The neurological deficits may be quite pronounced, depending upon the degree of cerebral tissue damage associated with the hemorrhage. These customarily include the usual signs of cerebral damage, including hemiparesis, hemisensory deficits, homonymous hemianopia, and dysphasia.

As with ruptured berry aneurysms, bleeding from an arteriovenous malformation may cause a number of changes in cerebrospinal fluid, including a bloody appearance. EEG often shows focal spike and slow-wave activity in the area of an arteriovenous malformation or possibly only focal slowing. Unlike aneurysms, arteriovenous malformations can frequently be identified by a CT scan, particularly when intravenous contrast enhancement is used. These lesions are also readily demonstrated by cerebral angiography. Serial angiograms may be helpful in identifying abnormal feeding arteries and veins draining the area, facilitating the feasibility of surgery and the approach to be used. Medical treatment for arteriovenous malformations following bleeding is essentially similar to that used for subarachnoid hemorrhage following rupture of an aneurysm. Surgical excision is performed when feasible, but if the lesion is in a critical location (the language area, for example) many surgeons are hesitant to operate. Microsurgical techniques are often used instead of a direct surgical excision (Sang & Wilson, 1975).

In addition, there are techniques which cause emboli within feeding vessels and thereby reduce the abnormal distribution of blood within the lesion and the resulting adverse consequences.

Many patients experiencing early symptoms of arteriovenous malformation without evidence of subarachnoid hemorrhage will show positive findings on neuropsychological examination. These findings frequently suggest the location of the lesion, although there is a great deal of variability between individual cases. Thus, neuropsychological diagnosis of arteriovenous malformation may be difficult for even the experienced neuropsychologist. A complicating factor appears to be the phenomenon of *"intracranial steal,"* which may occur in the presence of large arteriovenous shunts. In this situation the blood is shunted away from normal brain tissue to the area of the arteriovenous malformation. In a number of cases that have been examined neuropsychologically, the homologous area of the non-affected cerebral hemisphere shows mild neuropsychological dysfunction. Examination of the subjects following surgical repair of the arteriovenous malformation has shown improvement of function in this supposedly non-affected area. However, neuropsychological deficits related to the area of the arteriovenous malformation are usually more pronounced following surgery than pre-operatively; undoubtedly there is some inescapable damage to impaired (though partially functional) cerebral cortex at the time of operation.

Serial neuropsychological examinations usually show gradual improvement, sometimes reaching the pre-operative status. The neuropsychological examination is unquestionably of value because of its sensitivity to impaired brain functions, in both pre- and post-operative evaluation of patients with arteriovenous malformations.

## CEREBRAL HEMORRHAGE

A **cerebral hemorrhage** is a bleeding directly into the brain substance resulting from rupture of an artery, vein, or capillary. Cerebral hemorrhages range from devastating instances of damage to lesions affecting smaller areas with relatively milder damage. However, most patients with intracerebral hemorrhage (about 70%-80%) die as a result of the initial episode of bleeding.

About 20% of these hemorrhages occur in the posterior fossa (brainstem or cerebellum) and 80% occur in the cerebral hemispheres. The putamen is the most frequent site of *hypertensive intracerebral disease*. The characteristic pathologic anatomy is seen here so often that the site has warranted an eponym, "Charcot's quadrangle." This area includes the internal capsule medially, the putamen centrally, and the extreme capsule or insula laterally. The striatal branches of the middle cerebral artery are involved (Leech & Shuman, 1982).

These patients usually have prior evidence of vascular disease and, on autopsy, show pathological changes in other vessels that could eventually have led to intracerebral hemorrhage. Patients with long-standing hypertension develop degenerative changes in the muscle and elastic tissue of the blood vessel walls. These changes are often quite pronounced in the penetrating branches of the middle cerebral artery which supply the lenticular nucleus and internal capsule. These vessels may rupture if there is a sudden elevation of blood pressure. There may be numerous areas of vessel necrosis in persons with malignant hypertension and rupture is often preceded by papilledema, seizures, increased intracranial pressure, and transient neurological deficits. Some cerebral hemorrhages have been shown to be due to rupture of small anamolies of vessels located within the brain substance.

When a cerebral artery ruptures it releases blood into the brain substance under high pressure. There is widespread destruction of brain tissue in this immediate area and dissection of brain tissue along the planes of nerve tracts. In many instances the spread of blood may be quite extensive. If the patient survives the initial episode of bleeding there is rapid swelling of the involved cerebral hemisphere which reaches a maximum in about four to five days and then gradually subsides. The cerebral edema in its own right may cause additional damage through herniation of brain tissue, compression of the brainstem, and occlusion of additional cerebral arteries.

Many patients who develop cerebral hemorrhage have warning headaches, which usually are most severe upon awakening in the morning. Cerebral hemorrhages frequently occur during periods of physical exertion or excitement and are most common during the daylight hours when the patient is active. (Cerebral infarcts, on the other hand, often occur when the patient is sleeping or inactive.) The first manifestation of cerebral hemorrhage is severe headache followed by rapid impairment of consciousness and progression into stupor or coma. The neurologic deficits increase in severity and complexity as the mass of the hematoma expands, and there is clear correlation between the size of the intracerebral hemorrhage and the clinical severity: a small hemorrhage causes hemiparesis and hypesthesia; a moderate hemorrhage causes flaccid hemiplegia, hemianesthesia, hemianopia, and aphasia; and a massive hemorrhage causes coma, decerebrate rigidity, fixed and dilated pupils, absent eye movements and rapid death. With the increase in the hematoma's mass, intracranial pressure increases and headache, decreased alertness and vomiting ensue. Coma on admission to the hospital indicates a massive hemorrhage, markedly increased intracranial pressure, possibly a transtentorial herniation, and an exceedingly poor prognosis (Hier, David, Richardson, & Mohr, 1977).

## NEUROPSYCHOLOGY OF CEREBRAL VASCULAR DISEASE

Considering the great variability among individual patients that have cerebral vascular disease, it is not surprising that the higher-level aspects of brain functions in patients with CVD also show a considerable degree of variability. The deficits shown by these patients fall within the general range of neuropsychological functions that include (1) *input or receptive capabilities*; (2) *output or expressive capabilities*; and (3) the *three major areas of central processing* (verbal and language skills, temporal and spatial manipulatory abilities and abstraction, reasoning, and logical analysis). Neurological examination and diagnostic procedures frequently identify the input and output deficits of the patient in accurate detail. Unfortunately, higher-level aspects of brain functions are often relatively neglected in the neurological examination, even though they are tremendously important to the patient's overall quality of living.

Many patients who develop cerebral vascular lesions have "warning" attacks that may precede a sudden insult or stroke for a fairly extensive period of time. These prodromal episodes are referred to as **transient ischemic attacks** (TIAs). Some persons with gradually progressive conditions of cerebral vascular disease may have such attacks but never develop a focal thrombosis. When either focal or diffuse deterioration of the cerebral vessels occurs, it is likely that the results of neuropsychological examination will show impairment, even though the findings may be quite variable. We shall describe two patients; although both had cerebral vascular disease, their problems were quite different.

The first patient was 49 years old when he began experiencing transient episodes of numbness and weakness of his right upper extremity. At first he thought that perhaps he had limited the circulation in his arm by holding it in an incorrect position, and paid little attention to the difficulty. Even though these episodes continued to occur periodically, he ignored them because he seemed to be getting along fairly well in other respects. (The reader should note that persons with episodes of this kind not infrequently demonstrate neuropsychological evidence of generalized impairment of brain functions and, in some cases, even signs of focal deficit.) On the day that this man suffered a thrombosis involving the left middle cerebral artery, the first unusual thing that he was aware of was that he began dropping things with his right hand. About two hours later he noticed facial weakness on the right side and began to lose ability to communicate verbally.

By the time he was brought to the hospital the patient's speech ability had begun to return somewhat but he had a dull, frontal headache. During the course of the neurological examination his speech difficulties increased and by the end of the examination he was seriously aphasic and mumbling repetitive and unintelligible phrases. In fact, his stroke (with a developing right hemiparesis and right facial weakness) progressed under the direct observation of the

neurologist. Motor dysfunction was more pronounced in the upper than the lower extremity. Bilateral carotid angiograms indicated that a fairly extensive occlusion had occurred in the left middle cerebral artery.

The patient showed gradual improvement and was discharged about three weeks after the stroke occurred. He had shown some improvement in speech and the use of his right extremities but neuropsychological examination just before the time of discharge indicated significant impairment in two of the three major areas of central processing: language abilities and use of verbal symbols for communicational purposes, and abstraction, reasoning and logical analysis skills. Thus, in addition to the dysphasia and right-sided motor impairment, neuropsychological testing indicated that this man had significant losses in his basic problem-solving capabilities.

The patient had been employed as the director of a printing firm. The owner of the company was very sympathetic and appreciated the 25 years of service that the patient had provided as an employee and the contribution that he had made to the success of the firm. Consistent with this attitude, the owner decided that he would not hold the misfortune of a stroke against the patient and insisted that he return to work in his previous position.

Had the patient's problems involved only verbal communication and right hemiparesis it is possible that he might have been able to perform this job. However, his neuropsychological deficits were much more general: he was not able to keep several things in mind at the same time, he continually became confused, and it became apparent that he was not able to run the operation. At first he was given an assistant, but this did not work because the patient did not have the capability to use the assistant effectively. In a spirit of giving him every opportunity, the owner transferred the patient to positions having decreased responsibilities until finally the patient was attempting to work as an "ink-room assistant." By this time he was thoroughly demoralized, had lost all confidence in himself, and was not able to do any kind of job. It would have been a great advantage to the patient if his neuropsychological deficits had been realistically considered at the outset, a brain retraining program instituted, and the patient started occupationally at a level that he could handle so that he could have the opportunity of experiencing success rather than repeated failure as he attempted to regain his functional capacities.

A second patient with cerebral vascular disease had a rather different kind of problem. He was a 62-year-old man who had suffered from essential hypertension for a number of years. His internist was concerned because he had not been able to control the patient's blood pressure. At this point the patient was experiencing headaches, feelings of depression, and increasing anxiety concerning his ability to continue to function efficiently. The patient was a college graduate employed as the chief executive officer of a regional office of a national organization. It was clear that he was responsible for a large operation and that he had reached the point where he felt he was just not able to continue meeting his responsibilities. At this time his internist referred him for neuropsychological examination in order to assess higher-level aspects of brain functions, even though in most respects the physical and neurological examinations were within normal limits.

As expected, the test results indicated that this man had superior general intelligence levels. Both his Verbal and Performance I.Q. values were far above average. He did not show any signs of focal cerebral damage, but the indications of generalized impairment were severe. The patient had little remaining ability to analyze new and complex situations and reach meaningful conclusions. This loss in the area of abstraction and logical analysis undoubtedly was fundamental in contributing to his feeling of personal inadequacy in handling the affairs of his firm. He had good background abilities and many relevant experiences in the past, but little immediate adaptive capability either in relating these past abilities to immediate problems or in actually solving the immediate problems. In this case, the neuropsychological concomitants of diffuse cerebral vascular disease, which

were of critical significance, were not demonstrated by the medical and neurological evaluations. In most instances, integration of the neurological and neuropsychological findings constitutes the best approach in gaining a comprehensive understanding of the patient's problems and developing an approach for remediation and management.

Finally, it is important to emphasize that the absence of focal symptoms (such as hemiparesis, dysphasia, or homonymous visual field defects) does not serve as a valid basis for concluding that the brain disease or damage has left the patient unimpaired. While many patients show focal signs as well as generalized neuropsychological deficits, others show only the latter. Patients in this situation are often apprehensive, feel a complete lack of self-confidence, and become anxious, frightened, and depressed. In such instances it is not unusual for neurologists and neurological surgeons to conclude that all of the patient's difficulties relate to the manifestations of emotional distress merely because the examining techniques and methods in neurology fail to demonstrate positive findings. In fact, there is a tendency to attribute these symptoms to a psychiatric cause and fail to recognize the significance of generalized impairment of brain functions and the corresponding neuropsychological deficits. It is very clear that clinical assessment of the individual patient requires evaluation of any general as well as focal (specific) deficits, and that the physical neurological examination is directed principally toward focal signs.

# HEAD INJURY

Mortality and morbidity resulting from head injury is a major medical and neuropsychological problem. Trauma — the leading cause of death in youth and early middle age — is the third most common cause of death in the United States; it is exceeded only by vascular disease and cancer (U.S. Department of Health, Education, and Welfare, 1974). In death due to trauma, head injury contributes significantly in more than half of the cases. In patients with multiple injuries, the head is the part of the body most commonly injured and in fatal road accidents injury to the brain occurs in nearly 75% of the cases (Gissane, 1963). Although head injury occurs principally among younger persons, it still exceeds stroke as a cause of death in males aged 45-64 years.

Studies of patients who have sustained head injuries indicate that they have many pre-existing problems and do not appear to represent a cross-section of the population. Factors over-represented in this population include low socioeconomic status, alcoholism, a history of prior head injuries (probable accident-proneness), psychiatric problems, and neurological disorders.

## MECHANISMS OF TRAUMATIC INJURIES OF THE BRAIN

The initial impact of a blow to the head results in a temporary deformation of the skull with injury to the brain tissues resulting from compression or penetration, tension (or tearing the tissues apart), and shearing or sliding tissues over other tissues (including bone).

**Acceleration injuries** are those in which the head is struck by a faster-moving object. In such cases, the slower-moving contents of the skull may be damaged by sudden contact with bony prominences or the edge of dural membranes. Contusion (bruising) of the brain may occur in many locations, including the brain stem. The poles of the frontal and temporal lobes, as well as the orbital surfaces of the frontal lobes, are particularly vulnerable to injury of this type when they move in an anteroposterior and superoinferior direction because they strike bony ridges of the inner surface of the skull. A pressure wave is also established in acceleration injuries to the head. This pressure is greatest at the point of impact but may be a factor in producing injuries on the opposite side of the brain (*contrecoup injury*).

**Deceleration injuries** occur when the head is moving and strikes a fixed and solid object. Injury may occur at the point of impact or an opposite point (contrecoup damage). A fall on the back of the head, for example, may result in contusion of the both frontal and temporal lobes. Again, a pressure wave may be established at the point of impact with negative pressure in the area of injury and increasing pressure opposite the point of injury. Contrecoup injuries of the occipital areas are rare, probably due to the smooth contour and absence of bony projections on the inner side of the skull in this area.

A forceful impact to the head produces distortion of the skull, a change in the linear movement of the head (acceleration or deceleration), and frequently, rotation of the head. A sudden, forceful rotation of the head on the neck may produce shearing forces and resulting tearing of tissue, a mechanism that has been implicated as the major cause of contrecoup injuries (Ommaya, Grubb, & Naumann, 1970). Other movements of the brain within the cranial cavity may also set up shearing forces within the brain substance. These shearing forces may produce damage to blood vessels as well as brain tissue (Tomlinson, 1970).

These comments should make it clear that a blow to a particular point of the head may cause widespread damage to the underlying tissue and is not restricted to the point of impact. When a substantial force is delivered to a particular point on the skull the mechanisms of injury relate not only to deformation of the skull, penetration of the skull and direct tissue damage, but also to compression, tension, and shearing.

## TYPES OF HEAD INJURY

Gilroy and Meyer (1979) classify head injuries into three general categories: (1) skull fracture; (2) closed head injury without fracture; and (3) penetrating wounds of the skull and brain.

### Skull Fractures

Skull fractures generally fall into one of two categories: (1) *perforation of the skull or depressed fractures*, and (2) *comminuted or linear fractures*. About 70% of skull fractures are linear. Fig. 4–7 illustrates linear skull fractures.

### Head Injury Without Skull Fracture

Many persons sustain minor head injuries, with transient impairment of consciousness but without skull fracture, that resolve in a short period of time with complete recovery. It must be observed, however, that closed head injuries without skull fracture may result in severe and irreversible brain damage. Fatal brain damage can occur even without a skull fracture being present. The presence of a skull fracture, considered by itself, is of limited importance; the important point is to evaluate neurological and neuropsychological abnormalities in order to determine the clinical significance of the injury.

Autopsy studies of cases of severe closed head injuries have shown diffuse damage in the white matter, with disruption of axons apparently resulting from the shearing forces of the impact (Strich, 1970). Although the brain may appear normal at autopsy, microscopic examination shows lesions not only in the white matter but in other structures as well. Careful autopsy studies of patients who had sustained severe head injuries with primary brain stem damage showed evidence of more widespread diffuse damage extending beyond the brain stem in *every* case. A number of investigators (Mitchell & Hume-Adams, 1973; Reilly, Graham, Hume-Adams, & Jennett, 1975) reported that they were unable to find a single case of primary brain stem damage without associated diffuse damage. Oppenheimer (1968) studied patients who had recovered from relatively mild head injuries resulting in cerebral concussion and then ultimately died of unrelated causes. Neuropathological studies of these cases showed small microglial lesions diffusely distributed in the brain but not in the brain stem. In persons who had suffered cerebral concussion, it would seem possible that these residual lesions are the end result of small petechial hemorrhages.

It is apparent that the mechanisms and types of head injury may cause extensive damage throughout the brain, either as a result of direct or secondary damage of brain tissue and blood vessels. It is not surprising, therefore, that in persons who have sustained head injuries, the results rarely point to an area of specific, focal, discrete damage when significant neuropsychological deficit is found.

### Penetrating Wounds of the Brain

Many types of head injuries result in penetration of the brain and direct damage to the underlying brain tissue. In such injuries, pressure waves are set up by the penetrating missile and produce a profound change in brain stem function, with the combined effects being represented principally by increased intracranial pressure and reduced systemic blood pressure. If the injury is sufficiently severe, intracranial pressure may increase to the point that death occurs. In less severe cases brain stem centers again begin to function and a balance is restored, although increased intracranial pressure frequently remains high because of cerebral edema (Crockard, Brown, et al., 1977).

Open wounds of the head, with penetration through the skull into the brain, usually result in unconsciousness, although such injuries sometimes occur with little impairment of consciousness. When loss of consciousness occurs, the five stages of recovery of consciousness (*see* p. 215) are experienced and each stage, on the average, tends to be longer than in patients with closed head injuries. Some patients with injuries of this kind initially show no immediate loss of consciousness but gradually progress into coma over a period of several hours. After the penetrating head injury there is often an increase in intracranial pressure and shock with hypotension and the patient

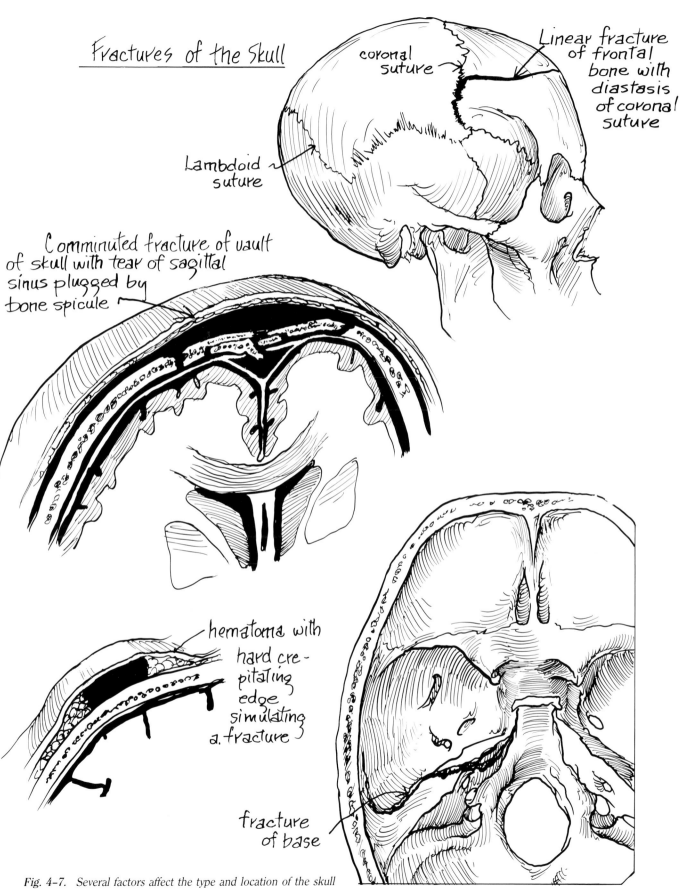

# Fractures of the Skull

coronal suture

Linear fracture of frontal bone with diastasis of coronal suture

Lambdoid suture

Comminuted fracture of vault of skull with tear of sagittal sinus plugged by bone spicule

hematoma with hard cre-pitating edge simulating a fracture

fracture of base

*Fig. 4–7. Several factors affect the type and location of the skull fracture, including the thickness of the bone, the force of the blow, and the patient's age.*

may be critically ill. These patients may be in a deep coma, with dilated pupils, a sluggish pupillary reflex and absence of reflex eye movements when the head is turned. Patients who survive may remain in a semicomatose state for several days or weeks before recovering consciousness. During this progression the patient may be quite restless, thrash about, show irritability, and be in a state of traumatic delirium which may last for several days or weeks. Upon reaching a stabilized condition, residual deficits are often present, including cerebral signs of dysphasia, hemiparesis or hemiplegia, homonymous visual field defects, emotional lability with temper outbursts and neuropsychological deficits. Impairment of eye movements and ataxia, associated with brain stem damage, are also frequently seen.

## DIVERSITY OF DAMAGE IN HEAD INJURY

As might be expected from the above description of the mechanisms of head injury, the underlying neurological damage is extremely variable and the resulting neuropsychological consequences are correspondingly variable. Head injuries may be penetrating or closed. In each case pressure gradients are established and may cause widespread damage of both gray and white matter. In addition, there may be direct damage of cerebral tissue from the force of the blow, tearing of tissues, and shearing of cerebral tissues against other tissues (including bone). Contusion, represented by rupture of capillaries in the cerebral cortex and white matter with resulting destruction of tissues, may also occur. Movement of the brain within the calvarium may damage blood vessels within the brain as well as those leading to or departing from the brain. Shearing effects may also damage cranial nerves. Autopsy studies of patients with severe head injuries have revealed that head blows may cause microglial scars, neuronal loss, axonal degeneration, loss of white matter, and long-term effects that can result in eventual formation of glial scarring or meningocerebral scar tissue formation. Fig. 4–8 shows some of the various types of damage from head injury.

## PATHOLOGICAL CONSEQUENCES OF HEAD INJURY

References have been made to some of the pathological changes produced by the forces that act upon the head and brain when they are struck by a significant blow. The pathologic sequelae may be quite varied, depending upon the force of the blow, penetration of the skull, and other factors.

A minor blow to the head may produce no brain injury whatsoever. Even a head injury sufficient to produce concussion is still viewed by some (Gilroy & Meyer, 1979) to be totally reversible, though a transient loss of brain function may occur. In this context it is important to recognize that the force of impact in head trauma ranges from mild to severe. Even though mild blows to the head may produce no damage, there is a point at which tissue damage will accompany a more severe blow. In addition, impact of the same force probably has a differential effect on the brains of individual persons. It is well known that clinical findings of deficit following head injury are variable from one person to another, even with head blows that seem to be approximately equivalent in force. Thus, it is fairly well established that the degree of impairment (judged by either neurological or neuropsychological evaluation) does not correlate perfectly with the estimated force of impact. For example, an individual may suffer severe focal damage to the brain with penetration and obvious tissue destruction and not even lose consciousness. Closed head injuries may produce prolonged periods of unconsciousness and neuropathological studies have indicated the frequent occurrence of microglial scars in the white matter and axonal damage. Severe head trauma is usually accompanied by loss of neurons in both the cerebral cortex and deeper nuclei. Diffuse cerebral atrophy may result from loss of neurons, degeneration of axons, and diminution of white matter. This decrease in brain substance is accompanied by enlargement (dilatation) of the ventricles (a condition referred to as *hydrocephalus ex vacuo*). Intracranial hypertension may also occur due to swelling of brain tissue as a direct result of the

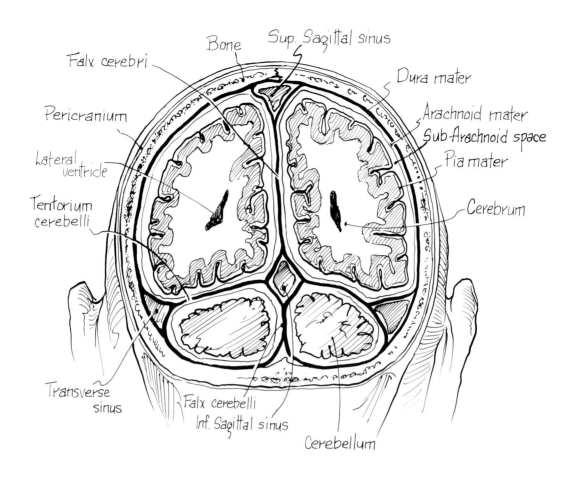

Falx cerebri
Pericranium
lateral ventricle
Tentorium cerebelli
Bone
Sup. Sagittal sinus
Dura mater
Arachnoid mater
Sub-Arachnoid space
Pia mater
Cerebrum
Transverse sinus
Falx cerebelli
Inf. Sagittal sinus
Cerebellum

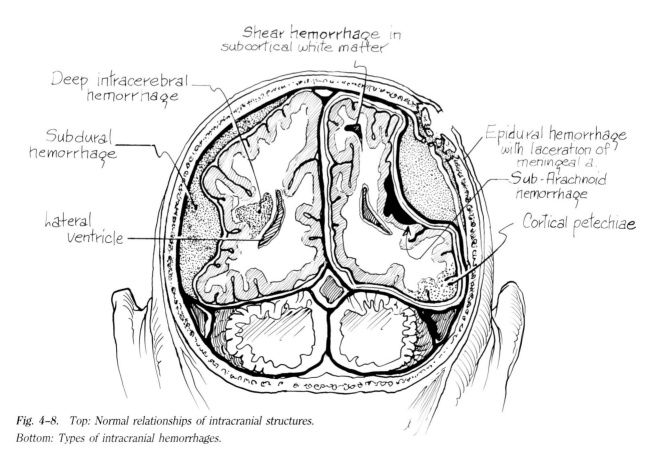

Deep intracerebral hemorrhage
Subdural hemorrhage
lateral ventricle
Shear hemorrhage in subcortical white matter
Epidural hemorrhage with laceration of meningeal a.
Sub-Arachnoid hemorrhage
Cortical petechiae

Fig. 4–8.   Top: Normal relationships of intracranial structures.
Bottom: Types of intracranial hemorrhages.

injury; it is often accompanied by increased pressure in the cerebral spinal fluid. Subarachnoid hemorrhage may cause scar tissue formation, interruption of the circulation of cerebral spinal fluid, and hydrocephalus. When subdural hematoma becomes chronic and is incompletely removed, the involved hemisphere may also show a degree of atrophy.

Contusion of the brain is represented principally by rupture of capillaries in the cerebral cortex and white matter and are seen as brownish scars at autopsy. Lesions of this type are particularly common in the frontal and temporal poles and the orbital surface of the frontal lobe, due to compression of the brain tissue in these areas and the bony projections on the orbital surface of the skull. When damage of this kind occurs, the necrotic tissue is removed by the phagocytic action of microglial cells. The surviving astrocytes proliferate and eventually form a glial scar or a scar involving both the meninges and the cerebral cortex (meningocerebral scar). Such scar tissue frequently causes spontaneous electrical discharges causing post-traumatic seizures. This occurs because the neurons included in the scar tissue formation suffer an alteration in metabolic function which results in abnormal electrical activity. Focal destruction of brain tissue may also occur in areas of intracerebral hemorrhage following head trauma. Thus, in cases of head injury, it is not unusual to find evidence of widespread as well as focal damage.

## GLASGOW COMA SCALE

The Glasgow Coma Scale has been studied in detail and is widely used to assess potential outcome in persons with head injuries. The wide usage relates to two factors: (1) it has proved to be a good indicator of outcome; and (2) it is simple to administer. In fact, most of the validational data has been gathered on persons who sustained severe head injuries shortly before the examination. The Glasgow Coma Scale assesses the patient's responsiveness in three modalities: motor response, verbal response, and eye opening. Several alternatives relating to the patient's performance are given in each of these areas and the subject is graded according to his best response. For example, in evaluating motor responsiveness, five categories are used ranging from no response to correct responses to the verbal commands of the examiner. The five possible alternatives in this category are (1) no response; (2) motor extension to a painful stimulus; (3) motor flexion to a painful stimulus; (4) ability to localize the painful stimulus; and (5) correct motor responses to the examiner's command.

The area of verbal responsiveness uses the following five categories: (1) no verbal response; (2) utterance of incomprehensible sounds; (3) verbal responsiveness but use of inappropriate words; (4) confusion in verbal communication; and (5) oriented and appropriate verbal responses.

Eye opening is assessed in four categories: (1) no eye opening; (2) eye opening in response to a painful stimulus; (3) eye opening in response to speech; and (4) spontaneous and normal eye opening.

## CLINICAL MANIFESTATIONS OF HEAD INJURY

Types of head injury may be classified according to clinical manifestations in a number of ways. It has already been noted that head injuries range from mild to severe and corresponding brain damage ranges from none to devastating. We should note that loss of consciousness and severity of brain damage correlate in certain ways, but their correlation is far from perfect. In fact, a significant degree of contusion or laceration of the brain may occur without loss of consciousness; in many instances the same occurs with severe penetrating injuries. The patient may feel dazed, mildly confused, light-headed, and have generalized motor weakness; such symptoms may even persist for an extended period of time. In cases of brain injury without loss of consciousness, headache is usually experienced for at least a number of days following the injury and the patient may show signs of irritability, poor concentration, impaired memory, and difficulty sleeping. In most cases the symptoms gradually abate, but in some instances recovery may take many months. Patients who suffer cerebral contusion and/or subarachnoid bleeding with loss of consciousness usually complain of a stiff neck and occipital headache.

The post-concussion syndrome — based upon subjective complaints of the patient — is difficult to define and has been questioned with regard to its validity. There is no doubt, however, that patients can suffer relatively mild closed head injuries that result in cerebral damage. The evidence for this conclusion is much better substantiated on the basis of neuropsychological than neurological findings. The head trauma may have caused only brief loss of consciousness or only confusion, etc. as noted above. However, the patient complains of headache, irritability, easy fatigue in both mental and physical activities, difficulty concentrating, and feelings of dizziness. Another symptom sometimes mentioned includes vertigo (when the inner ear or eighth nerve has been damaged).

In patients who suffer head injuries that cause loss of consciousness, the degree of impairment and stages of recovery have been divided into a number of categories (Gilroy & Meyer, 1979). The initial stage is *coma*, in which there is a complete paralysis of cerebral functioning but with preservation of activity of the medulla oblongata which subserves pulse, blood pressure, and breathing. However, the patient has no response to painful stimulation. The pupils usually react to light and reflex eye movements may still be present in response to head movements. In the second stage, *semi-coma*, the patient shows some reflex activity and begins to respond to painful stimuli by withdrawal. Stage three is referred to as *stupor*. The patient is restless but does not speak; gradually he begins to respond to simple commands but is irritable and seems to resent attention. In this stage some patients may become violent or delirious. In the fourth stage, *obtundity*, the patient begins to recover from extreme restlessness and go into a state of quiet confusion. The patient is able to respond to the examiner but is disoriented and does not seem to be very much aware of surrounding circumstances. The patient may talk excessively, and show a tendency toward confabulation in his verbal communication. The fifth stage is one of *full consciouness* and may be achieved gradually over a period of days, hours, or even months. At this point some additional insight about the severity of the head injury may be gained by determining the length of retrograde amnesia. This is done by finding out if the patient remembers the head blow and the extent to which his memory is impaired in the period of time preceding the injury. In less serious instances the events immediately preceding the head injury will be remembered but in severe cases the patient's memory may be totally absent for events even an hour or a whole day before the injury occurred. Neurologists customarily believe that eventual total recovery is to be expected in cases of concussion. However, neuropsychological evaluation has shown that a degree of improvement may continue for many months while still demonstrating some degree of deficit (Dikmen & Reitan, 1976).

## NEUROLOGICAL DIAGNOSTIC PROCEDURES IN HEAD INJURY

Diagnostic procedures used to evaluate brain damage in head-injured patients include skull x-rays, computed tomography, and electroencephalography. Cerebral angiography, once used frequently to evaluate head injury, has largely been replaced by computed tomography. Echoencephalography is sometimes used, particularly in instances of closed head injury, in an effort to identify a fluid collection (such as a subdural or epidural hematoma or, in more chronic cases, a subdural hygroma). Evoked sensory potentials have been shown to be of some use in evaluating the extent of head injury and the degree of abnormality of the evoked responses, recorded shortly after the injury, has been related to the degree of recovery.

## POST-TRAUMATIC SYNDROME (POSTCONCUSSION SYNDROME, POSTTRAUMATIC NEUROSIS)

As noted above, many patients who suffer relatively mild closed head injuries have persistent complaints of headache, irritability, a tendency to fatigue both physically and mentally, inability to concentrate, and feelings of dizziness or disturbance of equilibrium. The physical neurological examination is frequently negative and EEG findings are often non-contributory. In fact, neurological examination usually provides no objective evidence of damage of the brain. Thus, neurologists and neurological surgeons often conclude that the symptoms of the patient are not clearly related to gross structural damage of the brain, even though microscopic changes in nerve cells have been noted to occur in such cases.

The absence of definite neurological findings, coupled with the need for an explanation of the condition, has led many neurologists and neurological surgeons to conclude that the patient's complaints are due to emotional reactions to the head trauma and represent a post-traumatic neurosis. Nevertheless, patients who have sustained closed head injuries have a remarkable consistency in the configuration of their complaints although even this may be due to the fact that these are the "expected" reactions to head injury. It is generally recognized that there may be structural and physiological changes in the nervous system responsible for the clinical picture. Nevertheless, the absence of positive neurological evidence has led to the conclusion that the development and persistence of symptoms of the post-traumatic syndrome (postconcussion syndrome) are emotional in nature. Although recognizing the possibility of an organic basis in some cases, McLaurin and Titchener (1982), in discussing the mechanism of the neurotic response, say that the patient's "anxiety seeks discharge or containment through neurotic or occasionally psychotic symptoms, but mainly through personality change." They believe that the post-traumatic syndrome represents a complex interaction of neurophysiological, psychophysiological, and psychiatric factors plus additional factors which are unknown.

Obviously, the solution to this type of problem is to use examination techniques that are more sensitive to neurological damage or dysfunction combined with direct evaluation of the emotional status of the patient. Rather than depend upon the relatively insensitive techniques of clinical neurology, neuropsychological evaluation should be employed to identify possible significant (though perhaps mild) manifestations of cerebral damage. Further, the methods of clinical psychology used to evaluate emotional status are a valuable complement to neuropsychological testing. Thus, rather than presuming that the patient's problems are emotionally based because routine clinical neurological methods of evaluation are negative, it is more appropriate to take a direct and more sensitive approach to evaluation of brain-behavior relationships and combine this information with an evaluation of the patient's emotional status.

These considerations certainly do not alter the fact that many patients who have sustained head injuries may initially suffer symptoms that achieve secondary value in a neurotic framework or even with respect to potential litigation. However, head injured patients should be evaluated on objective evidence of deficit, as accomplished using comprehensive neuropsychological testing.

## POST-TRAUMATIC EPILEPSY

After head injury, it is not uncommon for the patient to develop epilepsy. In some cases, even minor head injuries have been identified as the basis for epileptic seizures. There are certain factors caused by the head injury more commonly associated with development of seizures. For example, epilepsy develops in about 60% of persons who sustain laceration of the brain resulting from a depressed skull fracture or a severe penetrating head injury (Ommaya, 1972). Intracerebral and subdural hemorrhages are associated with eventual epilepsy in about 40% of the cases; epidural hemorrhages are associated with only 10%. The location of the principal tissue damage is another significant factor. Lesions near the central sulcus, involving the motor area (and producing hemiplegia or hemiparesis) are more likely to cause seizures than lesions near the frontal or occipital poles. Russell and Whitty (1952) reported that 65% of patients with focal injuries in the middle part of the cerebral hemisphere develop seizures. Epilepsy developed in only 39% of patients with anterior frontal lesions and 38% of patients with lesions largely in the occipital area.

Epileptic seizures may begin at varying points in time following head injury. There is a significant association between the frequency of attacks and the persistence of seizures. Patients who have more than 10 seizures per year are likely to have a long-term seizure problem (Caveness, 1963).

The onset of epilepsy following head injury extends over a considerable period of time. Rasmussen (1969), studying a series of 265 patients, reported that 24% had their first seizure within six months of the injury; 43% within 12 months; 58% within two years; 66% within three years; and 78% within five years. In a series reported by Jennett (1965), 8% of the patients had their first seizure 10 or more years after the injury, with one case having an interval of 27 years.

It is estimated that 50% of patients who have had one or more seizures eventually stop having seizures. However, the earlier the seizures begin, the more likely they are to continue. Jennett (1969) reported that in one particular series, 25% of patients who had a seizure during the first week went on to develop persistent epilepsy; only 3% of patients who did not have seizures during the first week later developed epilepsy.

The pathophysiological changes responsible for development of epilepsy have not been fully described. However, Westrum, White, and Ward (1964) studied the morphology of experimental epileptic foci in animals and compared their findings with human biopsy specimens. Their results suggested that neurons in the epileptogenic foci have fewer synaptic endings on their dendrites than those in normal tissue and that this partial deafferentation might possibly lead to postsynaptic hypersensitivity of the epileptic neurons. It is also well known that the effects of head injury may include acute and chronic changes in cerebral circulation, development of gliosis and meningocerebral scar tissue, and alterations in the blood-brain barrier as well as glial-neuronal relationship factors (Jasper, 1970).

## ELECTRICAL INJURIES

Electrical shock may cause injury to the brain as well as other parts of the body. As with other insults,

the outcome may range from no discernible impairment or damage to death. Electricity clearly can damage living tissue and the human body can act as a conductor, carrying the current from the point of contact to the point of exit. Damage can occur if the nervous system (including the brain) is within the route taken by the current. In addition, concurrent damage to blood vessels may damage the vessel walls and cause delayed infarction resulting from diminished or interrupted blood supply.

Death due to respiratory arrest may occur if a sufficient quantity of the electrical current passes through the respiratory center. If respiratory arrest is followed by recovery of breathing, there is a possibility of anoxic encephalopathy. In persons with cerebral damage due to electrical injury the cerebral neurons appear to be particularly susceptible to damage, with various types of pathological changes occurring. Gilroy and Meyer (1979) state that when respiratory arrest has occurred for more than six minutes, the subject who recovers usually shows evidence of anoxic encephalopathy. In other instances, when the respiratory center is not specifically involved, indications of neuronal dysfunction may be manifested by generalized seizures followed by coma. These authors also note that a lesser current may produce temporary disturbances and confusion of the patient followed by full recovery. However, recovery in this condition is probably better evaluated through neuropsychological rather than neurological examination. Dysphasia and hemiparesis as well as organic dementia may occur. Parkinsonian symptoms and choreoathetosis have also been reported in patients sustaining brain damage due to electrical injury. Spinal cord damage and peripheral nerve injury are not uncommon in persons with severe electrical shocks

## TRAUMATIC BIRTH INJURIES

Traumatic injuries of the brain have been estimated to be responsible for about 10% of the deaths that occur at birth. Such injuries of the head during parturition include abnormal presentations, precipitated delivery, prolonged labor and the use of obstetric forceps. In children who sustain brain injuries at birth, anoxia is a major factor producing impairment. Trauma to the head may impair function of the medullary respiratory center resulting in anoxia and subsequent cerebral damage. The two principal types of trauma resulting in head injury during labor are (1) direct trauma from application of forceps; and (2) the use of other obstetric maneuvers and excessive compression or molding of the head within the birth canal. Injuries can occur to the scalp, skull, meninges (including the venous sinuses) or the brain tissue itself. Damage may be represented by hematomas directly under the skull, skull fracture, epidural hemorrhage, subdural hemorrhage, subarachnoid hemorrhage, and intracerebral hemorrhage. Traumatic hemorrhage at the time of birth may result in formation of a porencephalic cyst and probably is one of the major causes of this condition. Birth injuries may result in impairment of the individual's potential for development of normal brain-behavior relationships.

## "WHIPLASH" INJURIES

Although "whiplash" injuries involve damage to the cervical spine as a result of sudden hyperextension and flexion of the neck, these injuries may also cause brain damage (Ommaya, Faas, & Yarnell, 1968). In addition to spinal cord damage that may occur, whiplash injuries may also involve the vertebral arteries, causing possible occlusion of these vessels and ischemia of the brain stem and occipital areas. The linear acceleration produced by the extreme movement of the head may also result in concussion and contusion of the brain stem and brain.

After a whiplash injury the patient usually does not lose consciousness but, after a short period of time, has a feeling of weakness and unsteadiness and sometimes ataxia, vertigo, and vomiting. These symptoms may be due to ischemia of the brain stem. Patients frequently develop occipital headache which may spread to the temporal areas within a relatively short period of time after the injury. Pain and tenderness in the neck area may disappear after a few days, but the headache often persists for weeks or even months.

## NEUROPSYCHOLOGICAL MANIFESTATIONS OF HEAD INJURY

As noted above, head injuries may cause brain damage ranging from very mild to very severe. Even with focal destruction of brain tissue, there are diffuse effects. In some cases, of course, the effects may be principally diffuse (rather than focal) in nature. Thus, a variety of aspects of head injury interact in the individual case. Neuropsychological findings in head injury also are quite diversified. A number of studies, as well as clinical experience, has indicated that in cases of head injury, neuropsychological testing is more sensitive to brain damage than the neurological examination and EEG. Thus, if positive neurological findings are present, it is entirely likely that neuropsychological deficits will be found. It is more difficult to postulate any type of consistent relationship between EEG abnormalities and neuropsychological findings, except that underlying characteristics of the traumatic brain lesion may be relevant with respect to both sources of information. It is common to find generalized involvement in patients with traumatic brain injuries demonstrating only evidence of focal damage from a neurological or neurosurgical point of view. For example, on neuropsychological testing, a person with a depressed skull fracture and evidence of contusion underlying the fracture very probably will show evidence of both the focal area of tissue damage as well as diffuse involvement.

As noted above, many patients with closed head injury fail to demonstrate any objective evidence of cerebral damage from neurological examination, EEG, computed tomography, and other neurological diagnostic tests. Many such cases show unequivocal evidence of neuropsychological impairment, often with the particular types of changes being entirely typical of craniocerebral trauma rather than brain damage resulting from any other etiology. These patients are often bewildered and upset by the negative neurological findings, realizing themselves that they have suffered some degree of deficit. Thus, a confusing discrepancy exists when, on the one hand, the physician congratulates the patient for not sustaining any permanent injury and, on the other hand, family, friends, teachers and the patient himself all recognize that impairment has occurred. If the patient insists that he or she has sustained some loss, a psychiatric basis for the complaints may be suggested, or, in other cases, if litigation is involved, the motive of financial gain may be proposed. In many such cases, neuropsychological examination has clearly indicated that the relative insensitivity of neurological evaluation may be a definite handicap in understanding the patient's impairment and in discerning the true circumstances. In fact, unless a patient with head injury shows positive signs on the neurological examination or definite EEG abnormalities, it is likely in clinical practice that a definite conclusion of "no brain damage" will be reached.

An example of the problem implicit in negative neurological findings in persons with closed head injuries was shown in the case of a graduate student in Speech and Hearing Sciences. This young woman had sustained a significant head injury, was unconscious for several weeks, but regained consciousness and had no positive neurological signs or EEG abnormalities. Therefore, a conclusion was reached that she had suffered some temporary brainstem impairment that resulted in a loss of consciousness but had no permanent brain injury with recovery of consciousness. She was advised to return to graduate school and resume her studies where she had left off. However, it soon became apparent to the patient that she did not have the academic aptitude or ability that she had before the injury. In fact, her professors also noticed that she did not do as well as she had before. Some of them leaned in the direction of the neurological findings, urging her to make greater efforts and do better. Other professors felt that she had sustained a brain injury and, in the patient's own words, began treating her like a "brain-injured child." These reactions were quite distressing, but her major problem was that she was not able to do as well in her courses as she had before and actually developed strong feelings of guilt because she had been told by specialists that she had not sustained any permanent injury.

Finally, neuropsychological examination was performed and showed clear and convincing evidence of cerebral damage, which provided a framework within which a realistic approach to the patient's problems could be developed. Recognition of her areas of deficit, together with counseling to overcome the adverse effects of the negative neurological findings, eventually helped the patient make realistic progress within the framework of her capabilities, both in terms of graduate school as well as in her self-image and personal assessment.

The subtle but very real deficits in higher-level brain functions that occur in many persons with closed head injuries are generally susceptible to a degree of spontaneous improvement in time (Dikmen & Reitan, 1976). However, there is a great deal of individual variability in the degree of spontaneous improvement. In addition, impairment before this improvement occurs can constitute a significant problem for the patient if he/she is encouraged to resume normal challenges and responsibilities prematurely. Finally, it is definitely advantageous to identify the particular kinds of deficits shown by a patient in complete detail, especially considering the developing possibilities for brain re-training. However, it is necessary to identify the areas of neuropsychological dysfunction that require retraining in order to develop a program that is appropriate to the patient's needs (Reitan & Wolfson, 1985).

# INFECTIONS OF THE BRAIN

In general, the brain and spinal cord are well protected against the entry of bacteria, viruses, fungi, and toxic substances by the skin, mucous membrane, muscle, bone, and meninges. The blood-brain barrier also functions to restrict entry of adverse substances to the brain. However, because antibody production within the nervous system is not particularly active or effective, and the passage of antibodies into the brain is hindered by the blood-brain barrier, relatively mild infections of the brain may develop into meningitis or brain abscesses. It appears that the mechanisms to counter infection within the brain are less effective than those existing elsewhere in the body. In addition, the cerebrospinal fluid is almost ideal as a culture medium for growth of infectious agents. Thus, once infections become established in the brain, they may constitute a significant clinical problem.

There are a number of ways in which brain infections may occur. Direct infection may be caused by penetrating wounds of the head. Although a rare occurrence, the cerebrospinal fluid may become infected through poor technique or use of contaminated needles during lumbar puncture. Direct infection may also occur without traumatic penetration by way of direct extension from nearby infections, such as sinusitis or mastoiditis. An infectious agent may enter the brain along nerve trunks or through the blood stream. Arterial supply may carry infectious agents or infection may occur by by-passing the blood-brain barrier through the choroid plexus into the cerebral spinal fluid. Finally, retrograde infection may occur through venous blood flow.

Infections of the brain may involve entry of bacteria, viruses, and fungi. Infections are frequently identified by (1) their anatomical location or the structures involved; (2) the type of virus; or (3) the type of infection. In this section we will briefly review epidural abscess, brain abscess, thromboses of the dural sinuses, cavernous sinus thrombosis, meningitis, neurosyphilis, fungal infections, and viral infections (including slow-virus infections).

## EPIDURAL ABSCESS

An abscess is a localized collection of pus. A cranial epidural abscess usually results from extension of an adjacent infection into the epidural space. The initial infection is often chronic sinusitis, acute or chronic mastoiditis, or osteomyelitis of the skull. These lesions are usually small because the dura mater is firmly attached to the inner table of the cranial cavity. However, this kind of infection may progress through various stages and become a brain abscess.

In some instances, an epidural abscess may become sufficiently large to cause headache, contralateral focal motor seizures, hemiparesis, drowsiness, stupor, and even papilledema. Cranial nerve involvement (especially signs of irritation of the fifth and sixth cranial nerves) may also be present.

Plain skull films may show areas of clouding of paranasal sinuses, indications of mastoid process infections, or changes suggesting osteomyelitis of the skull. Cerebrospinal fluid studies may also be abnormal. Computed tomography may reveal these lesions as an area of reduced density between the inner table of the skull and the brain.

## BRAIN ABSCESS

Brain abscess presents a difficult clinical problem. Mortality is high, but surgery can reduce the mortality significantly. A brain abscess presents the greatest danger to the patient not because of the infection but because of the related mass effect. An abscess is more likely to be fatal in patients who have progressed to a stage of brain stem compression before surgical drainage. One-third of patients die before surgery can be performed, either because of the disease's fulminant course or because the abscess is not diagnosed. Middle ear and mastoid infections used to be fairly common causes of brain abscesses, but there has been a definite reduction in their frequency. The incidence of brain abscess has decreased since the introduction and systematic use of antibiotic drugs. However, there is some current evidence that the incidence has stabilized or perhaps even shown a slight increase in recent years. Fig. 4–9 illustrates some of the characteristics of abscesses.

As noted above, a brain abscess may be caused by a direct spread from middle ear, sinus, or bone infections; bacteria entering the brain through cortical venous vessels carrying infection from the middle ear or the paranasal sinuses; osteomyelitis of the skull; infectious lesions of the skin of the face; or an abscess around an infected tooth. Penetrating wounds of the skull may be responsible for brain abscesses, particularly when foreign matter has been driven into the brain. Improved neurosurgical care and the use of antibiotics has reduced the incidence of such abscesses.

In cases of chronic pulmonary infections, septic material from the lungs may enter the pulmonary veins and, through systemic circulation, cause an abscess in the brain. Septic emboli may also arise directly from the heart in acute and subacute bacterial endocarditis. In congenital heart disease, emboli sometimes bypass the lungs, enter the aorta, and, through cerebral arterial circulation, cause brain abscesses. In many cases the etiology of the brain abscess is unknown, although symptoms of a space-occupying lesion of the brain are present. The abscess may be discovered during surgery for suspected brain tumor. Except for the abscesses of the temporal lobe as a complication of otitis media and in the cerebellum and brain stem resulting from mastoiditis, the most common sites of brain abscess are the frontal and parietal lobes. Eighty percent of brain abscesses occur in the cerebrum and 20% occur in the cerebellum. Brain stem and spinal cord abscesses are rare. A wide range of bacteria, fungi, yeasts and other organisms have been isolated from brain abscesses.

Brain abscesses that develop from either arterial or venous circulation generally begin at the junction of the gray and white matter. The infection spreads principally into the white matter and involves the gray matter less, probably because the white matter has a relatively poorer blood supply and a less rapid response to inflammation. Therefore, brain abscesses tend to be found deep within the hemisphere rather than immediately below the surface. The brain's first reaction to an abscess is edema and congestion. Central necrosis and liquifaction follows with the formation of pus. Various tissues proliferate to form a fibroglial capsule. When an abscess extends toward the cortex, meningitis results; when it extends toward the ventricles, ventriculitis results. Rupture into the ventricles is usually catastrophic.

Brain abscesses may occur at all ages but are commonly associated with congenital heart disease in children and adults between the ages of 20 and 50 years. The initial clinical manifestations may be quite varied depending principally upon the location of the abscess and its possible multi-focal nature. Focal neurologic deficits, seizures, or both will be seen in 30%-40% of patients. There is a 3:1 male predominance. Sometimes an abscess simulates a rapidly growing intrinsic tumor, such as a glioblastoma multiforme. In other cases (especially chronic brain abscess), there is little or no evidence of increased intracranial pressure, focal neurological deficits are well-defined, and the course appears to be slowly progressive. In such instances the abscess mimics some meningomas, slow growing astrocytomas, or subdural hematomas. There may be few localizing neurological signs, particularly if the abscess is in the anterior frontal or occipital area. The patient may show signs of rapidly increasing intracranial pressure, including headache, vomiting, obvious intellectual impairment, and severe papilledema.

The same symptoms also occur with multiple abscesses; focal and bilateral signs of neurological deficit and rapid progression of deterioration may also be present. EEG generally shows abnormal changes with marked focal slowing around the site of the abscess. Studies of cerebrospinal fluid are generally non-contributory. In fact, because of intracranial hypertension, lumbar puncture may be dangerous. Computed tomography is the most definitive procedure in diagnosis of brain abscesses.

Surgical treatment is usually necessary in order to drain the abscess. If the primary focus of infection can be identified, it should also be treated with appropriate antibiotics. Single abscesses can usually be treated successfully surgically and, in some early

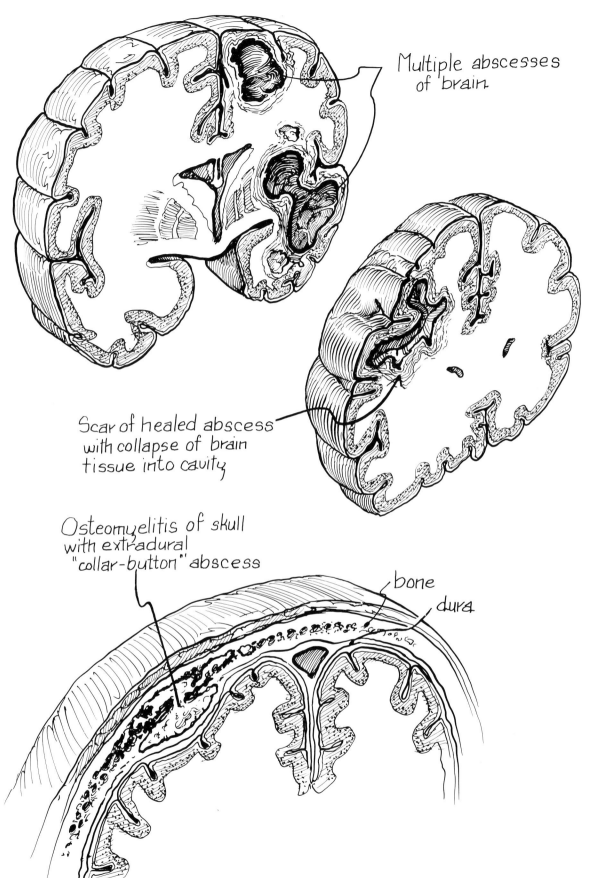

Multiple abscesses
of brain

Scar of healed abscess
with collapse of brain
tissue into cavity

Osteomyelitis of skull
with extradural
"collar-button" abscess

bone

dura

*Fig. 4–9.* Top: *Multiple abscesses of the brain are frequently metastatic and may develop from a lung abscess, osteomyelitis, or a urinary tract infection.*
Middle: *An abscess may cause disintegration of white matter and consequent collapse of brain tissue into the cavity.*
Bottom: *A "collar-button" abscess is caused by a thrombophlebitis spreading along the diploe and eroding the skull bone.*

cases in which central necrosis and abscess formation has not yet occurred, the infection may be resolved using aggressive antibacterial therapy. Abscesses are multiple in 5%-20% of cases. If a person has multiple abscesses or an abscess which has caused unconsciousness, the prognosis is very poor. Morbidity following a brain abscess is also a problem. One-half of the survivors will have neurologic symptoms. Paralysis is common, and seizures are seen in 30% of survivors.

## THROMBOSIS OF THE DURAL SINUSES AND CAVERNOUS SINUS THROMBOSIS

The dural sinuses are composed of strong, rigid layers of dura mater attached to the skull. They receive the venous drainage of the brain by way of the cerebral veins. A **thrombus** is an aggregation of blood factors (primarily platelets and fibrin) frequently causing vascular obstruction at the point of its formation. Thrombosis is the development of a thrombus. Thrombosis of the dural sinuses and cortical veins is usually a complication of infection of the scalp, skull, face, middle ear, mastoid air cells, paranasal sinuses, or nasopharynx, but may also occur in association with other conditions, such as heart disease and heart failure, conditions causing severe dehydration (e.g., fever), conditions related to hypercoagulation of the blood (occurring after some instances of surgery or childbirth), post-traumatic states following closed head injuries, cerebral arterial thrombosis or hemorrhage, and blood dyscrasias (particularly leukemia).

Clinical symptoms associated with thrombosis of the superior longitudinal (sagittal) sinus include many of the manifestations of intracranial disease, such as severe headache, seizures, hemiparesis or hemiplegia, homonymous hemianopia, dysphasia, confusion and loss of orientation. Thrombosis of the cavernous sinus has a highly characteristic clinical picture, largely because of the structures that pass through this sinus. The patient may complain of fever, headache, nausea and vomiting, and demonstrate signs of involvement of the third, fourth, sixth and the ophthalmic divisions of the fifth cranial nerves. If the ophthalmic veins are obstructed the patient may have edema of the orbit and eyelids with ptosis and edema of the surrounding periorbital structures. Obstruction of the venous return of blood from the eye may produce hemorrhage, edema of the retina, and papilledema with impairment or loss of vision. Involvement of these structures results in paralysis of the external eye muscles and pain in the eye which radiates over the area above the eye to the forehead and scalp. Initially there may be excess lacrimation; later this may be reduced and the cornea may be insensitive to pain. The thrombosis may spread through the intercavernous sinuses, resulting in bilateral cavernous sinus thrombosis and bilateral clinical manifestations.

## MENINGITIS

**Meningitis** is a condition of bacterial infection of the cerebrospinal fluid with inflammation of the pia mater and arachnoid tissue, the subarachnoid space and, to some degree, the superficial tissues of the brain. The spinal cord is also involved. Meningitis was fatal before the introduction of antibiotic drugs, but there has been a marked reduction in both mortality and morbidity.

Many different organisms have been identified in the production of acute purulent meningitis. These organisms seem to flourish in the cerebrospinal fluid because it provides an ideal culture medium. In addition, circulation of the cerebrospinal fluid spreads the infecting organisms throughout the subarachnoid space. Thus, although focal lesions may occur in some instances, the usual picture is one of general involvement of the central nervous system. There are striking differences in the bacteria associated with infection in different age ranges. The incidence of certain agents causing meningitis is higher in neonates and infants than children and adults. Even when comparing younger children with older children and adults the frequency of a particular bacteria causing meningitis varies. Over 70% of all cases of meningitis occur in children under five years of age (CDC, 1979). Twenty percent of cases occur in people over 70 years of age; only 10% occur in the ages between 5 and 70 years.

The infection may reach the brain by a number of routes, including direct implantation of bacteria (via an open head wound); direct extension from infectious processes of the middle ear, paranasal sinuses, the scalp, or the face; implantation through the blood stream by extension from cortical thrombophlebitis; extension from abscesses involving the extradural or subdural spaces or the brain tissue itself; and through access to the brain secondary to cerebrospinal fluid rhinorrhea (leakage of cerebrospinal fluid through the nose).

The infection in *acute bacterial meningitis* spreads rapidly through the subarachnoid space and the ventricular system and causes an acute inflammatory response. An inflammatory exudate accumulates in the cisterns around the base of the brain and may become particularly thick over the superior aspects of the convexities of the hemispheres, in the choroid plexus, and the lining of the walls of the ventricular system. This exudate causes the meninges to have a cloudy or milky appearance. A gradual obstruction of ventricular flow and absorption develops, leading to increased intracranial pressure and dilatation of the ventricular system, which may last for several weeks. Inflammation of arteries and veins may occur and cause thrombosis, edema in the vicinity of these vessels, and degeneration of neurons. Thus, in acute purulent meningitis, there is involvement of the brain tissue and the condition may be regarded as a superficial encephalitis.

The clinical onset is usually rapid; fever and headache are followed by drowsiness, confusion, and loss of consciousness. Nuchal rigidity is demonstrated in 80% of patients, though it is often absent in children. In some cases the onset may be slowly progressive over a period of several days with accompanying signs of upper respiratory tract infection. In other patients an acute onset of fever, headache, and nuchal rigidity may be followed by acute shock with hypotension and tachycardia due to an overwhelming septicemia (pathogenic bacteria and associated toxins in the blood).

Early diagnosis and prompt treatment using appropriate antibiotics are important determinants of the clinical course. The mortality and residual morbidity is greater in instances of pneumococcal meningitis and in patients who are severely ill at the time of admission to the hospital.

*Pneumococcal meningitis* is a type of purulent meningitis. Although it may occur at any age, it occurs principally among adults. There are a number of predisposing factors, including splenectomy, sickle cell disease, and conditions that produce an altered immune response. It may also be seen as a complication of otitis media, mastoiditis, or paranasal infections and debilitating conditions, such as chronic alcoholism. The mortality rate in this condition seems to be quite variable in different locations, ranging from 17% to 60% in various locations. This variability may well reflect differences in patient populations. For example, the mortality rate is very high in chronic alcoholics with pneumonia. Death is usually associated with acute hydrocephalus resulting from the inflammatory exudate.

*Meningococcal meningitis* generally occurs among persons living in confined and overcrowded conditions. Outbreaks in military camps, especially when people have been crowded together, have been reported and probably result from transmission of nasopharyngeal droplet infection. Infection of individuals may also occur in the winter months when there is an increased spread of infections of the upper respiratory tract. Many persons with these infections have an acute nasopharyngitis and septicemia may produce a mild systemic illness and a rash resembling rubella. Low-grade fever and mild systemic symptoms may persist for many weeks. However, if the patient develops acute purulent meningitis, there is usually a rapid onset with high fever, vomiting, stiff neck and symptoms of encephalitis, leading to coma. There is also a rash involving the skin and mucus membranes. Some patients may have a very rapid progression to coma, shock and death within 24 hours. The onset may be more gradual in other cases, and the prognosis is then considerably better.

Before the introduction of streptomycin in 1947, *tuberculous meningitis* invariably followed a fatal course, usually within about three months of onset. With the drugs currently in use, most patients recover. The best prognosis occurs among patients who, despite indications of meningeal irritation, do not lose consciousness or rational behavior and have no focal neurological signs or evidence of hydrocephalus. These patients nearly always recover with antituberculous therapy. Other patients become confused from the illness and have focal neurological signs, such as paresis of extraocular muscles or hemiparesis of the extremities. More than 80% of these patients appear to make a good recovery. When the illness causes stupor and coma or complete delirium, or if the patient has profound neurological deficits, the prognosis is poor. Less than 50% of these patients survive and residual and permanent brain damage may occur.

Tuberculous meningitis is found in persons with primary tuberculous infections elsewhere in the body, particularly in the lungs. The onset is gradual and is characterized by a low-grade fever, headache, and stiff neck. Children often appear to be listless and irritable, have a low-grade fever, and complain of fatigue, poor appetite, and vomiting. Adults frequently complain of malaise, weight loss, muscular pains (particularly in the back), low-grade fever and inability to concentrate. In some cases the degree of mental confusion is pronounced, with hallucinations, delusions, and uncontrolled excitatory behavior. Later the patient may become obtunded, irritable when aroused, and show signs of papilledema, cranial nerve palsies, mild hemiparesis and epileptic seizures.

Some patients with tuberculous infection develop *tuberculomas* (space-occupying lesions of the brain). Tuberculomas usually occur supratentorially (and are multiple in about 60% of patients), but may also occur in the cerebellum. These lesions may be diagnosed by computed tomography and treated by surgical excision and a full course of antituberculous treatment.

## Neurosyphilis

**Neurosyphilis** is a condition caused by invasion of the nervous system by *Treponema pallidum*. Syphilis may be divided into three stages: primary syphilis, secondary syphilis and syphilitic meningitis, and tertiary syphilis. In *primary syphilis*, although symptoms are not usually evident, there is a rapid dissemination of the *Treponema* throughout the body, probably including the central nervous system to some extent. *Acute syphilitic meningitis* occurs most commonly in the secondary stage but also has been observed to develop during the tertiary stage many years after the primary infection. Acute meningitis with secondary syphilis causes the usual symptoms of fever, headache, nausea, vomiting, cranial nerve palsies, rigidity of the neck, and occasional hyperactivity of deep tendon reflexes and extensor plantar responses. Patients may show striking mental changes, including delirium and confusion. In these cases the patient is probably suffering from encephalitis and inflammatory changes of the arteries in addition to meningitis.

Approximately 6%-7% of persons with untreated primary or secondary syphilis develop symptoms of neurosyphilis that may be divided into the following categories: chronic basal meningitis and meningovascular syphilis (about 38% of the cases), general paresis (about 32%), tabes dorsalis (about 27%) and gumma of the brain (about 3%). There has been a steady decline in the incidence of neurosyphilis, largely because of effective treatment of syphilis in the earlier stages.

**Chronic basal meningitis** due to syphilis is usually demonstrated by sudden onset of diplopia (due to involvement of the third and sixth cranial nerves), followed by paralysis of other cranial nerves. Trigeminal neuralgia and bilateral facial palsy may also be present together with eighth nerve signs of tinnitus, vertigo and deafness. Involvement of the tenth and twelfth cranial nerves may cause difficulty in swallowing and enunciating and wasting of the tongue muscles. The patient may have both chronic basal meningitis and syphilitic arteritis, with symptoms of occlusive thrombosis of blood vessels and infarction in the brain or brainstem. Such lesions may produce any of the focal signs usually associated with thrombosis of blood vessels of the brain.

**General paresis** is a condition characterized by progressive deterioration of the brain due to syphilitic infection. The condition may be viewed as a subacute encephalitis with diffuse thickening of the meninges, atrophy of the brain and dilatation of the ventricular system. Microscopic examination shows diffuse infiltration of the meninges with lymphocytes and plasma cells. The cerebral cortex shows a loss of neurons, proliferaton of astrocytes and an increase in microglial cells. A diffuse syphilitic arteritis is also present.

The onset of clinical manifestations of general paresis may be abrupt or gradual. The condition is characterized by progressive mental deterioration leading to dementia. Changes cover the entire range of mental functions, including loss of recent memory, impairment of judgement, changes in temperament and personality (including irritability, emotional lability, and manic episodes), deterioration of personal grooming, apathy and mental obtundity, and eventual disorientation with paranoid delusions or hallucinations. Physical signs include a coarse tremor, an increase of deep tendon reflexes, deterioration and slurring of speech, and generalized or focal seizures followed by a long period of post-ictal confusion.

**Tabes dorsalis** (locomotor ataxia) develops in about 25% of persons with neurosyphilis, although the frequency of new cases is definitely declining. The disease affects both the dorsal nerve roots and the posterior column of the spinal cord and is generally thought of as an effect of syphilis that is limited to the spinal cord. However, our experience in neuropsychological examination of patients with disorders supposedly limited to spinal cord functions suggests that there is a general element of central nervous system dysfunction, including the brain. The spinal cord of patients with tabes dorsalis shows thickening of the meninges, particularly in the dorsal regions, and atrophy of the dorsal nerve roots and posterior columns.

A number of clinical manifestations characterize tabes dorsalis. First, the patient often complains of sharp, stabbing pains, particularly involving the lower extremities but sometimes in other locations. These pains may develop years prior to other neurological symptoms. Patients with tabes dorsalis also experience sudden attacks of epigastric pain, nausea and vomiting, which may last from a few hours to several days. Locomotor ataxia usually begins before the diagnosis is definitely established. Patients have difficulty functioning in the dark or when their eyes are closed and may even lose their balance. Loss of tactile sensation in the feet and numbness or tingling in other areas of the body, particularly around the mouth, are not uncommon. A loss in bladder sensation and loss of reflex contraction of the bladder is sometimes seen. The contractile tone of the internal sphincter eventually decreases and results in urinary incontinence. A loss of sensation and reflex activity of the genital organs occurs in both males and females, leading to a diminution of interest in sexual activity.

Other infectious conditions, probably of an infective nature, sometimes affect the nervous system. They include conditions such as sarcoidosis, adhesive arachnoiditis, tetanus, brucellosis and psittacosis.

## FUNGAL AND PARASITIC DISEASES

Parasitic and fungal diseases are among the most common illnesses in the entire world and constitute an enormous health problem. At any one time, these diseases afflict hundreds of millions of people and are the cause of death of an estimated three million persons annually.

Parasitic and fungal diseases usually produce initial symptoms that involve pulmonary and gastrointestinal functions; the brain is rarely the first organ to be affected.

In parasitic diseases the body (host) is invaded by an organism which then lives upon or within the body tissues. Use of the term "parasitic disease" has usually implied that these organisms are either protozoa or helminths (worms). Fungi are common in the environment although relatively few are pathogenic.

A great number of fungal and parasitic infections which may invade the central nervous system have been identified. Fungal infections include aspergillosis, cryptococcosis, histoplasmosis, actinomycosis, mucormycosis, cerebral nocardiosis, coccidioidomycosis, blastomycosis, candidiasis, and clodosporiosis.

There are many parasitic infections of the central nervous system, including toxoplasmosis, cerebral amebiasis, cerebral malaria, cysticercosis, trypanosomiasis, and a number of diseases caused by invasion of the larval stages of trematodes and nematodes such as echinococcosis, schistosomiasis, paragonimiasis, trichinosis, and angiostrongyliasis.

Only a few of these diseases will be described in this chapter.

*Cryptococcus neoformans* is a yeastlike organism that causes **cryptococcosis**. This organism produces an infection of the lungs, kidneys, lymph nodes, and may also invade the central nervous system of man. Prior to 1956, the year effective drug treatment became available, meningitis associated with the condition was almost invariably fatal. The organism is apparently inhaled with dust and enters the body through the respiratory system. The organism has been isolated from feces of sparrows and pigeons. Clinical manifestations of cerebral involvement with this disease, which are usually gradual in onset, include headache, nausea, and vomiting. In addition, the patient develops unsteadiness of gait, extreme sensitivity to light (photophobia), blurred vision, and pain behind the eyes. Fever and stiff neck occur in only about 50% of the cases. As the disease progresses there may be psychological manifestations including impaired memory, agitation and uncontrolled behavior, and personality changes. Cranial nerve dysfunction, papilledema, and changes in deep tendon reflexes are among the later findings.

Despite the fact that several effective pharmacological agents have been identified and the number of deaths has been strikingly reduced, the mortality rate still approaches 40%. An additional group of patients (about 25%) suffers relapses following chemotherapy.

**Histoplasmosis** is a widely distributed mycotic (fungal) infection that appears to be world-wide in its distribution but is most heavily endemic in the midwestern United States. The majority of cases are asymptomatic. The disease is usually confined to the lungs but when it becomes disseminated the likelihood of involvement of the central nervous system is increased to a 10%-25% incidence.

Probably about 95% of persons who develop histoplasmosis have a relatively mild illness which resembles viral infection and is characterized by fever, coughing, and sometimes chest pain. Recovery, even without treatment, generally occurs in 10 to 14 days. Another form of the disease, usually limited to the lungs, may produce definite pulmonary symptoms and resembles tuberculosis. Cerebral involvement produces symptoms that are similar to a number of mycotic infections. Indications of meningitis (headache, nuchal rigidity, and possibly seizures) may occur; occasionally the patient will show signs of a mass lesion affecting the brain with typical focal neurological signs.

Despite aggressive therapeutic procedures, a mortality rate approaching 25% occurs with infection of the central nervous system. The central nervous system component of histoplasmosis is manifested as meningitis and the resulting obstructive hydrocephalus may persist long after the actual infection is overcome. Deaths from histoplasmosis occur most commonly in adults in the older age ranges and infants.

**Aspergillosis** is a disease caused by only a few of the large number of species of the *Aspergillus* group. The disease is found principally in persons who have contact with dust, grain, birds, and animals. Although cerebral involvement is rare, aspergillosis is still one of the more commonly encountered mycotic infections of the central nervous system. The fungus enters the body through the respiratory tree and may involve only the respiratory system or become disseminated to various sites, including the skin, kidney, brain, gastrointestinal tract, and eye. Brain involvement in the acute disseminated form usually occurs in infants and may progress rapidly to death. The more chronic form, which may affect people of any age, sometimes presents with symptoms and signs suggesting a brain tumor or brain abscess; other patients have headache, neck pain, and cranial involvement suggesting meningitis. The infection may involve arteries, producing inflammation that may lead to aneurysms, subarachnoid hemorrhage, or thrombosis of the internal carotid or middle cerebral arteries.

As noted above, a large number of parasitic diseases may also involve the central nervous system with the infections due to protozoa and helminths. **Toxoplasmosis** is one of the most common protozoan infections in human beings. This disease is caused by *Toxoplasma gondii*, an intracellular parasite dependent upon its host for life, and may produce a wide spectrum of diseases in both mammals and birds. However, the vast majority of toxoplasmic infections in human beings do not produce symptoms and show no evidence of corresponding clinical disease. However, when a pregnant woman becomes infected with toxoplasmosis the organism may be transmitted to the fetus through the placenta and can result in severe damage to the developing brain. The majority of these children survive but often are mentally retarded. After having been infected with toxoplasmosis and transmitting the disease congenitally to a child, the mother is immune and infection of any future children through the placenta will not occur.

The clinical manifestations do not form a consistent picture. In some instances the course is very rapid, and may lead to death as a result of encephalitis. Other cases follow a protracted and chronic course. Most patients with brain involvement show some degree of impairment of alertness, confusion, and even partial or complete coma. Meningeal signs of headache, stiff neck, and seizures sometimes occur. Various focal neurological deficits are present in more than 50% of these patients.

Most patients with toxoplasmosis of the brain do not survive unless they are treated. The prognosis is improved if diagnosis is prompt and chemotherapy is started early. However, patients who are debilitated and have a depressed immuno-response system have

more serious illnesses, a more rapid course, and a prognosis that is less encouraging.

**Cerebral malaria** is another condition that occurs in association with infection by the malarial parasite, occurring in 1%-2% of patients with this illness. Patients who develop cerebral infection have usually had symptoms of malaria for more than a week and then suddenly have a pronounced relapse with high fever, disorientation, confusion, and at least somewhat impaired consciousness. Sometimes these symptoms are immediately preceded by a generalized epileptic seizure. The patient may develop stupor followed by coma and may have a variety of symptoms of brain involvement, including hemiparesis, hemisensory loss, unilateral hyperactivity of deep tendon reflexes and other signs. Complete neurological recovery is expected in most patients who are given prompt and adequate therapy.

Several species of amebae may infect human beings but only one is considered pathogenic and causes **amebiasis**. Hepatopulmonary and intestinal forms of the disease are relatively common, but cerebral involvement is rare. Development of amebiasis nearly always requires ingestion of the cystic form of the organism and persons living under non-hygienic conditions develop this disease most frequently. Many patients are asymptomatic. The disease is often characterized by dysentery with diarrhea, weakness and prostration. Antibiotics are often effective in the acute stages.

**Trypanosomiasis** is a disease that has two major types — the African and the American diseases. African trypanosomiasis is often referred to as sleeping sickness. Both of these diseases are parasitic and cause extensive neuronal damage and serious neurological consequences.

A number of parasitic diseases are caused by infestation with the larval stage of worms. **Cysticercosis** is such a disease and, when the brain is involved, may show dramatic clinical manifestations. The disease is caused by the pork tapeworm and infection rates are highest among populations whose dietary habits include eating raw or inadequately cooked pork that contains the larvae of the organism. Fruits and vegetables may also be contaminated with the organism. The onset of clinical symptoms may take a considerable period of time after ingestion of the organism; symptoms may begin within months of infection or may be delayed for years, averaging a period of about five years. Studies have suggested that 80% of infected persons will show symptoms within seven years. No specific treatment is available though certain experimental studies have noted promising results. The prognosis is poor because the majority of brain lesions are multiple and not amenable to operative excision. Thus, the usual clinical course is one of progressive deterioration and eventual death.

**Echinococcosis** is an infection caused by the larval stage of the dog tapeworm, *Taenia echinococcus*. It is believed that the disease is contracted through direct contact with feces of dogs but the usual hosts may also include wolves and foxes. Cattle, sheep, hogs, and human beings may serve as intermediate hosts. Involvement of the central nervous system is relatively rare and healthy individuals may be protected by the normal defense mechanisms of the body. Debilitated persons, however, develop symptoms of the infection much more readily. Cerebral echinococcosis is much more predominant in children than adults. The organism produces cysts in various organs of the body, including the liver, lungs, and brain. Cysts of the brain are more common in the white matter than the gray. The clinical manifestations include signs of increased intracranial pressure (headache, vomiting, and papilledema) and, as the disease progresses, mental changes and the complete range of focal signs of both cerebral and cerebellar involvement. Seizures occur in approximately 10% of children with brain infections and are even more frequent in adults. In addition, the course of the disease is more rapid among adults than in children.

The prognosis is variable depending upon factors such as the number of cystic lesions and the location and size of the lesion(s). However, most lesions are single and a total surgical removal, using meticulous technique and the utmost care to avoid further con-

tamination and remove the cyst completely, can be accomplished.

**Schistosomiasis** refers to an infection caused by trematodes, also known as blood flukes because they inhabit the circulatory system. These worms can produce lesions throughout the human body, including the brain and spinal cord. Many mammals, including man, can be affected. The organisms are excreted in urine or feces. When these eggs find their way into fresh water they invade certain snails and then are transformed into their infective larval form. If direct contact with the larvae is made while bathing, swimming, or working in infected water, the larvae are capable of penetrating human skin. This disease is primarily endemic to Africa, South America and Asia, and may involve nearly 90% of certain indigenous populations. Schistosomiasis principally infects young people and children; the average age is less than 30 years. Central nervous system involvement with schistosomiasis, estimated to affect 2%-4% of the patients with the disease, is relatively rare. Additional evidence suggests that even when the eggs are present in the brain, possibly more than half of the patients will remain asymptomatic.

Usually, acute cerebral manifestations initially appear with signs of meningitis and encephalopathy, including headache, pyramidal tract symptoms, disturbances of alertness, and personality changes.

**Trichinosis** is caused by the invasion of the larval form of *Trichinella spiralis*. The majority of human infections of this nematode can be traced to eating inadequately cooked pork and pork products, although hosts other than pigs have also been implicated (rabbits, walruses, foxes, and bears). Usually, trichinosos is first manifested by onset of gastrointestinal symptoms which appear within 48 hours of ingestion of the infected meat. Central nervous system involvement is estimated to occur in 6%-17% of patients having gastrointestinal symptoms of the disease. The most frequent clinical presentation is that of a localized encephalitis with varying degrees of meningitis. Headache, neck pain, and impairment of alertness and cognitive ability characterize the early stages of the disease and cranial nerve deficits may be noted as the disease progresses. Without treatment there is progression of neurological deficits, including focal signs and severe generalized motor dysfunction. Treatment with corticosteroids often produces dramatic improvement, shown not only in central nervous system symptoms but in other systems as well. The longer the central nervous system phase of the disease persists without treatment, the more significant the morbidity and the higher the mortality rate. With early, appropriate, and effective treatment, the mortality rate is negligible.

Many other parasitic and fungal infections, some of which invade the brain and spinal cord, have been described. The interested reader is referred to Baker (1970), and Trelles (1978) for further information and detailed descriptions.

## VIRAL ENCEPHALITIDES

The **viral encephalitides** is a group of diseases in which there is direct invasion of the central nervous system and the meninges by any of a large number of identified viruses. St. Louis encephalitis is the most common viral encephalitis in the United States and over the years outbreaks have occurred in the southwestern, south central, and southeastern states. This virus was isolated from the brain in 1933 and confirmed by isolation of the virus from the mosquito in 1941. Since that time a large number of additional viruses which cause other forms of encephalitis have been isolated. In the majority of cases of encephalitis it is possible to identify the virus through serologic tests and tissue culture methods using human cell tissue culture specimens of cerebrospinal fluid, blood, urine, feces, and throat flora.

The pathological changes in viral encephalitis include destruction or damage to neurons; the presence of intranuclear inclusion bodies (one type of inclusion body is seen in neurons and oligodendroglial cells and another type in anterior horn cells of the spinal cord); and edema and inflammation of the brain and spinal cord with cuffing of polymorphonuclear leukocytes and lymphocytes around blood vessels. There is also inflammation of small blood vessels (angitis) with thrombosis and proliferation of astrocytes and microglia. Often there is wide-spread destruction of the white matter by both the inflammatory process and thrombosis of blood vessels.

Gilroy and Meyer (1979) indicate that there are two distinct syndromes caused by viral infections of the brain, identified as **aseptic meningitis** and **encephalitis**. *Meningitis* refers principally to inflammation of the meninges; *encephalitis* implies viral invasion of the tissue of the brain and spinal cord. Aseptic meningitis can result from infection by a wide variety of viruses and results in a mild inflammation of the meninges. Any of the viruses that invade the central nervous system can probably give rise to aseptic meningitis, but the most common viruses are Coxsackie B, mumps, ECHO and lymphocytic choriomeningitis viruses. The onset may be sudden or gradual; there is moderate elevation of temperature, headache, stiff neck, vomiting, and a general feeling of illness and weakness which usually lasts about 10 days. There is no specific treatment for aseptic meningitis except for the use of analgesics (particularly to control headache) and bedrest. Intravenous fluids may be necessary if there is a significant degree of vomiting (and consequent dehydration). Full recovery usually occurs within a period of a few days to a few weeks, although some patients complain of fatigue and malaise for a few months after the illness.

A large number of viruses which cause encephalitis have been identified. Among those that infect human beings, it is conventional to differentiate them into those carried by arthropods and those that are not. In addition, "slow virus infections," in which the infection continues and produces progressive disability over a period of many months or years, have been recognized. These infections were first clearly demonstrated in a disease known as *kuru*, and have also been demonstrated in Jakob-Creutzfeldt disease and subacute sclerosing panencephalitis (in which a measles or measles-like virus has been isolated). There is no effective treatment for these slow viral infections and, over the period of months, the course of the disease often progresses to death.

Some viral agents cause very severe and rapidly progressive signs and symptoms which may lead to death; others cause only mild or even subclinical infections. Of course, with any particular type of virus, variability among individual patients also occurs. In viral illnesses the onset is usually rather abrupt. The patient develops a high fever, headaches, drowsiness, irritability, and possible obtundity, stupor, or coma. Nuchal rigidity and muscle pains are common. Frequently, the patient also has nausea and episodes of vomiting. Epileptic seizures are not uncommon and motor deficits and cranial nerve palsies may also be present. There is a tendency among neurologists to feel that many patients with viral encephalitis recover completely in time; however, residual neurological deficits are definitely noted in some patients. It is not uncommon to find clear evidence of neuropsychological impairment of cerebral functions even when the results of the neurological examination are negative.

The arthropod-borne viruses are carried by mosquitoes and ticks and may infect human beings. There are a number of types of viruses. Mosquito-borne viruses include Western equine encephalitis, Eastern equine encephalitis (usually considerably more severe than the Western variety), Venezuelan equine encephalitis, St. Louis encephalitis, Japanese B encephalitis, West Nile encephalitis, Murray Valley (Australian X) encephalitis, yellow fever, dengue, and California encephalitis. Tick-borne encephalitis is caused by the bite of an infected tick or by drinking infected goat's milk. A number of viruses may be responsible. Illness may range from minimal symptoms to severe illness and death. When the illness is severe, diffuse brain damage may result in those who survive.

A considerable number of additional viruses have been identified, including rabies, poliomyelitis, coxsackie A, coxsackie B, herpes simplex, herpes zoster, ECHO, mumps, measles, encephalomyocarditis, infectious mononucleosis, influenza, infectious hepatitis, and others.

**Rabies** is a viral infection transmitted through the bite of a rabid animal. These are usually dogs, but bats, weasles, skunks, wolves, cats, jackals, foxes, squirrels, racoons, and ermine have all been identified as being capable of infecting human beings. The virus is communicated along peripheral nerves from the point of entry to the central nervous system and produces an encephalomyelitis. The entire brain and spinal cord are involved in inflammatory changes; the dorsal root ganglia and the brain stem particularly are highly infected. Relatively less inflammation tends to occur in the cerebral cortex, hippocampus, and the cerebellum.

The incubation period is usually 21 to 60 days. The first signs of the disease often include increased pain and numbness at the site of the bite, fever, and a general feeling of malaise. Next, the patient often becomes hypersensitive to stimuli, such as noise or light touch. The patient also begins excessive sweating, salivation, lacrimation, and constriction of the pupils. The pharyngeal muscles spasmodically contract on contact with fluid, and a forceful expulsion occurs when the patient attempts to drink. Muscular involvement may cause respiratory arrest and cyanosis. Seizures are common, and although death may occur at this stage, the patient usually progresses into a state of apathy, stupor, and coma before expiring.

Rabies is usually fatal and no specific treatment is available after the disease has developed. However, supportive care has lead to survival and apparent recovery in some cases. The most effective treatment is vaccination before the clinical symptoms develop. Thus, it is important that the animal be kept under observation for about 10 days if there is any suspicion of rabies. If the animal is still healthy at the end of that time, the bitten person does not require vaccination. In earlier forms of vaccine, there was sometimes a devastating post-rabies vaccine encephalomyelitis that occurred. However, a duck embryo vaccine is now available and serious reactions are extremely rare.

**Herpes simplex encephalitis** constitutes about 10% of cases of viral encephalitis in the United States and appears to be increasing in frequency. This disease affects all age groups. In older children and adults it is not uncommon for one side of the brain to be considerably more involved than the other. This is a severe infection and terminates in death within a few weeks in about 80% of the cases. If recovery does occur there usually are marked neurological deficits. Pathological changes in the brain are characteristic of viral encephalitis. The clinical picture is similar to other viral infections causing encephalitis, but develops quite rapidly and causes severe symptoms and early neurological manifestations. No specific medication is available and treatment is mainly supportive, consisting principally of attempts to control intracranial pressure caused by edema.

**Herpes zoster** (shingles) and **varicella** (chicken-pox) are caused by the same virus. It appears that herpes zoster is a long-term result of latent reactivation of earlier exposure or illness with varicella or represents a new infection by the virus in a patient who is only partly immune. A viral encephalomyelitis which follows varicella may occur 1 to 21 days after the rash. Lethargy, seizures, headache, and nuchal rigidity are the characteristic symptoms. With evidence of cerebral involvement, the mortality is about 35%. When symptoms are referable to cerebellar infection (lethargy, headache, ataxia, nystagmus, scanning speech and nuchal rigidity) the prognosis is much better.

Either sex may be affected by herpes zoster. This disease is rare in children. The posterior ganglia are particularly involved and the disease causes pain and a vesicular skin eruption in the sensory distribution of affected nerves.

**Infectious mononucleosis** is very probably caused by viral infection and consists of a mild febrile illness, sore throat, and involvement of the lymph glands. Enlargement of the spleen and a rash may be present. Only about 5% of cases show evidence of involvement of the central nervous system. Usually the indications of brain involvement are relatively mild, but cases have been reported in which the onset was abrupt and included seizures, focal signs of cerebral damage, cranial nerve palsies, vertigo, slurring of speech, cerebellar ataxia and other brain stem signs, spinal cord involvement causing paraplegia, and progression to stupor and coma.

**Coxsackie viral infections** (Types both A and B) occur predominantly in children. Type A infection may cause aseptic meningitis, acute cerebellar ataxia, convulsions on one side of the body followed by hemiplegia and possible permanent motor deficit. Type B viruses also cause aseptic meningitis with an overall clinical picture very similar to poliomyelitis. Although deaths have been reported with extensive damage of the nervous system, most patients improve rapidly.

**Cytomegalovirus infection** (salivary gland virus) produces a systemic disease of newborn infants and causes severe brain damage. If the child survives to the age of 6 months, mental retardation and microcephaly are often observed.

The incidence of **poliomyelitis** has been greatly reduced since a vaccine was developed in 1953. Poliomyelitis virus produces subclinical infection in most patients. In fact, 95% of infected persons show no significant symptoms; systemic infection is present in 3%; aseptic meningitis in 1%; and paralytic poliomyelitis in 1%. When the brain is involved there is an initial inflammatory response in the meninges resembling aseptic meningitis. The virus shows a strong predilection for motor neurons of the spinal cord, the motor nuclei of the brain stem, neurons of the substantia nigra, hypothalamus, and cerebellar nuclei, and sometimes the precentral gyri (motor area) of the frontal cortex. The percentage of patients with poliomyelitis who had apparent cerebral involvement was always low, but fortunately the incidence has been reduced even further with use of vaccines.

Over 40 types of **ECHO viruses** have been identified. Infants and children are particularly susceptible to infection. These viruses usually cause a febrile illness that may be accompanied by a skin rash, infantile diarrhea, and upper respiratory infections. When the nervous system is involved the child may show evidence of aseptic meningitis. The virus seems to have a predilection for the brainstem and cerebellum and cerebellar signs and ataxia are common clinical manifestations.

**Measles encephalitis** is reported to occur in only about 1 of 1,000 cases of measles. However, this is very probably an underestimate. EEG abnormalities, for example, have been reported in about 50% of patients with measles (Pampiglione, 1964).

When measles encephalitis develops it usually appears on the fourth or fifth day following the onset of the rash. The initial fever (which may have subsided) returns and the patient complains of headache and shows evidence of cranial nerve palsies, dystonic movement disorders, cerebellar involvement, and hyperactivity of deep tendon reflexes. The mortality rate is about 10% and, among those who survive, many show evidence of cerebral damage and post-encephalitic epilepsy.

The **mumps virus** usually produces an infection of the salivary glands about 18 to 21 days after exposure. In addition, the virus may infect the testes and surrounding tissues, prostate, ovaries, thyroid, pancreas, and the nervous system. In the majority of cases, the nervous system infection is subclinical. A small percentage of these patients develop symptoms of aseptic meningitis with headache, stiff neck, and a mild degree of confusion. The prognosis in mumps encephalitis is usually good.

There is a group of microorganisms, parasitic in arthropods, that sometimes infect man. These include *epidemic typhus* (louse vector), *scrub typhus* (mite vector), *murine typhus* (rat flea vector), and *Rocky Mountain spotted fever* (tick vector). These rickettsial diseases almost invariably invade the nervous system and cause particular damage to the endothelium of small blood vessels, which become swollen and thrombosed. Degenerative changes of nerve cells in the vicinity of the occulsion occur secondary to diminution of blood supply. Glial scars may be scattered throughout the nervous system after this illness, and are caused by astrocytic proliferation within the damaged tissues.

The **typhus infections** include the characteristic signs of encephalitis (severe headache, mental dullness, delirium, stupor, coma, and nuchal rigidity). In addition, seizures, involuntary movements, hemi-

plegia, and deafness may also result. Although there may be recovery of these specific deficits, generalized impairment is frequently present as a residual effect.

**Rocky Mountain spotted fever** is now found throughout the United States and is increasing in frequency. Two-thirds of the patients are children. Infected patients usually show evidence of fever, rash, headache, gastrointestinal symptoms, prostration, and muscle pains. The rash, which begins on the third or fourth day, involves the ankles and wrists and spreads to the palms and soles of the feet. The rash then progresses up the limbs and may finally involve the body and face. Both the general and focal neurological signs associated with encephalitis are frequently present. The mortality rate with rickettsial diseases previously was high, but has been considerably reduced with the use of antibiotic and steroid therapy supplemented by good supportive care.

**Cat-scratch disease**, believed to be caused by a virus, is manifested by fever, skin lesions, and tenderness of lymph glands. Encephalitis, though uncommon, may follow the initial illness in 1 to 5 weeks. The onset with seizures and coma is usually abrupt, although the illness is relatively brief and recovery is usually complete in a neurological sense. However, the patient may continue to complain of at least mild neurological deficits for several months.

As mentioned earlier, slow virus infections have been clearly established in several conditions including kuru, Jakob-Creutzfeldt disease, and measles. **Subacute sclerosing panencephalitis** follows a history of measles infection in early childhood. Pathological changes of the brain are diffuse, involving both gray and white matter. Many patients show a fairly rapid progression with a mean of nine months from onset of the disease to death. Other patients show a more chronic course, with instances of remission that may even last for several years only to be followed by a relapse and further progression. The incidence of SSPE is very low, and may be even further reduced through effective use of measles vaccination.

For many years **Jakob-Creutzfeldt** disease was classified as a degenerative disease of the nervous system in which deterioration was extremely rapid and death usually occurred within a few months to 1-2 years. Recently, research studies have demonstrated that this condition can be transmitted to laboratory animals. Transmission from one human being to another has also been recorded, suggesting that the disease is caused by a viral infection.

Persons with Jakob-Creutzfeldt disease show widespread damage in the central nervous system and a number of concomitant symptoms. The earliest signs are usually lapses of memory which progress to include confusion, dysphasia, and deterioration in personal grooming. Several types of the disease have been identified, but they vary principally in prominence and severity of one kind of symptom compared with another.

Customarily, the patient develops a fixed facial expression, stooped gait, and a parkinsonian type of tremor. Cerebellar signs, including ataxia, slurring of words, and an intention tremor are frequently present. Myoclonic jerks, choreiform movements, spasticity, rigidity, and seizures may also occur. Some patients show pronounced signs of involvement of the occipital cortex with a number of manifestations of visual deficit which may lead to complete cortical blindness. Because of evidence that human-to-human transmission occurs, all patients who are suspected of having Jakob-Creutzfeldt disease should be kept in isolation, using septic precautions and isolation procedures. No specific treatment has been developed and the only treatment that can be given is directly oriented toward relief of symptoms.

There are many other viral diseases in which the infectious organism may invade the nervous system. It is apparent, however, that most patients with viral illnesses do not have central nervous system complications. It is likely that viral infections of the brain are under-diagnosed and that neurological examination is insufficient to elicit evidence of cerebral impairment in many cases, even when it has occurred. Aguilar and Rasmussen (1960), for example, have shown the presence of typical encephalitic pathological changes in patients subjected to surgical anterior temporal lobe excision for treatment of epilepsy, even though the clinical history of the patient did not include identification or diagnosis of encephalitis. The reader who is interested in additional details regarding the neurological aspects of viral encephalitis is referred to Baker (1962) and Fields and Blattner (1958).

# DEMYELINATING DISEASES
## INCLUDING MULTIPLE SCLEROSIS

If demyelinating diseases are defined as conditions in which there is breakdown or deterioration of myelin, a number of diseases can be included in this category, even though the degree of neuronal damage varies. Multiple sclerosis fits the category most closely if the definition requires injury and deterioration of myelin with preservation of axons. In a more general definition, however, the category would include the leukodystrophies, lipid storage diseases, acquired allergic and infectious diseases that result in breakdown of myelin, a group of viral diseases, and a group of degenerative diseases (Gilroy & Meyer, 1979).

The **leukodystrophies** include a number of familial diseases which occur most commonly in infancy and childhood as well as conditions resulting in abnormal metabolism and formation of myelin. These diseases are associated with a degree of destruction of axons, relative preservation of nerve cells, and absence of inflammation.

The most common of these conditions is **metachromatic leukodystrophy (MLD)**, an inherited autosomal recessive trait characterized by a genetically determined enzymatic defect. In the relatively adult form of this disease the patient shows a gradual intellectual deterioration, episodes of moodiness and withdrawal, possible delusions and hallucinations, and outbursts of rage. This condition is frequently given a psychiatric diagnosis incorrectly. Because leukodystrophies are quite rare we will not discuss them in detail in this volume.

**Lipid storage diseases** with cerebromacular degeneration were previously referred to as "amaurotic familial idiocies." **Cerebromacular degeneration** results from accumulation of lipid in the ganglion cells of the retina. The fovea is usually free of ganglion cells and appears as a dark purple or cherry red spot. Other diseases in this category, previously described on the basis of age of onset and clinical symptomatology, are now identified in terms of the chemistry of the stored material or by the enzyme deficiency which represents the metabolic abnormality. Conditions affecting lipid storage occur very rarely in adults.

**Tay-Sachs disease** is the result of an enzyme deficiency that leads to accumulation of material in the neurons of the retina and central nervous system. This disease causes a deterioration of myelin and neurochemical changes in the structure of myelin. Tay-Sachs is an inherited disease with onset nearly always in infancy. The child is normal at birth but by the age of six months demonstrates a typical triad of symptoms: (1) cherry red macula; (2) an exaggerated startle response to sound; and (3) psychomotor arrest. Speech is rarely attained. The child's vision deteriorates into wandering nystagmus and eventually blindness results. Convulsions usually develop in the child's second year; death usually occurs by the age of three.

**Niemann-Pick disease** is a sphingomyelin lipidosis, a rare condition probably inherited as an autosomal recessive trait. There are several forms of the disease, differing in the degree of enzyme impairment, the age of onset, and the degree of nervous system involvement. This disease usually begins at about six months of age and is characterized by atrophy and widening of sulci without ventricular dilatation. It is clinically manifested by progressive dementia and blindness with eventual complete unresponsiveness. Most affected children die by the age of four years.

A number of other diseases which attack myelin have been associated with viral infections, including postvaccinal encephalomyelitis, postinfectious encephalomyelitis and postinfectious polyneuropathy (Guillain-Barré syndrome). In addition, diseases such as subacute sclerosing panencephalitis (SSPE), which appears to be due to a measles virus, and other viral encephalitides (including herpes virus) are associated with demyelinization. Still other demyelinating diseases show a rather progressive degenerative course and may be associated with systemic diseases. Thus, it is clear that demyelination as a prominent feature characterizes the pathological nature of a considerable range of inherited and environmentally induced illnesses.

## MULTIPLE SCLEROSIS

Multiple sclerosis (MS) is a disease in which there are areas of demyelination scattered throughout the brain and spinal cord. The symptoms of multiple sclerosis are extremely variable because of the widespread nature of the lesions. This variability of symptoms, and indications of a disseminated disease of the central nervous system, are major factors characterizing the illness. There is also a definite tendency for the signs and symptoms to relapse and remit in multiple sclerosis. Because the cause of multiple sclerosis is unknown (although a number of theories exist), no specific treatment is available and current treatment is aimed toward relief of symptoms. In general, the course of the disease is progressive, although there is great variability in this respect.

Although multiple sclerosis is the most common of the demyelinating diseases, it still affects only 50-60 persons per 100,000 population. This illness is somewhat more common in women than in men and is known as a disease of the young adult. It is rarely seen in persons below 15 years of age, occurs with greatest frequency in about the 30-35 year age interval, and is diagnosed infrequently in older adults.

Epidemiological studies have indicated that multiple sclerosis is more common in some geographic areas than others. The prevalence appears to be highest in Europe and the northern hemisphere in latitudes between 65 degrees and 45 degrees north. An increased incidence is again noted between the same latitudes in the southern hemisphere, covering New Zealand and southern Australia. There also appears to be some racial factors. Multiple sclerosis has been reported to be relatively rare in Japan and extremely rare in Korea, and to have a lower frequency among Japanese Americans than the rest of the U.S. population. Racial and geographic differences have suggested the possibility that certain foods may contribute to the development of multiple sclerosis, but this hypothesis has not been established.

A familial connection is suggested by findings that the risk of developing multiple sclerosis is increased about 20 times over that of the general population if a sibling has the disease and about 12 times if a parent is affected. About 10% of patients with multiple sclerosis have a positive family history. If one member of identical twins has the disease, there is a 20%-25% chance that the other twin will develop the disease. Among fraternal twins, however, the likelihood is reduced to 15%. Although results of this kind suggest the possibility of some genetic influences, it must also be remembered that the probability of infection by a common agent might also be increased among twins and among other family members.

A number of additional factors have been suggested as being influential in the development of multiple sclerosis. Both trauma and allergic reactions have been implicated as causes of MS in some patients. However, these factors have not been substantiated or confirmed. Clinical reports have suggested that the relapse rate in women who already have multiple sclerosis is increased during pregnancy. There appears to be some increase during the first three months after the birth of a child, but the data are variable. Although some patients have reported that their symptoms increase in hot weather or when they take a hot bath, changes in temperature generally do not seem to be a significant factor.

Etiological factors in multiple sclerosis have not been identified and theories outnumber facts. However, at the present time the principal theories include the postulates that multiple sclerosis is a result of a slow virus infection, an autoimmune deficiency, or a combination of both. The existence of viruses that produce symptomatology and degenerative changes months or years after the infection has been acquired has been well established in the disease known as kuru, both in transmission among human beings and to other primates. As noted in the chapter on infectious diseases, slow-virus infections also produce subacute sclerosing panencephalitis (SSPE), progressive multifocal leukoencephalopathy and Jakob-Creutzfeldt disease. A number of the pathological and biochemical characteristics, as well as the epidemiologic factors and the course of the disease, would be compatible with a theory of viral infection. The autoimmune theory also has support, particularly derived from development of an experimental animal model of allergic encephalomyelitis that has relapsing characteristics (Raine & Stone, 1977). There is some evidence of altered cellular immunity in multiple sclerosis which could be related to the destruction of myelin (Knight, 1977). The two theories may be integrated by recognizing that a viral infection may initiate an autoimmune reaction.

Although the brain usually appears grossly normal in acute cases of multiple sclerosis, some atrophy of the cerebrum may be present in chronic multiple sclerosis. Areas of demyelination are scattered throughout the white matter with invasion of the adjacent cerebral cortex. Although the plaques of demyelination occur rather generally, they are predominantly found around the ventricles. Lesions in the brain stem have their greatest frequency around the cerebral aqueduct (aqueduct of Sylvius) and beneath the floor of the fourth ventricle. Plaques also involve the spinal cord. Although grossly the plaques often appear to be rather sharply defined, microscopic examination shows that they gradually fade into normal tissue. As the waste products of breakdown of myelin are carried away by microglial cells there is a proliferation of astrocytes. This results in an increase in glial fibers, eventual formation of a glial scar, and impairment of enzymatic activity in the affected area. There is considerable degree of variation among patients in terms of the intensity and extent of the myelin breakdown.

The clinical symptoms of multiple sclerosis are variable both in individual patients and between patients. This is to be expected because of the scattered location of plaques in all parts of the central nervous system. There is a general tendency toward a pattern of relapse and remission of specific symptoms in about 90% of patients with multiple sclerosis; the remaining patients have a course of progressive deterioration.

Multiple sclerosis strikes young adults who, in most cases, have previously been healthy. It is not uncommon for patients to initially go through a period of vague complaints, feelings of fatigue, loss of energy, intermittent and occasional blurring of vision, headache, unsteadiness in gait and possible loss of control in movement of the extremities and muscle and joint pains. Such feelings may continue intermittently for variable periods of time before more specific and definite symptoms appear. Symptoms of MS can often be categorized into one of four areas: (1) motor weakness; (2) ataxia of gait and coordinated movements; (3) distinct episodes of blurring of vision and/or diplopia; and (4) specific feelings of numbness in various parts of the body. There is however, a considerable degree of inter-individual variability. Initial complaints may also include episodes of vertigo and vomiting, urinary urgency and incontinence. Although rare, seizures may sometimes occur in patients with multiple sclerosis.

Symptoms of motor weakness may be vague and difficult to define or they may represent initial complaints that progress rapidly to paraparesis or paraplegia. Deep tendon reflexes are often hyperactive, extensor plantar responses occur, and the muscles have an increased tone. Abdominal reflexes are often absent. Somatosensory symptoms may include brief periods of numbness and tingling, often in a localized area. Patients may experience warmth, coldness, or a burning sensation in a limb or other parts of the body. Ataxia as well as loss of vibration and position sense may occur in affected limbs. Some patients, upon flexing the head and neck, have a sensation of electrical shock running down the spine to the legs and feet.

Optic or retrobulbar neuritis is often present in the early stages of multiple sclerosis. It has been estimated that at least 25% of patients with multiple sclerosis show temporal pallor of the retina within five years of the onset of the disease. The symptoms include blurred vision, impairment of color vision, pain behind the eye(s), headache, and progressive loss of visual acuity that may, in a few cases, lead to blindness. Homonymous visual field losses, though very unusual, may occur and later resolve.

During the course of the disease many patients show clinical signs of brain stem involvement, including cranial nerve signs of diplopia, impairment of conjugate eye movements, paresis of individual extrinsic eye muscles, and nystagmus. Additional cranial nerve signs may include facial numbness, feeling of pain or loss of pain sensitivity, facial weakness, loss of taste, difficulty enunciating, impairment of ability to swallow, nystagmus, slowing of rapid alternating hand movements, and ataxia. In some patients spinal cord involvement with corresponding sensory and motor difficulty, especially involving the lower limbs, appears to be the major clinical manifestation. Such patients may need a wheelchair for ambulation but often are able to use their upper extremities effectively.

The diagnosis of multiple sclerosis is based essentially upon evaluation of the history and results of clinical neurological examination. Cerebrospinal fluid findings are often helpful but not definitive. Nystagmus can frequently be induced or enhanced in patients with multiple sclerosis by raising the body temperature. Visual, auditory, and somatosensory evoked potentials are abnormal in a high percentage of patients. In many cases, computed tomography shows decreased density that probably represents areas of sclerosis. Many patients have diffuse ventricular dilatation and cortical atrophy. However, none of these procedures is absolutely definitive in the diagnosis.

Gilroy and Meyer (1979) cite the importance of neuropsychological testing in patients with multiple sclerosis. Reitan (1964) performed "blind" evaluation of Halstead-Reitan Neuropsychology Battery protocols for a group of 112 patients with definite but diversified neurological diagnoses, including 16 patients with multiple sclerosis. On the basis of the neuropsychological test results alone he correctly classified 15 of the 16 patients with multiple sclerosis. Nevertheless, neuropsychological testing cannot be considered an adequate or routine diagnostic procedure for this disease; there appears to be too much variability among the patients and overlap of the neuropsychological findings with patients having other conditions. Thus, the principal value of neuropsychological evaluation is to perform a detailed assessment of the intellectual and cognitive deficits of these patients that will aid in their management, rehabilitation, and assessment of the rate of progression of the disease.

Several publications have been oriented specifically toward consideration of the evidence necessary for reaching a definite diagnosis of multiple sclerosis (Brown, Beebe, Kurtzke, Loewenson, Silberberg, & Tourtellotte, 1979; Poser, Paty, Scheinberg, McDonald, Davis, Ebers, Johnson, Sibley, Silberberg, & Tourtellotte, 1983; Poser, Paty, Scheinberg, McDonald, & Ebers, in press; Schumacher, Beebe, Kibler, Kurland, Kurtzke, McDowell, Nagler, Sibley, Tourtellotte, & Willmon, 1965). Conclusions representing the consensus of a study group attempted to provide definitions that could generally be applied as well as establish criteria of definite multiple sclerosis and probable multiple sclerosis (Poser, Paty, et al., 1983). The deliberations were based upon consideration of detailed historical and clinical symptomatology, immunological observations, cerebrospinal fluid tests, neurophysiological procedures (including visual, brain stem auditory, trigeminal, and somatosensory evoked potential measurements), the evoked blink reflex, a variety of physiological and psychophysiological procedures, neuropsychological assessment, tissue imaging procedures (such as computed tomography and nuclear magnetic resonance), and urological studies of bladder, bowel, and sexual dysfunction. The basic purpose was to improve and achieve greater consistency in diagnosis of multiple sclerosis, particularly to foster improved group composition for research purposes.

Several investigators have developed rating procedures for evaluation of disability and severity of illness in multiple sclerosis (Kurtzke, 1955; Kurtzke, 1961; Kurtzke, 1965; Kurtzke, 1970; Kurtzke, 1983; and Mickey, Ellison & Meyers, 1984). These investigations have resulted in the development of the Kurtzke Disability Status Scale, the Kurtzke Functional Systems Scales, and the Illness Severity Score.

The approach in developing these procedures has been based fundamentally upon neurological evaluation of patients with multiple sclerosis and the validity of the ratings has been correlated with evaluations independently done by one or more neurologists. The Illness Severity Score (Mickey, Ellison & Meyers, 1984) was viewed by the authors as a "finer-grained version of the Kurtzke Scales" that combines Kurtzke scales with evaluations of the phase (active-inactive) and course (relapsing versus progressive) of the illness. Scales of this kind may definitely be valuable in evaluating the clinical status of individual patients. However, considering that these scales are based principally upon neurological evaluations, they would not necessarily correspond with results of neuropsychological evaluation which includes assessment of intellectual and cognitive abilities.

No specific laboratory test for diagnosis of multiple sclerosis has been discovered and the diagnosis is essentially based upon clinical evaluation. Steroid therapy, with both adrenocorticotropin (ACTH) and corticosteroids as well as immunosuppressive therapy have been studied. A diet high in polyunsaturated fat (vegetable oil supplement) has also been tried as an attempt to restore possible depletion of linoleate levels in the brain. Although somewhat better clinical results have been reported in treated than with control groups, these treatments cannot be considered specifically effective in multiple sclerosis. Of course, symptomatic treatment (physical therapy, care of bladder and bowel function, prevention of decubiti) is necessary in many cases.

## NEUROPSYCHOLOGY OF MULTIPLE SCLEROSIS

As noted above, no laboratory test has been devised to definitely diagnose multiple sclerosis; the diagnosis is based upon careful serial clinical examinations supplemented by several other tests and procedures. There is considerable degree of variability in both the history and symptomatology among patients with multiple sclerosis. The majority of persons with MS also show a considerable variability (remission and relapse) in their own courses. Despite this diversity, neuropsychological studies have shown a fairly consistent picture of deficit in patients with multiple sclerosis (Goldstein & Shelly, 1974; Ivnik, 1978; Jambor, 1969; Knehr, 1962; Matthews, Cleeland, & Hopper, 1970; Parsons, Stewart, & Arenberg, 1957; Peyser, Edwards, Poser, & Filskov, 1980; Reitan, Reed, & Dyken, 1971; Ross & Reitan, 1955; and Staples & Lincoln, 1979). Confirmation of neuropsychological deficit, particularly using the Halstead-Reitan Battery, has recently been reported by Heaton, Nelson, Thompson, Burks, and Franklin (1985). These investigators also showed that persons who have the chronic-progressive type of multiple sclerosis were more significantly impaired than those afflicted with the relapsing-remitting form of the disease.

The clinical picture characteristic of patients with multiple sclerosis will generally show relatively normal general intelligence measures, adequate performances on tests that require alertness and concentrated attention over time, fairly good ability in dealing with tasks that require keeping several aspects of the situation in mind at the same time, good ability in complex tasks of reasoning, logical analysis, and abstraction, striking deficits in motor areas that may affect both primary motor functions and complex psychomotor tasks, and scattered sensory-perceptual losses. It is not uncommon to observe a specific deficit on the Picture Arrangement subtest of the Wechsler Scale in conjunction with the motor, psychomotor, and sensory-perceptual deficits. It would seem difficult to use a pattern of this type for individual diagnosis; however out of a group of 112 patients with various neurological diagnoses, Reitan (1964), using only the results from the Halstead-Reitan Battery, was able to correctly identify 15 of 16 patients with multiple sclerosis. Thus, it would appear that there is a fairly characteristic neuropsychological configuration of test results in multiple sclerosis. We must emphasize though, that neuropsychological examining methods cannot be used to diagnose the disease.

Initially, the neuropsychological deficits that

characterize persons with multiple sclerosis usually involve motor and sensory-perceptual problem-solving tasks; other abilities are relatively spared. As the disease progresses there is a corresponding deterioration of neuropsychological functions, both in the initial areas of impairment and extending to include other areas. A great deal of variability exists in this regard. Some patients show minimal additional impairment with progression of time and others, in the chronic-progressive group, develop much more generalized impairment. It is especially important to note that abstraction, reasoning, and logical analysis abilities are often relatively spared in persons with multiple sclerosis. These patients can use this remaining ability with great ingenuity in solving their adaptational problems. Many patients, even with significant motor problems, are able to continue functioning in a very productive manner for many years although their motor problems may have become quite handicapping.

As with other diseases involving impairment of brain functions, it is extremely important that neuropsychological assessment be performed to evaluate the strengths as well as the weaknesses of the individual patient. The neuropsychological profile of persons with multiple sclerosis only partly coincides with the neurological picture. Heaton, Nelson, Thompson, et al. (1985) have shown that disability ratings based upon the clinical neurological examination were highly correlated with motor and sensory performances, but that clinical neurological examinations were inadequate in predicting the patients' cognitive status.

# ALZHEIMER'S DISEASE

It has been estimated that up to 4.5% of the population over the age of 65 suffers from severe dementia: intellectual deterioration accompanied by personality disorganization and inability to carry out the normal tasks of daily living (Katzman, 1976). This estimate increases to 11% if mild cases of dementia are included. However, these percentages do not include the "normal" losses in memory and learning ability that occur in a much larger percentage of the population after late middle age. Furthermore, among persons over 65 years of age, approximately 60% of those who are demented have been reported to have Alzheimer's disease (Tomlinson, Blessed, & Roth, 1970). Although senile dementia of the Alzheimer's type (SDAT) is the most common of the age-related neurological disorders that cause dementia (an estimated incidence of 500,000 persons among those over 65 years of age), other conditions are of definite frequency and significance.

Atherosclerotic vascular disease is second to Alzheimer's disease as a cause of dementia in the aged. Approximately 10%-20% of demented patients over 65 years show evidence of ischemic infarction (in the absence of neurofibrillary changes) as the major neuropathological findings, indicating that vascular rather than primary neuronal disorder is present (Tomlinson & Henderson, 1976; Corsellis, 1962). Additional conditions which show age-related neurological disorders (including dementia) are Huntington's disease, Creutzfeldt-Jakob disease, Pick's disease and Parkinson's disease. Idiopathic normal pressure hydrocephalus is also associated with dementia in the elderly.

The etiology of Alzheimer's disease is unknown, although many studies have identified evidence of widespread neuronal losses and other pathological changes. Post-mortem examinations of the brains of persons with Alzheimer's disease indicate that their brains weigh less than the normal brain and show generalized atrophy with widening of the sulci and diminished size of the gyri. Diffuse ventricular dilatation due to atrophy of both the gray and white matter also occurs. Impaired function of certain essential intracellular enzymatic systems have been reported, resulting in interference with neurotransmitter functions. Several reports have indicated that enzymatic function involved in the synthesis of acetylcholine is reduced and hypotheses that Alzheimer's disease represents failure of the cholinergic system have been formulated. There have also been reports of increased concentrations of aluminum and manganese in the brains of Alzheimer's patients and that neurotoxic effects of these metals may contribute to neuronal loss.

The research of Coyle, Price and DeLong (1983) suggested that Alzheimer's dementia was a result of selective degeneration of acetylcholine-releasing neurons that project from certain forebrain nuclei. This study and others (Davies, 1979; Rossor, Garrett, Johnson, et al., (1982) suggest a fairly uniform distribution of cortical abnormalities of the cholinergic system except possibly in the very elderly. Foster, Chase, Mansi, Brooks, Fedio, Patronas and DiChiro (1984) studied regional cerebral glucose metabolism using positron emission tomography as an index of neuronal activity in normals as compared with patients clinically diagnosed as Alzheimer's disease. Glucose metabolism in patients with Alzheimer's disease was far below that of normal subjects and the pattern of hypometabolism, though similar for both cerebral hemispheres, showed definite regional variations. The frontal and anterior temporal areas were relatively spared whereas the posterior parietal cortex and contiguous temporal and occipital areas were most deficient. The regional variations measured bring into question the "cholinergic" hypothesis of Alzheimer's disease.

The major pathological findings in Alzheimer's disease include cortical atrophy with evidence of diffuse marked neuronal loss; intraneuronal deteriorative changes; neurofibrillary tangles; extraneuronal neuritic (or senile) plaques; and granulovacuolar degeneration. Persons aged 65 years or less having these neuropathological changes and dementia are referred to as having *presenile dementia*; if they are 65 or older, the diagnosis is *senile dementia*. There are no changes in the neuropathological correlates of the dementia in accordance with this age separation, but the incidence of these neuropathological changes in normally aging persons beyond the age of 65 causes a problem of overlap in the older age group. In fact, the term *Alzheimer's disease* has been recommended for use in persons 65 and younger whereas *senile dementia of the Alzheimer type* (SDAT) has been advised for persons 65 and older.

Since motor deficits and other focal neurological signs are essentially absent during the initial stages of Alzheimer's disease, it is often clinically distinguishable from other neuronal degenerative diseases and from multi-infarct dementia. Clinically, Alzheimer's disease is defined as a progressive, generalized loss of intellectual functions, particularly involving recent memory (which is often the initial or presenting complaint). General alertness is relatively preserved and in the early stages there are no positive findings on the physical neurological examination. In later stages, however, abnormal neurological signs may appear. A relatively high incidence of incontinence and gait disturbance is present in more advanced cases of Alzheimer's disease, and this makes the distinction from normal pressure hydrocephalus difficult.

Certain problems exist in differentiating normal aging from presenile and senile dementia. Many authorities hold to the notion that the normal memory and learning problems of advancing age are subject to differentiation from the kinds of problems shown by persons with Alzheimer's disease and that it is probable that Alzheimer's disease represents a distinct pathological entity which is different from merely accelerated aging. However, differentiating the clinical and neuropathological changes in Alzheimer's disease from cases of accelerated normal aging is not a simple matter. Microscopic studies of the cerebral cortex in persons demonstrating normal aging indicates the presence of neuritic plaques in approximately 15% of normal persons by age 50, in 50% by age 70, and in 70% by age 90 (Tomlinson & Henderson, 1976). However, the actual number of plaques per unit of area

is reported to be much lower among normal subjects than those with Alzheimer's disease. Of course, this finding only dissociates the frequency of plaque counts of nondemented (normal) subjects from subjects suffering from dementia. Such a comparison does nothing to establish the limits of senile plaques in normal subjects compared with demented subjects nor identify a meaningful cutoff point.

The same situation exists for neurofibrillary tangles. A majority of normal persons beyond the age of 65 shows evidence of such changes and, by age 90, few persons have no neurofibrillary tangles, although the presence of these neuropathological changes have been identified in certain areas of the brain as being 6 to 40 times more frequent in Alzheimer's disease than in age-matched controls (Ball, 1976). Again, however, the established association is with dementia versus no dementia, a cutoff frequency has not been identified, and the type of change is essentially the same in normal aging and Alzheimer's disease. Thus, a very definite problem exists in specific neuropathological characterization of Alzheimer's disease compared with normal aging, with the data relating to *frequency* rather than *type* of neuropathological involvement.

Some studies have indicated a correlation between the frequency of senile plaques, neurofibrillary tangles, and granulovacuolar degeneration and the patient's ability to perform activities of daily living as well as psychometric tests (Blessed, Tomlinson, & Roth, 1968). The association between quantitative measures of dementia and of senile change in the cerebral gray matter of elderly subjects, however, is far from perfect.

Brody (1955) showed that there was no correlation between age and glial cell counts; however, there is a highly significant correlation, roughly linear in nature, between neuronal loss and age during the third through the ninth decades, representing a mean attrition of about 50%. In addition, there appears to be as much variability in neuronal counts per unit of cortex from senile Alzheimer's disease patients as from same-age control subjects. Terry (1977) has found an equivalent mean neuronal loss per unit area of frontal and temporal cortex in patients with senile dementia and persons undergoing normal aging. Ball (1977), however, found that normal aging was accompanied by a gradual, progressive loss of neurons in the hippocampus but a more severe loss was consistently present at all age levels in patients with Alzheimer's disease.

Thus, Alzheimer's disease is a condition characterized by memory loss, disorientation, agitation, dysphasia, psychotic manifestations, incontinence, general dyspraxia, hemiparesis and reflex changes, gait disturbances and other manifestations of central nervous system dysfunction associated with aging (Katzman & Karasu, 1975). In individual cases these clinical deficits are often not closely correlated with pathological changes of the brain seen at autopsy.

A number of studies have related clinical diagnosis of Alzheimer's disease to eventual neuropathological findings at autopsy. The results have shown that clinical diagnoses are not very accurate, with the neuropathological findings corroborating clinical diagnosis as follows: Green, Stevenson, Fonseca and Wortes (1952)—47%; Sim and Sussman (1962)—67%; Smith, Turner and Sim (1966)—58%; Tomlinson, Blessed and Roth (1970)—50%; Bowen, Sim, Benton, Haan, Smith, Neary, Thomas and Davison (1982)—58%; and Davies, Katz and Crystal (1982) — 46%. It would appear that only about 50%-60% of patients with a clinical diagnosis of Alzheimer's disease actually have the condition.

Alzheimer's disease occurs with approximately equal frequency in men and women. Hereditary factors have not definitely been implicated, even though cases may occur within the same family. Early symptoms of the disease include various kinds of mental changes which show up in rather pronounced form on neuropsychological examination with the Halstead-Reitan Battery but are usually undiagnosed in neurological examination. Symptoms may include inappropriate behavior and verbal comments, a tendency toward grandiosity and some evidence of euphoria, spells of irritability and deterioration in occupational performances. Depression and withdrawal may be present and mask deterioration of intellectual and cognitive abilities. Complaints about memory and judgment- often made by family members — will frequently bring

the patient to professional attention. The patient often denies having any problems. In fact, the patient may sometimes present uncritical though elaborate and complex rationalization of his/her behavior. The disease progresses to development of additional mental changes, including paranoid ideas, withdrawal and diminished verbal communication with others, dysphasia, irritability, and sometimes even physical assaults on close associates such as family members. At this point there are relatively minimal (if any) motor or sensory deficits.

The disease progresses until the patient is obviously demented. Facial expression is fixed, blinking is infrequent, there are sucking and licking movements of the tongue, posture becomes semiflexed with generalized rigidity and slow movements, and the patient is confused, untidy, unable to care properly for himself/herself, and is often dysphasic and dyspraxic. Seizures and myoclonic jerks may occur in some cases. Patients often show a general apraxia, being unable to use instruments (even such as a pencil) with any degree of proficiency. The patient may have difficulty in walking and getting out of a chair and eventually becomes bedridden and incontinent. The patient usually dies from pneumonia or urinary tract infection. The reported course is about 5-6 years from onset to the time of death, but it is likely that unrecognized (though significant) deficits have long preceded the diagnosis.

There is no specific treatment for Alzheimer's disease, although the use of drugs may help control combative, agitated, or paranoid behavior. In addition, nutritional needs of the patient must be carefully met and family counseling is often of benefit in dealing with the distressing symptoms shown by the patient.

The pathological findings in patients diagnosed as having Alzheimer's disease differ in *frequency* rather than *type* from similar findings among normally aged persons. Despite these problems of scientific definition, deterioration of higher-level brain functions among the elderly is a problem of great and increasing significance.

# PICK'S DISEASE

The clinical manifestations of Pick's disease are similar to those seen in Alzheimer's disease and a differential clinical diagnosis cannot be made. Both diseases involve progressive deterioration and dementia; however, the histopathological involvement and the areas of atrophy show differences in the two conditions.

Microscopic examination of the brains of persons having Pick's disease shows a pronounced loss of neurons in the areas maximally affected (usually the frontal and temporal lobes). The disease is maximal in the outer three layers of the cerebral cortex. Surviving cells in these layers of the cortex frequently have inclusion bodies which have a characteristic appearance and are known as Pick's cells. Pyramidal cells in parts of the hippocampus show a granulovacuolar deterioration and there is a definite proliferation of astroglial cells in affected areas. Senile plaques and neurofibrillary tangles, which are prominent in Alzheimer's disease, are usually absent or infrequent in Pick's disease.

In gross examination the brain shows marked atrophy of the frontal and temporal lobes, usually to a similar degree on both sides. Occasionally, though, either the frontal or temporal lobe is more involved than the other. The frontal lobe shows maximal atrophy in the orbital areas, including the inferior frontal gyrus. The temporal lobe is usually principally involved in the area of the temporal pole, the anterior part of the superior temporal gyrus, and the inferior and middle temporal gyri. Although these are the areas usually maximally involved, atrophy of the parietal lobe has been described by some investigators. In addition, atrophy of the subcortical nuclei including the globus pallidus, caudate nucleus, putamen, and thalamus has been noted. Cerebral atrophy, even to a pronounced degree, occurs in some cases.

The course is one of gradual progression leading to severe dementia. No specific treatment has been identified.

# PARKINSON'S DISEASE

Although a great deal has been learned in recent years about the underlying physiological and neuro-chemical mechanisms as well as the characteristic pathological changes in Parkinson's disease, this condition is diagnosed through clinical examination. Diagnosis depends upon identification of a triad of symptoms reflecting motor disorders: (1) tremor; (2) rigidity; and (3) bradykinesia. These manifestations of dyskinesia will be described in more detail below.

Parkinson's disease usually begins after the age of 50 years and afflicts about 1% of the population in this age range. Estimates suggest that at any given time there are about 300,000 persons with Parkinsonism and 40,000 new cases per year in the United States. Obviously, this disease represents a major health problem in the older age ranges. There are about four cases in males to every three cases in females. It seems likely that there will be an increasing number of persons with Parkinson's disease as our population ages. However, many of the recent and current cases appear to result from the large number of cases of encephalitis lethargica that occurred from about 1916-1926, and it seems that the incidence of encephalitis-related cases is currently decreasing.

There are certain early signs that may suggest the development of Parkinson's disease, although the classical syndrome consists of tremor, rigidity, and bradykinesia. In the very early phases the patient may have diminished swinging of the arms on one or both sides when walking and diminished movements when sitting. For example, the patient may sit in a rather motionless position with his feet planted squarely in front of him. The patient may also demonstrate the *glabellar tap sign*. To elicit this sign the patient is tapped lightly over the glabella (the smooth area of the frontal bone just above the midpoint between the eyebrows) from behind in order to avoid visual cues. In the normal patient, blinking accompanies the initial taps but rapidly subsides; the patient with Parkinson's

disease will continue to blink in response to each tap. Another early sign is the absence of bodily movements while sleeping.

The fundamental pathophysiological factor in Parkinson's disease is a depletion of dopamine in the brainstem and basal ganglia. Alpha and gamma motor neurons are influenced in their activity at different levels in the nervous system. However, one of the most active systems, which includes excitatory and inhibitory effects on motor neurons, is mediated via the corpus striatum. Dopamine is produced in the neurons of the pars compacta of the substantia nigra and arrives at the corpus striatum via the axons of the nigrostriatal pathway. Dopamine concentration is significantly decreased in the three structures of the corpus striatum (caudate nucleus, putamen, and globus pallidus) in patients with Parkinson's disease. Since dopamine is necessary for the normal functioning of the excitatory pathways to the gamma motor neurons, a loss of this neurotransmitter releases unrestricted inhibition of the gamma neuron. A resulting imbalance in the activity of the alpha and gamma motor systems (a depression of gamma activity and an increase of alpha activity) apparently produce the tremor, rigidity, and bradykinesia of Parkinson's syndrome.

Tremor is the most frequent initial symptom of Parkinson's disease and customarily has a 3-5 cycles/second rate. The tremor is usually present at rest. It may be temporarily inhibited with voluntary action, but appears more prominently as the action continues. In patients who show minimal tremor, the abnormality may be more clearly manifested by having the patient hold his arms in front of his chest with index fingers pointing at each other but not quite touching. The tremor disappears during sleep. In addition to the usual evidence of a pronounced tremor, the other classical signs (rigidity and bradykinesia) are also present, at least to a degree. If the patient does not have these symptoms, many neurologists do not feel that the condition represents Parkinson's disease.

The muscle tone of both antagonistic and protagonistic muscle groups is increased in Parkinsonism and gives the muscles a plastic quality when they are passively stretched. During passive stretching the muscles may also alternately relax and contact, which produces the phenomenon know as *cogwheeling*. For example, with passive movement of an extremity there is free movement between five and ten degrees but then a tonic contraction of the stretched muscle occurs. Regular contraction and relaxation of the muscle follows as the stretching continues. Rigidity is also manifested by limitation of arm swing when walking as well as limitation of "wrist flop" when the relaxed forearm is passively moved forward and backward. Parkinsonian patients who have rigidity also complain of painful muscle cramps in the extremities and severe fatigue. The latter probably results from the additional effort necessary to achieve voluntary movement in a rigid muscle. In these patients there is no loss of muscle bulk or obvious weakness of individual muscles and deep tendon reflexes are normal.

Rigidity almost certainly interferes with adequacy of functional motor activities, but bradykinesia is a separate component of the syndrome. *Bradykinesia* refers to slow movement and difficulty in initiating voluntary movements. The slowness is particularly prominent when the patient attempts to begin a voluntary act or to engage in repetitive activities. Testing is performed by having the patient make a fist, place each finger in sequence on the thumb in rapid succession, tap his toes at a rapid pace, and wiggle his toes. Bradykinesia is frequently evident in handwriting, with progressive diminution in the size of the letters and micrographia. The midline musculature of the body is also involved. The patient may tend to freeze in position and be unable to resume any additional movement. Bradykinesia of the midline musculature is frequently the cause of falls.

A distinction is frequently made between involvement of the musculature of the limbs and midline structures in patients with Parkinsonism. Surgical treatment of Parkinson's disease (which has now been replaced by medical treatment in most cases) was much more effective for relief of symptoms involving the extremities. Midline symptoms include an expressionless face, loss of modulation of speech and progressive diminution of volume to a monotone as speech continues, inability to protrude the tongue beyond the outside border of the lips, slow movements of the tongue and associated slurring of speech and general disturbances of trunk mobility causing abnormalities of gait. A festinating gait pattern (involuntary increase in the speed of walking) appears and the upper part of the body is bent forward. The patient may also have a restriction of upward gaze, extrinsic eye muscle impairment which causes difficulty in convergence of vision, limited blinking of the eyes, difficulty opening the eyes, and upward deviation of the eyes due to tonic contraction of extraocular muscles, lasting from several minutes to several hours (*oculogyric crisis*). In addition, the patient may have bradykinesia of the pharyngeal muscles and great difficulty in swallowing. The patient is sometimes unable to clear saliva from the throat and it drains out through the lips. Certain autonomic changes have also been described and include unusual sweating, very oily skin, constipation, and urinary urgency.

In his original description of this disease, Parkinson noted the dyskinesias that are customarily present but explicitly excluded intellectual deterioration. More recent studies (Pollock & Hornabrook, 1966; Selby, 1968-1969; Hoehn, Crowley & Rutledge, 1976; and Marttila & Rinne, 1976) have estimated that one-sixth to one-third of patients with Parkinsonism show evidence of significant intellectual deterioration and dementia. More detailed neuropsychological studies (Reitan & Boll, 1971) have shed some light on the conflicting opinions (no intellectual deterioration versus significant impairment) that goes beyond an explanation that dementia tends to be present only in the more advanced and severely disabled patients. Neuropsychological examination with the Halstead-Reitan Neuropsychological Test Battery indicates that general intelligence as measured by the Wechsler scale often continues to be quite intact despite the fact that the patient shows significant impairment on tests that are more immediately sensitive to the brain and even severe deficits in the area of reasoning, abstraction, and logical analytical abilities (Category Test).

The basic pathological change in Parkinson's disease is manifested by degeneration of some neurons in the substantia nigra and a degree of melanin depigmentation. However, most patients do not have striking pathological abnormalities. Surviving cells in the substantia nigra contain inclusion bodies that are rich in sphingomyelin, known as Lewy bodies. Lewy bodies as well as neuronal degeneration may also occur in other locations, including the locus ceruleus, oculomotor nucleus, dorsal nucleus of the vagus nerve, and the spinal cord and sympathetic ganglia. In many patients there are diffuse pathological changes involving the basal ganglia, thalamus, brainstem and cerebral cortex. In fact, cerebral atrophy is about twice as common in patients with Parkinson's disease as in control subjects of the same age. Ventricular dilatation also occurs in some cases (Selby, 1968-1969).

A number of patients develop idiopathic Parkinsonism (manifestation of the disease with unknown cause). It is generally agreed that in some cases encephalitis may precede the development of Parkinsonism, with a few patients developing signs and symptoms of the disease in the acute phase; however the majority who appear to make a complete clinical recovery develop Parkinsonism months or years later. Post-encephalitic Parkinsonism is thought to be related to the increased incidence of encephalitis that occurred from about 1916-1926. There probably have been a continuing smaller number of new cases of postencephalitic Parkinsonism over the years. Some authors definitely feel that arteriosclerosis may be a cause of Parkinsonism (Gilroy & Meyer, 1979), whereas others (Ojemann & Ward, 1982) state explicitly that atherosclerosis does not seem to be a cause of Parkinsonism despite the classic references to idiopathic, postencephalitic, and atherosclerotic types. Those who believe in the existence of atherosclerotic or arteriosclerotic Parkinsonism cite the coexistance of symptoms of occlusive cerebral vascular disease and a history that usually includes hypertension and transient ischemic episodes or a history of definite focal neurological deficits resulting from

lacunar infarcts in the pons and basal ganglia. Eadie and Sutherland (1964) have pointed out that patients with Parkinsonism have an incidence of atherosclerotic disease elsewhere in the body that is either normal or lower than normal. Schwab and England (1968-1969) do not believe that discrete ischemic lesions are found frequently in cases with Parkinson's disease and that the infrequent instances of such lesions of the basal ganglia have not been directly associated with occurrence of Parkinsonian symptoms.

The Parkinson's syndrome seems, at least to some extent, to be a matter of definition; if there is any deviation, either in terms of having a greater or fewer number of symptoms than the classical triad (Parkinsonian tremor, rigidity, and bradykinesia) the patient does not have the diagnosis of Parkinson's disease. Instances of Parkinsonism with clinical manifestations have been reported in other situations: following traumatic brain injuries (especially involving severe injury to the brainstem); with parasagittal meningiomas; with gliomas of the basal ganglia and midbrain; with toxic effects of manganese and carbon monoxide; and in patients with adverse effects of phenothiazines and reserpine. Parkinsonism resulting from these conditions, however, often has additional signs of nervous system disorder. In some cases familial factors also appear to be contributory. However, dyskinesias may occur in a number of other syndromes, including dystonia musculorum deformans, choreoathetosis (including Huntington's chorea and Wilson's disease as well as choreoathetosis due to other causes), cerebellar tumors, multiple sclerosis, and movement disorders associated with senility.

There is a considerable degree of individual variability in the signs and symptoms manifested by patients with Parkinson's disease. In addition, the symptoms are variable from one time to another in the same patient. Either emotional or physical stress tends to exacerbate the symptoms.

Nevertheless, despite the wide variance in symptomatology, there have been reports that particular manifestations characterize patients with post-encephalitic Parkinsonism. Patients may demonstrate symptoms of the oculogyric crisis, blepharospasm (spasmodic and frequent blinking of the eyelids), or retraction of the eyelids that is so extreme and prolonged that it may cause inflammation of the corneas. Nystagmus is frequent and paralysis of the medial extrinsic eye muscles may impair accommodation of vision. Respiration is often irregular and impaired pulmonary function may increase the risk of pneumonia. Some patients with post-encephalitic Parkinsonism have been reported to develop psychotic behavior as well as dementia.

Patients with **arteriosclerotic Parkinsonism** are thought to manifest symptoms associated with the occurrence of small strokes, including a gait consisting of short steps, difficulty swallowing, poor enunciation of complex words, and episodes of crying.

The course of Parkinson's disease is variable and the symptomatic manifestations are individualistic. About 10% of patients with Parkinsonism have symptoms that involve the extremities of only one side of the body and even though progression of these symptoms occurs, they never spread elsewhere. An additional group of less than 10% will begin with unilateral symptoms and then have sudden and rapid progression to other parts of the body. About 20% have a rapid and malignant form of the disease. The majority of patients, however, have symptoms that begin on one side of the body and gradually and relentlessly progress to involve the other side and midline structures. Two-thirds of patients with Parkinson's disease will be disabled within 10 years of diagnosis. The symptoms progress faster when the onset occurs at a younger age. Patients with Parkinson's disease have a death rate that is nearly three times that of comparable control subjects. In patients with Parkinsonism, pneumonia is the principal cause of death, followed by urinary tract infections.

The standard treatment of Parkinson's disease is replacement therapy with levodopa. Dopamine is unable to pass the blood-brain barrier; however, levodopa can pass the blood-brain barrier, be converted to dopamine in the brain, and replenish the depleted dopamine supply in the brainstem and basal ganglia. Levodopa is often supplemented by drugs which block extracerebral dopa-decarboxylase activity and thus enhance the uptake of levodopa by the brain and thereby reduce the amount of levodopa that must be administered daily. In addition, this combined therapy reduces the toxic side effects of levodopa and produces more rapid and consistently progressive relief of symptoms. The most common side effects of levodopa are nausea, vomiting, and occasional mental confusion. The patient may also experience the "on-off" phenomenon, in which there is a sudden change in the nature of the symptoms and resultant unevenness in the response to medication. It appears that therapy has to be discontinued in about 25%-30% of patients either because of lack of therapeutic response or because of adverse side effects.

Before the use of levodopa, the treatment of choice for Parkinsonism was to place surgical lesions in the ventrolateral thalamic area. This procedure produced immediate complete relief of tremor and rigidity in the contralateral extremities in 70%-90% of patients with unilateral symptoms. Relief of symptoms in the upper extremity is more frequent than in the lower extremity. Often the symptoms progressed to the other side of the body, and a second operation on the contralateral side of the brain was necessary. Bradykinesia, as well as midline symptoms, did not appear to be as much improved by thalamotomy as tremor and rigidity that involved the extremities. The festinating gait of the patient was sometimes made worse by the surgery, particularly when lesions had been placed in both ventrolateral nuclei of the thalamus.

# NEUROPSYCHOLOGY OF PARKINSON'S DISEASE

Although there is a considerable degree of variability in the neuropsychological deficits found in patients with Parkinson's disease, these patients generally show a fairly consistent pattern. General intelligence — as measured by the Wechsler Scale —

is relatively intact, particularly in terms of verbal intelligence. As would be expected, evidence of dyskinesia appears prominently on the motor tests in the Halstead-Reitan Battery. It is not uncommon to see (1) evidence of tremor in the patient's drawings of figures such as a square, cross, and triangle; (2) indications of bradykinesis in the patient's writing (often manifested by micrographia and deterioration as the writing progresses); (3) poor performances on a complex psychomotor task (Tactual Performance Test); and (4) deficient performances on measures of primary motor ability (Finger Oscillation Test).

In addition to these manifestations, most patients with Parkinson's disease also show generalized impairment of cerebral functioning, demonstrated by elevated Impairment Indexes. A striking example of generalized impairment frequently occurs on the Category Test, which is often performed very poorly. This finding indicates that patients with Parkinson's disease often have significant impairment of abstraction, reasoning, and logical analysis skills. In fact, clinicians who are not familiar with the neuropsychological characteristics of this illness are frequently surprised to see persons with such good verbal intelligence perform so poorly on the Category Test. Experienced neuropsychologists are well aware that such disparities in performances can occur with persons having cerebral disease or damage.

The higher-level pattern of brain impairment in patients with Parkinson's disease has very definite implications. It is not uncommon for neurologists to express disappointment when the quality of life for these patients does not improve as their motor symptoms resolve following successful treatment with medication. The same type of disappointment had previously been voiced by neurological surgeons who observed alleviation of dyskinesia following thalamotomy but found that the patient did not return to normal activities of daily life.

The one aspect of intellectual and cognitive behavior that is probably the most apparent in casual contact with these patients concerns verbal intelligence. It is not uncommon for a person with ade-

quate verbal intelligence to be judged as intellectually normal even though there may be profound deficits in other areas of functioning. Also, in a general sense, verbal intelligence is probably the area most resistive to deterioration in cases of slow and gradual diffuse biological impairment of the brain. The areas of neuropsychological functioning which most readily reflect impairment with brain disease (i.e., abstraction, reasoning, and logical analysis) are often the most difficult to discern on the basis of casual contact. Nevertheless, losses in these areas are of great significance in practical aspects of adaptation to problems in everyday living. A person who is not able to understand complex situations or relationships between events and circumstances and is not able to draw reasonable conclusions on the basis of readily available observations is hardly in a position to "pick up the pieces" and reorganize his/her life in a meaningful manner.

The essence of these comments is that the neuropsychological picture in Parkinson's disease extends far beyond the elements of neurological diagnosis. Although medication may improve the dyskinesia, the neuropsychological deficits are likely to be unaffected. In instances of brain disease it is important to recognize that the neuropsychological deficits constitute an important additional dimension over and beyond the neurological description of the illness. If the patient has striking neuropsychological impairment (even though it is not obvious on the basis of verbal intelligence), it is entirely unlikely that he/she will be able to function normally even if the dyskinesia is resolved. Every patient with Parkinson's disease should receive a thorough neuropsychological evaluation in order to assess the full extent of his/her brain-related intellectual and cognitive capabilities. Only with complete information of this kind can error be avoided in assisting the patient to regain abilities when possible and to adapt to deficits as necessary.

# HUNTINGTON'S CHOREA

Huntington's chorea is a hereditary condition. Although it usually begins after the age of 30 it has been described even in young children. It is characterized by progressive development of choreoathetotic movements and deterioration of intellectual and cognitive abilities. There is a strongly positive family history and the disease is transmitted as an autosomal dominant trait with nearly complete penetrance. Symptoms of clumsiness, slowness of finer movements, and a tendency to drop objects may be present for several years before the development of involuntary choreoathetotic movements.

As the disease progresses, the patient develops irregular, rapid, jerking movements of the fingers and wrists and recurring slower movements, of a dystonic and writhing nature, of the upper extremities. The patient's gait is characterized by a tentative, jerking type of movement and ataxia is present in the lower limbs, neck, and trunk. A characteristic type of grimacing of the face is present together with involuntary movements of the tongue. Dementia usually precedes the development of these choreoathetotic symptoms, but in some cases may precede them. Deterioration of intellectual and cognitive functions is progressive and may be profound. In neuropsychological examination it is difficult to dissociate the patient's motor limitations from intellectual deficit in tasks that require use of the upper extremities, but generalized neuropsychological impairment is clearly present (Boll, Heaton, & Reitan, 1974; Caine, Ebert, & Weingartner, 1977).

Huntington's disease involves a deficiency of the neurotransmitter gamma-aminobutyric acid (GABA) in the basal ganglia as well as other neurochemical defects. The brain shows cortical atrophy (especially involving the frontal lobes) and dilatation of the ventricular system. Changes in the basal ganglia are demonstrated particularly by marked atrophy of the caudate nucleus and putamen associated with a striking loss of neurons in those nuclei. There is also a significant gliosis, especially in the caudate nucleus.

Neuronal loss also occurs in other areas, including the thalamus and subthalamic nucleus, the dentate nucleus and cerebellar cortex as well as the cerebral cortex. Treatment with drugs has shown some effect in decreasing involuntary choreoathetotic movements, but, as noted above, the disease is progressive in nature.

# TOXIC AND METABOLIC DISORDERS

There are many types of toxic and metabolic disorders that may have adverse effects on brain function. These include abnormalities of water and electrolyte balance, including hypo- and hypernatremia (depletion of sodium or excessive sodium in the blood often associated with fluid intake); hypokalemia (loss of intracellular potassium); and hyper- and hypomagnesemia. Cerebral anoxia and anoxic encephalopathy, which can result from many causes, may also impair brain functions.

A wide range of endocrine abnormalities may also be significant in producing signs and symptoms of neurological deficit, including diabetes mellitus, hypoglycemia, hyperglycemia, hypothyroidism, hyperthyroidism, hypoparathyroidism, hyperparathyroidism, and disorders of liver and pancreatic functioning. Illnesses and lesions that cause hormonal abnormalities of hypothalmic-hypophyseal relationships are also included in this group.

A number of diseases and conditions are also of significance in their effect on brain functioning, including hemoglobinopathies and blood dyscrasias, polycythemia, leukemia, Hodgkin's disease, multiple myeloma, macroglobulinemia, cryoglobulinemia, the non-metastatic effects of carcinoma, the porphyrias, Wilson's disease, amyloidosis, adult celiac disease, fibrous dysplasia of the skull, and benign intracranial hypertension. Failure of major organs, including the liver (hepatic encephalopathy), kidneys (uremic encephalopathy), and the pancreas (pancreatic encephalopathy) may also cause brain deficits. Certain toxins are well known for their adverse effects on brain functions. These include ethyl alcohol (in prolonged continuous use), methyl alcohol, and heavy metals and industrial toxins such as lead, arsenic, manganese, mercury, bismuth salts, carbon tetrachloride, methyl bromide, insecticides, thalium sulfate and toluene.

Finally, a number of substances ingested by human beings (for therapeutic as well as other reasons) may have an adverse effect on brain functions. These include oral contraceptives, phenothiazine and antipsychotic drugs, quinidine, barbiturates, antibiotics, vincristine (used in the treatment of cancer), anticholinergic drugs, bromide, and gold (used in the treatment of rheumatoid arthritis). It is apparent that there are many toxic substances and metabolic disorders that may have an adverse neurological effect. We shall not attempt to describe each of these in complete detail, but they will be mentioned briefly. The reader will find more comprehensive treatment of these subjects in the references noted in the text.

## WATER INTAKE AND ELECTROLYTE IMBALANCE

**Hyponatremia** is a deficiency of sodium in the blood. The most common situations in which hyponatremia is observed are those cases of dehydration or edema in which salt has been lost in excess of water or water has been retained in excess of salt. Hyponatremia is seen in patients given excessive amounts of water or other liquids (including psychiatric patients who are compulsive water drinkers). The condition may also be associated with heart failure, hepatic cirrhosis, and adrenal insufficiency. Clinically, hyponatremia is referred to as *depletional hyponatremia*, in which there is a low level of sodium and of body fluids (dehydration) and *dilutional hyponatremia*, in which there is a low level of serum sodium but a high level of body sodium and body fluids (edema). Patients with hyponatremia may have symptoms of fatigue, nausea, vomiting, and abdominal cramps. Some patients may progress to manifestations of confusion, delirium, epileptic seizures, and coma. Brain damage may occur and be fatal in some patients.

**Hypernatremia** is an excess amount of sodium in the blood. It reflects loss of water in excess of salt or administration (or ingestion) of salt in excess of water. It occurs particularly in children who have suffered severe dehydration. In an attempt to achieve rehydration, cerebral edema may occur. There can be a number of other causes of hypernatremia. The brain complications may be severe and include increasing somnolence, stupor, and coma leading to decerebrate rigidity. Seizures may also occur. About one-third of these patients expire, one-third show definite residual neurological abnormalities and one-third seem to recover.

In **hypokalemia** the intracellular potassium escapes into the extracellular space. Physiologically, potassium deficiency impairs neuromuscular function. The patient complains of muscle weakness and fatigability. In severe cases a total flaccid paralysis may occur. In some instances the patient may reach a state of confusion, impaired consciousness and delirium which may lead to coma. Profound hypokalemia may be caused by an adrenocortical adenoma. Potassium deficiency may also occur in patients receiving cortisone. In general, conditions which lead to potassium deficiency may also result in magnesium depletion.

Either too much or too little of the magnesium ion, which is mainly intracellular, may interfere with the proper function of many enzymatic systems. **Hypomagnesemia** does not usually occur in persons with a normal diet because magnesium is present in most food. It has been observed in small infants fed a diet limited to milk. When related to deficiency disease, it is most commonly associated with protein-calorie malnutrition. Other potential causes include malabsorption syndrome, alcoholism, cirrhosis of the liver and diabetic acidosis. Magnesium deficiency causes an increase in neuromuscular activity. Thus, the clinical signs may include confusion, irritability, a state of agitation, muscle twitching, and hallucinations and coma. Seizures and other symptoms that sometimes occur in alcoholic withdrawal may be influenced by a transient hypomagnesemia.

**Hypermagnesemia** may occur in renal failure resulting from ingestion of substances containing magnesium salts, usually in the form of antacids. Increased ingestion of magnesium may result in lethargy, coma, respiratory failure and even death.

## CEREBRAL ANOXIA AND ANOXIC ENCEPHALOPATHY

A number of factors may contribute to cerebral damage as a result of oxygen deficiency. **Anoxia** (deficiency of oxygen) can be classified as anoxic anoxia, stagnant anoxia, anemic anoxia, and histotoxic anoxia. There is considerable overlap in these categories.

*Anoxic anoxia* generally refers to diminished oxygen in the arterial blood despite normal ability of the blood to contain and carry oxygen. It may be due to respiratory obstruction, paralysis of respiratory muscles (caused by conditions such as poliomyelitis, cervical spinal cord lesions, myasthenia gravis, and amyotrophic lateral sclerosis); dysfunction of the respiratory center in the brainstem (due to infectious damage, poisoning, cerebral hemorrhage, trauma or severe electrical shock); impaired lung function (from various etiologies); ingestion of gases that produce anesthesia; and oxygen deficiency due to high altitude exposure. *Stagnant* or *hypokinetic anoxia* is a generalized or localized oxygen lack due to deficiency in volume of blood which occurs in cardiac failure or arrest, shock, arterial spasm, thrombosis or other conditions causing reduced circulation of blood. *Anemic anoxia* is a deficiency in the oxygen-carrying power of the blood such as may occur with carbon monoxide poisoning or blood loss. In *histotoxic anoxia* the oxidative processes of tissues are depressed or abolished, as in cyanide poisoning.

The brain is dependent upon a continuous supply of oxygen and neurological symptoms may appear if oxygen consumption is reduced by more than 30%. The symptoms and impairment caused by hypoxia vary widely among individuals, depending upon a number of factors including duration of hypoxia, body temperature, blood pressure, and the cerebral metabolic rate for oxygen. Because the metabolic rate is higher for the gray matter, when symptoms occur they usually reflect cerebral cortical damage to a greater extent than damage to the white matter. The metabolic rate is generally reported to be somewhat lower for the occipital, parietal, and temporal cortex and the basal ganglia and cerebellum than for the cortex of the frontal lobes. The brainstem has a still lower metabolic rate and neurons in the medulla are reported to survive oxygen deprivation the longest. As might be expected, the first clinical signs reflect impairment of higher-level neuropsychological functions, followed by perceptual and visual difficulties, loss of consciousness, and decorticate and decerebrate motor manifestations. If the anoxia is not reversed, progressive paralysis of cranial nerve function, respiratory failure and death will result.

The course following anoxia is variable. In some cases death may occur very shortly after the anoxic episode. In other instances, a period of coma will be followed by signs of diffuse brain damage. Death may occur within several days or not for several months. In some patients, however, a period of coma is followed by apparent recovery over a period of two to three weeks, after which the situation takes an adverse turn with progressive development of neurological deficits that may result in death or serious neurological residual deficit. In patients who expire, the brain shows acute congestion and diffuse dilation of blood vessels. There are scattered petechial hemorrhages and sometimes large hemorrhages throughout the central nervous system. In some cases certain areas show striking necrosis, including the gray matter of the cerebral cortex. However, other patients, especially those who seem to be recovering and then deteriorate, have been described as having damage predominantly in the white matter with widespread demyelination in the cerebral hemispheres.

The residual deficits in patients who recover from anoxic episodes may range from none to severe and include intellectual impairment, generalized rigidity with a mild parkinson-like tremor, severe brain dysfunction with involuntary movements, myoclonic jerks, and decerebrate rigidity. Permanent deficits are not unusual.

## ENDOCRINE ABNORMALITIES

Peripheral neuropathy with demyelination and axonal loss that can involve both the somatic and autonomic nervous systems occurs frequently in diabetes mellitus. Children, and sometimes adults, often show wide fluctuations in blood glucose levels and occasional hypoglycemic reactions with confusion and coma.

Clinical neuropsychological examination not uncommonly shows evidence of diffuse cerebral dysfunction in persons with diabetes mellitus. Approximately 30% of patients with cerebral atherosclerosis who have been studied have been found to have diabetes mellitus. Thus, in some patients, the basis of diffuse neuropsychological dysfunction is probably related to an accelerated degree of cerebral atherosclerosis.

**Hypoglycemia** (deficiency of sugar in the blood) is a metabolic disorder that can be caused by a number of factors, including hyperfunction of the islets of Langerhans (which secrete insulin) or injection of an excessive quantity of insulin. Glucose and oxygen support brain metabolism and the symptoms of glucose deficiency are very similar to those of anoxia. The onset may be somewhat slower because there is no store of oxygen in the brain. Initial symptoms include acute fatigue, restlessness, malaise, marked irritability and weakness. In severe cases, hypoglycemia may cause seizures, mental confusion, delirium, coma, and possibly death. Irreversible degeneration of neurons may occur, particularly in the gray matter of the brain. Residual impairment of brain functions varies greatly; however, changes are thought to be reversible except when coma has developed.

**Hyperglycemia** (an increase of blood sugar) may cause acute cerebral involvement and is a common complication in juvenile diabetes.

**Hyperthyroidism**, the excessive production of thyroid hormone, may result in thyrotoxicosis and a range of neurological manifestations, including peripheral neuropathy and muscular dysfunction with weakness, spasticity, hyperactive reflexes, and extensor plantar responses. There may be progressive weakness of the extrinsic eye muscles as well as weakness in muscles of chewing, swallowing, and talking. Cerebellar ataxia has also been reported. Sensory function is usually relatively unimpaired. Signs of brain dysfunction may include a general feeling of apprehension, irritability, emotional instability, and excessive activity.

**Hypothyroidism**, an inadequate production of thyroid hormone, may result in *cretinism* in children. In adults this condition is known as *myxedema*. There are many causes of myxedema, including an iron-deficient diet and hypofunction of the anterior pituitary gland. Neurological manifestations include slowness of movement and a general disinterest in motor activity, headache, and mental apathy. The patient may have a number of complaints, including intolerance to cold, impaired hearing, hoarse voice, neuralgia, muscular weakness, dry skin, puffiness around the face, and dry and brittle hair. This condition responds well to replacement therapy using dessicated thyroid or other hormonal preparations. Myxedema has been studied neuropsychologically (Reitan, 1953) and deviations from control subjects have been documented.

**Hyperparathyroidism** is due to an abnormal increase in function in one or more of the parathyroid glands with an increase in production of parathyroid hormone. The majority of these patients have an adenoma of one or more of the parathyroid glands with the principal result being hypercalcemia. Neurological manifestations may vary considerably but often include headache, weakness, fatigability, and a general feeling of anxiety. In more rapidly progressive cases the patient may develop rigidity, tremor, disorientation, and hallucinations and delusions that appear to be psychotic manifestations. Unless the tumor is identified and removed, coma and death may follow in a short period of time.

**Hypoparathyroidism** may also cause neurological symptoms, which essentially result from hypocalcemia and high phosphorous levels. Hypocalcemia causes extreme excitability of neurons with muscle spasms and epileptic seizures. Headache, paresthesias of the face, fingers, and toes, and increase in intracranial pressure may occur. There may also be neuronal degenerative changes as well as calcification of the basal ganglia (often demonstrable on computed tomography before being visible on plain skull films).

## DISTURBANCES OF HYPOTHALAMIC-HYPOPHYSEAL RELATIONSHIPS

The **hypophysis** (pituitary gland) is often referred to as the governing endocrine gland because it secretes several very important hormones which regulate the functioning of the thyroid, gonads, adrenal cortex, and other endocrine glands. Thus, it is of great significance in the growth and maturation of the individual. Dysfunction of the posterior lobe of the hypophysis results in diabetes insipidus. The hypophysis is attached to the hypothalamus by a stalk and complex relationships between the hypothalamus and hypophysis are of significance in the development of certain neurological disorders.

**Diabetes insipidus** results from insufficient secretion of antidiuretic hormone (vasopressin) due to lesions of the hypothalamus or posterior pituitary lobe. This condition may follow trauma, tumors, neurosurgical operations, infections, and inflammatory conditions. When impaired hypothalamic control results in excessive secretion of antidiuretic hormone, the patient may develop water retention, hyponatremia, and renal salt loss. Muscular weakness and decreased reflexes occur initially and, in severe cases, may progress to signs of bulbar palsy, stupor, convulsions, and extensor plantar responses. Injury to the hypothalamus may impair temperature control resulting from abnormal vasomotor activity and cause high body temperatures (hyperthermia). Eosinophilic adenomas of the anterior lobe of the pituitary gland cause **giantism** in children and **acromegaly** in adults. **Cushing's syndrome** may be produced by tumors of the anterior lobe of the pituitary gland or adrenal gland and results in obesity, hypertension, hypernatremia, diabetes mellitus, hypokalemia, increase in body hair, fatigue and weakness.

**Panhypopituitarism** may result from tumors involving the hypothalamus and pituitary gland such as chromophobe adenoma or craniopharyngioma, as well as other causes. This condition is characterized by weakness, dryness of the skin, premature aging, weight loss, signs of hypothyroidism and hypoadrenalism, loss of axillary and pubic hair, impotence in the male and amenorrhea in the female, sensitivity to cold, and episodes of hypotension and hypoglycemia.

## DISORDERS OF BLOOD, LYMPH AND BONE MARROW

The **hemoglobinopathies** are genetically determined conditions in which the red blood cells (erythrocytes) contain an abnormal hemoglobin. **Sickle cell anemia** is an example of these conditions. It appears that neurological abnormalities in sickle cell disease have been underestimated and Gilroy and Meyer (1979) state that about 25% of these patients have such complications. The neurological symptoms may be quite varied, and include repeated episodes of optic nerve involvement followed by optic atrophy and blindness, sudden deafness, other cranial nerve palsies, hemiparesis, seizures, meningeal irritation, subarachnoid hemorrhage, and progression to coma. These patients are at risk for cerebral infarction and repeated focal cerebral vascular lesions may cause severe neuropsychological deficits. The average age of the patient at the time of the stroke is 10 years.

**Polycythemia**, in which there is a continued elevation in red blood cell count, hemoglobin content, and circulating blood volume, may also have cerebral complications. Cerebral blood flow is greatly reduced in this condition because of increased viscosity of the blood and the risk of cerebral thrombosis is increased. These patients frequently report symptoms of headache, dizziness, blurred vision, sleepiness, and lethargy. The clinical neurological examination is often within normal limits but the patients may complain of transient ischemic episodes.

**Leukemia** is a progressive, malignant disease of the blood-forming organs, characterized by distorted proliferation and development of leukocytes and their precursors in the blood and bone marrow. The nervous system is affected with leukemia of both chronic and acute types in about 25% of cases. Infiltration of many organs occurs, including the nervous system, as a result of neoplastic proliferation of white blood cells. Intracerebral hemorrhage (particularly in the white matter) may occur in acute leukemia. Meningeal infiltration by leukemic cells is quite common in children and may produce intracranial hypertension, headache, vomiting, and papilledema. Computed tomography may show widening of the sutures. In fact, cerebral atrophy may occur in cases treated with standard procedures, including intrathecal methotrexate and radiation therapy of the head. Of course, many brain-related symptoms may occur. An increasing number of children treated for acute lymphocytic leukemia are reported to eventually develop mental retardation or impaired intellectual functions, learning disabilities, epilepsy, etc.

**Hodgkin's disease**, a neoplastic involvement of lymphoid tissue, may also spread to involve other organs of the body, including the central nervous system. Approximately 10% of patients with Hodgkin's disease demonstrate neurological complications. Direct invasion of the brain or spinal cord is very rare and the neurological symptoms are usually produced by non-metastatic effects. Encephalopathy with axonal swelling and gliosis has been reported. Involvement of nerve tissue generally shows a good response to irradiation or chemotherapy.

**Multiple myeloma** is a malignant neoplastic condition that arises from plasma cells of the bone marrow. This disorder may be represented as a single tumor, called a *plasmacytoma*, or as a disseminated neoplastic condition. In the rare event that a plasmacytoma involves the brain directly, symptoms may include cranial nerve palsies and seizures. However, the most common type of neurological complication is probably a sensorimotor peripheral neuropathy. An increase in serum gamma globulin may occur secondarily to multiple myeloma, leukemia, and other conditions. Neurological symptoms of this condition are a result of increased serum viscosity, resulting in slow movement of the blood in small vessels. This, in turn, produces hypoxic changes resulting in headache, loss of alertness, and, in some cases, frankly psychotic behavior. Other patients may manifest transient ischemic attacks with a variety of temporary signs of brain involvement. Deterioration of visual functions is relatively common as a result of papilledema or hemorrhages of the retina or vitreous substance.

Cryoglobulinemia is a condition in which gamma globulins are precipitated by a fall in body temperature. An increased viscosity and sludging of the blood occurs with consequent thrombosis of smaller vessels. It is found in association with pathogenic conditions such as multiple myeloma, leukemia, and certain forms of pneumonia.

## DISEASES WITH METABOLIC ABNORMALITIES THAT MAY AFFECT THE NERVOUS SYSTEM

Porphyria is an inherited metabolic disease in which porphyrins are retained in the tissues. There are two main types: erythropoietic porphyria, which does not have neurological manifestations and hepatic porphyria, which may cause serious brain damage. Hepatic porphyria is due to disturbance in liver metabolism such as occurs following hepatitis, poisoning by heavy metals, certain anemias, and other conditions. Porphyria is associated with an increase in production of delta aminolevulinic acid and porphobilinogen, the porphyrin precursor.

Pathological studies have shown diffuse neuronal loss in the cerebral cortex and focal areas of infarction. The neurological manifestations of hepatic porphyria are extremely varied and may include motor manifestations ranging from peripheral weakness to a rapidly progressive involvement with flaccid quadriparesis and respiratory failure, various manifestations of brain stem involvement, seizures, temporary or permanent visual losses, and behavioral changes, including excitement, agitation, delirium, and hallucinations. In patients with latent forms of the disease, certain substances may precipitate porphyria attacks, including barbiturates, alcohol, sulfonamides, estrogen, and exposure to industrial solvents. Obviously, patients with porphyria should avoid such substances.

Wilson's disease is an inherited condition characterized by generalized neuronal degeneration. It is associated with abnormal copper metabolism and probably results from toxic effects of copper in the cerebral tissues. In this disease there is also an increase in deposition of copper in liver cells, causing at least mild cirrhosis of the liver. Deposition of excess copper (which is brownish-green) is also found in the outer limits of the cornea, next to the sclera (Kayser-Fleischer ring). The brain may appear to be grossly normal or show some degree of cortical atrophy. Microscopic examination shows diffuse neuronal degeneration throughout the gray matter with secondary gliotic changes. Widespread atrophy of the brain may be present, particularly involving tissues of the motor system.

Incidence of Wilson's disease is equal in males and females and the age of onset varies from 5 to about 40 years. In general, an early onset has a worse prognosis. The description of Wilson's disease by neurologists customarily emphasizes motor disorders including generalized rigidity, bradykinesis, dysarthria, and a mask-like facial appearance. The patient's gait resembles that of Parkinson's disease, with a forward stoop and an absence of arm swinging. Tremor may be present but it is often mild or absent entirely. The condition is more rapidly progressive in children with Wilson's disease and motor difficulties are characteristically dystonic in nature. Untreated cases show progressive impairment, including emotional lability, epileptic seizures, progressive muscular weakness, cirrhosis of the liver, and eventual dementia. Without treatment, death usually occurs within four or five years following the onset of symptoms. Ten-year survival occurs in some patients who have had a later onset of the disease. Treatment methods have been developed for inhibiting absorption of copper from the intestinal tract and promoting excretion of tissue copper into the urine.

Amyloidosis is a metabolic disorder marked by deposition of amyloid in organs and tissue. It is thought to be the result of disturbed endogenous protein metabolism. Amyloid is a white insoluble protein substance that is translucent and colorless. The clinical and pathological lesions in amyloidosis occur in conjunction with the site of deposition of amyloid. Deposits have not been described in the brain and spinal cord but have been shown to occur in the choroid plexus, pia mater, and lining of central nervous system blood vessels. The condition may result in axonal degeneration probably due to toxic metabolic processes.

**Adult celiac disease** is a chronically progressive form of intestinal malabsorption resulting in a cumulative multiple vitamin deficiency. Diffuse neuronal loss has been observed in the cerebral cortex, basal ganglia, hypothalamus, cerebellum, brain stem, and anterior horns of the spinal cord. Symptoms of chronic diarrhea and weight loss may be present for many years before neurological manifestations begin. The patient may develop ataxia, numbness of the hands and feet and progressive impairment of memory and intellectual deterioration.

**Fibrous dysplasia of the skull** is a metabolic abnormality in which there is replacement of bone by fibrous tissue. In some cases the disorder is generalized but in other instances it is limited to a single bone. The skull is involved in more than 50% of cases and the frontal and sphenoid bones are often affected. Visual loss may occur if the optic nerve is compressed as the fibrous growth increases in size. Precocious puberty and an increased incidence of seizures have been reported to occur with this condition. The neuropsychological effects are similar to any slowly developing extrinsic growth that compresses brain tissue. As with meningiomas, focal signs may occur in the context of relatively mild generalized impairment.

**Benign intracranial hypertension** (also referred to as pseudotumor cerebri) is a condition in which cerebral spinal fluid pressure is increased without evidence of infection, an intracranial growth, or hydrocephalus. Although the condition may be caused by a number of factors, the intracranial hypertension usually resolves itself spontaneously. The patient often complains first of dizziness and a feeling of light headedness or unsteadiness; occasionally nausea

and vomiting occur. Lethargy and blurring of vision are not uncommon. Clinical neurological examination shows papilledema but few other specific signs. However, patients with benign intracranial hypertension not uncommonly demonstrate generalized neuropsychological impairment; specific focal signs are usually not present.

## ORGAN DISEASE OR FAILURE

Certain organs are intimately involved in metabolic processes; disease or failure of these organs may seriously affect brain functions. **Hepatic encephalopathy** has been organized into three categories: 1) *acute hepatic coma*, characterized by sudden and intense hepatic failure (usually due to viral or toxic hepatitis) and a high mortality rate; (2) *hepatocerebral degeneration syndrome*, due to long-standing liver disease and demonstrating a slow progression and a generally poor response to treatment; and (3) *reversible hepatic encephalopathy*, which occurs in patients with cirrhosis and often has a specific identifiable cause.

All cases of liver failure which cause hepatic coma and hepatic encephalopathy are the result of the liver's inability to detoxify metabolites. This has an adverse effect on many cerebral metabolic processes and portal venous blood, carrying neurotoxic substances absorbed directly from the gastrointestinal tract, is shunted into the systemic circulation. Thus, when the liver is unable to detoxify foreign substances and they enter the systemic circulation, an acute and profound disturbance of neuronal metabolism occurs, resulting in coma.

In reversible hepatic encephalopathy a number of other metabolic disturbances are present. The brain may show some neuronal loss with diffuse gliosis. However, in acute hepatic coma, which has a sudden onset and carries a high mortality rate, the brain does not show any abnormalities on gross examination. In this condition there may be rapid development of delirium, stupor, and coma with a number of additional signs of brain dysfunction. In hepatocerebral degeneration a progressive dementia accompanied by rigidity, spastic paraparesis, and hyperactive reflexes may occur and eventually terminate in hepatic coma. Reversible hepatic encephalopathy is associated with confusion and varying levels of alertness and consciousness. Obvious intellectual impairment may be present even when the patient is alert and shows no focal neurological signs. Drowsiness, slurred speech, and other neurological signs, including seizures, may occur. Neuropsychological evaluation is capable of identifying signs of generalized cerebral dysfunction even in patients who have much milder evidence of liver failure and who demonstrate no intellectual impairment on clinical neurological examination.

**Renal failure (uremia)** may cause complex metabolic disorders. In addition, complications of dialysis may also relate to brain dysfunction. Uremic encephalopathy probably stems from chronic acidosis with secondary metabolic changes that affect neuronal function. The early signs are increased fatigue, impairment of alertness, and difficulty concentrating. The condition may progress to stupor, a variety of neurological signs, and eventual decerebrate posturing and coma.

Although dialysis has been successful in treating patients with chronic renal failure, it may also lead to many complications, including encephalopathy. This condition may develop immediately following dialysis and is probably due to cerebral edema. **Progressive dialysis encephalopathy**, beginning from 14 months to 7 years after the start of dialysis treatments, may also occur and lead to progressive dementia, focal neurological deficits, seizures, and death.

**Pancreatic encephalopathy** may occur during the course of acute pancreatitis. Brain involvement may be due to other factors associated with acute pancreatitis, such as hypoxia resulting from pulmonary fat embolism or fat embolism of the brain. This illness begins with the typical symptoms of pancreatitis: sudden onset of abdominal pain, nausea, constipation, and rigid abdomen. In the ensuing one to five days the patient may develop mental confusion, disorientation, hallucinations, focal neurological signs, seizures, stupor, coma, and, in some cases, death.

## ADVERSE EFFECTS OF HEAVY METALS AND INDUSTRIAL TOXINS

Several heavy metals and industrial toxins have been shown to have an adverse effect on nervous system functioning. There is an increasing amount of lead released into the environment and blood levels of lead have been rising throughout the world. It is reported that more than 15% of preschool children in urban areas have blood level concentrations that exceed the acceptable upper safety limit. Although such paint is no longer available for interior decorating, **lead** poisoning in children still occurs as a result of ingestion of lead paint. Lead poisoning may result from many other sources, including car exhaust, burning car batteries, industrial cutting of lead-painted steel with acetylene torches, lead mining operations, gasoline sniffing, and ingestion of lead-contaminated distilled whiskey. **Arsenic** ingestion may result from eating fruits and vegetables contaminated by sprays, certain paints and plasters, medicinal preparations, and insecticides and rodenticides. **Manganese** poisoning may result from working in ore-crushing mills and steelmaking plants where manganese ore is used for hardening steel. Workers are exposed through inhalation of dust from the environment.

**Mercury** poisoning is now relatively rare but may be seen in persons who inhale mercury vapor while preparing dental amalgam. However, more persons ingest organic mercury compounds while using fungicides, weed killers, and seed disinfectants. Eating meat from animals that had been fed with mercury-contaminated grain may also be a cause. **Bismuth salts** are sometimes used for treating constipation and toxic encephalopathy has been reported in some cases. Because of its solvent properties, **carbon tetrachloride** has been used in cleaning clothes and is commonly used in fire extinguishers. Toxicity to this substance is enhanced when it is used in conjunction with alcohol. If working with carbon tetrachloride one should be careful not to be exposed to the fumes in an enclosed place because of the dangers of inhalation. **Methylbromide** is used as a fumigant, an insecticide, a refrigerant, and in fire extinguishers. Although colorless and nearly odorless, it may produce effects if inhaled.

**Organophosphorus compounds** are used extensively throughout the world as agricultural insecticides. Parathion has been responsible for cases of accidental poisoning and death. Ingestion of cooking oils or fats contaminated with other organophosphorus compounds may also have serious consequences. **Thallium sulfate** was previously used as a depilatory agent and dusts containing thallium are produced in some industrial processes. Poisoning with thallium has been reported. **Toluene**, an organic solvent, is extensively used for industrial purposes. This substance is contained in glue and contact cements that are available in toy and hardware stores and has been used extensively by glue sniffers. The effects of heavy metals and industrial toxins on the nervous system have been documented in many instances. There is some degree of variability in the reported symptoms and their sequence of development. However, personality and behavioral changes are frequently the initial symptoms. Patients also complain of headache, visual symptoms of various kinds, vertigo, ataxia, and feelings of numbness. Motor involvement and peripheral neuropathy are also fairly common. In some cases the toxic effects may lead to dementia and death.

## VITAMIN DEFICIENCIES

Neurological deficits due to vitamin deficiencies are fairly common although certain of these disorders have decreased in frequency because of better nutritional standards. **Vitamin A deficiency** has been reported to cause hydrocephalus, mental retardation, and cranial nerve palsies, but this deficiency is relatively rare except in children with malabsorption diseases.

**Thiamine (Vitamin B$_1$) deficiency** is a major cause of *Wernicke's encephalopathy*. It is also the principal factor in the development of beriberi, peripheral neuropathy, and retrobulbar neuritis. This deficiency occurs in conditions of starvation, inadequate diets or severe gastric disturbances. In some cases, the heart enlarges and fails and edema of the limbs develops.

Many neurologists believe that the neurological manifestations of Wernicke's encephalopathy are due principally to these nutritional deficiencies rather than a direct neurotoxic effect of alcohol ingestion. The neurological manifestations relate principally to impairment of higher cerebral functions, and include loss of critical judgement, excitement or depression (depending upon individual reactions), and paranoid behavior. In addition, memory is impaired and the patient may show slurred speech, ataxia of gait and the upper limbs, dilated pupils, and increased respiratory rate. Coma may result from acute intoxication but death is rare.

**Nicotinic acid deficiency** is a major factor in the development of *pellagra*, a disease characterized by severe protein malnutrition and a deficiency of other vitamins in addition to niacin. Pellagra is endemic in some parts of the world and may occur secondary to gastrointestinal diseases and alcoholism. Severe niacin or nicotinic acid deficiency may result in morphological changes of cells in the cerebral cortex as well as the basal ganglia and most of the nuclei of the brain stem, consisting of isolated neuronal changes characterized by cellular chromatolysis without associated glial or vascular changes. The major clinical features are diarrhea, dermatitis (a scaly brown rash on those parts of the skin exposed to light), and dementia. Early signs of brain dysfunction include headache, insomnia, irritability, and symptoms of anxiety or depression. Sometimes the patient is disoriented and delirious, has hallucinations, and shows signs of an acute psychosis. Seizures are also relatively common. A progressive dementia may ensue unless early treatment is instituted.

**Pantothenic acid deficiency** may be contributory in Wernicke's encephalopathy, beriberi, and pellagra. This deficiency causes paresthesia in the lower limbs with the so-called "burning feet" syndrome. **Vitamin B$_6$ deficiency** (pyridoxine) may also contribute to the symptoms of pellagra. A lack of this vitamin, which usually occurs in infants, may cause severe epileptic seizures.

**Vitamin B$_{12}$ (cyanocobalamin) deficiency** affects

the spinal cord principally in its neurological manifestations; in advanced cases it may show patchy areas of demyelination and axon degeneration in the white matter of the cerebral hemispheres. The patient is frequently a middle-aged, white-haired woman who complains of numbness and tingling in the fingers and toes, soreness of the calves (due to peripheral neuritis), and unsteadiness in walking, particularly in the dark (due to posterior column degeneration). There is a slightly yellowish tinge to the tongue, which is frequently shiny and sore (*superficial glossitis*). Plantar reflexes may be exaggerated if the pyramidal tract degeneration predominates. The majority of patients show mental changes such as forgetfulness, lack of alertness, suspiciousness and perhaps paranoid ideas, and irritability progressing to generalized dementia. Vitamin $B_{12}$ deficiency leads to pernicious anemia. A small dose of parenteral $B_{12}$ usually corrects the vitamin deficiency but much higher doses are necessary to treat the neurologic lesion. The polyneuritis generally improves; the symptoms of spinal cord disease may only partially recover if they have been present for a long time.

## NEUROLOGICAL EFFECTS OF INGESTED SUBSTANCES AND MEDICATIONS

Many chemical substances, often used for medical purposes, can cause neurological deficits. A number of these will be mentioned briefly.

**Oral contraceptives** have been studied in some detail following individual reports of cerebral vascular lesions. The physiological changes induced by oral contraceptives include salt and water retention and an increased tendency to formation of thromboses. Research evidence suggests that the risk of circulatory disease increases with relation to the length of time that oral contraceptives have been used and that the risk is greater in women over 35 and those who are habitual cigarette smokers. Some investigators have reported that women who suffer from migraine headaches have increased symptoms when using oral contraceptives; but there have been other studies that claim improvement in migraine symptoms in women taking oral contraceptives. Some reports have shown an increase in the incidence of acute strokes in young women using oral contraceptives but other researchers have failed to confirm this finding.

**Phenothiazine** and **antipsychotic drugs** have found a very useful place in treatment of the mentally ill; however, certain neurological side effects which involve abnormal movements are not uncommon. These fall in three categories: acute dystonia, tardive dyskinesia, and parkinsonism.

*Acute dystonia* is characterized by abnormal posturing of the trunk or an extremity. Dystonia usually occurs shortly after administration of a phenothiazine. Motor manifestations include extended contraction of muscle groups. The head and eyes may be deviated upward or to one side and the patient may not be able to use muscles for speech. There may be bizarre, grotesque movements of the pelvis and shoulder and difficulty with gait. The tongue may protrude and the neck may be maintained in an abnormal posture. These symptoms are sometimes mistaken for tetanus and the muscle tonicity may be sufficiently pronounced to cause dislocation of the jaw.

*Tardive dyskinesia* involves involuntary movements of the mouth, tongue, and lips together with choreoathetoid movements of the trunk and extremities that may persist for months or years. Tardive dyskinesia is a side effect of several antipsychotic drugs and usually does not occur until weeks or months after treatment is initiated.

*Parkinson-like symptoms* frequently occur in patients taking phenothiazine drugs. Symptoms may include a mild bradykinesis to generalized rigidity, lack of facial expression, flexed posture, and a typical parkinsonian gait. Tremor may occur in some cases but is less frequent than the above reactions.

**Quinidine**, used for the control of cardiac arrhythmias, has been reported to cause progressive dementia resembling Alzheimer's disease. Rapid recovery has occurred when administration of quinidine has been discontinued.

Ingestion of **barbiturates** is a common cause of death by poisoning. In barbiturate intoxication cerebral blood flow and metabolism are reduced. Moderate barbiturate intoxication resembles alcoholic intoxication in many respects. In severe intoxication the patient is comatose and tendon responses are greatly reduced or absent. Respiration is reduced and respiratory arrest may occur. Blood pressure falls because of involvement of the vasomotor center and the patient may develop shock. Renal failure may also result.

**Antibiotics** can cause severe toxic effects involving the brain and produce a variety of symptoms. Dysfunction of the auditory and vestibular divisions of the eighth nerve as well as optic neuritis and muscular weakness may occur. Some antibiotics may cause seizures; others cause tremor, mental confusion, impaired function of the respiratory muscles and flaccid paralysis of the extremities. Acute psychotic manifestations with visual hallucinations have also been reported.

Drugs used to treat leukemias and lymphomas may also cause toxic neurological manifestations, including seizures, muscular atrophy, peripheral neuropathy, and intellectual slowing.

**Anticholinergic drugs**, including atropine, scopolamine, belladonna, tricyclic antidepressants and phenothiazines all may produce brain changes that result in a wide variety of symptoms, including a dry mouth, blurred vision, dry and flushed skin, striking increases in body temperature, weak and rapid pulse, agitated, restless, anxious and confused behavior, visual hallucinations, ataxic gait, slurred and thick speech, and impairment of intellectual functions.

**Acute bromide intoxication** is manifested by impaired cognition and memory, drowsiness, irritability, and emotional disturbances that may include delusions and hallucinations with coma following ingestion of large doses. A variety of neurological signs may be present, including motor incoordination, tremors, cerebellar signs, and decreased deep tendon reflexes.

**Methyl alcohol poisoning** causes depression of the central nervous system in a manner similar to ethyl alcohol. In addition, it also causes severe metabolic acidosis and has a specific toxicity for the optic nerves.

Eight to 36 hours after ingestion the patient may complain of headache, vertigo, vomiting, abdominal pain and blurring of vision. The visual symptoms may progress to blindness with optic atrophy. Cerebral spinal fluid pressure is often elevated as a result of cerebral edema. Although the patient usually recovers from the acute intoxication, the optic nerve damage may be permanent and result in a significant loss of visual acuity or blindness.

Rheumatoid arthritis is sometimes treated through chrysotherapy and this can cause a **gold encephalopathy**. Neurological manifestations may include cranial nerve palsies, seizures, memory deficits, and intellectual impairment.

# EFFECTS OF ALCOHOL

Following ingestion of alcoholic beverages, ethanol is usually absorbed into the bloodstream through the walls of the stomach and the upper small intestine. It is then distributed to all parts of the body, including the brain, because there is no blood-brain barrier to ethanol. A small amount of ethanol may be discharged from the body through breathing, sweating, etc., but the detoxification process occurs principally through metabolic degradation by oxidative enzymes of the liver. The amount of alcohol in the body is usually estimated by determining blood alcohol levels. Levels above 100 mg ethanol/100 ml blood are usually associated with some noticeable effects, such as a change in mood and a feeling of being "high," especially in non-habituated persons; 150 mg/100 ml often results in a moderate degree of incoordination; 200 mg/100 ml results in frank intoxication; 300-400 mg/100 ml usually produces stupor or coma, and levels above 500 mg/100 ml are often fatal.

## Pathological Effects of Alcohol

There is general agreement (Adams & Victor, 1981; Krigman & Bouldin, 1983) that neurological disorders due to or associated with ingestion of alcohol fall into several categories: (1) *acute alcoholic intoxication*, including drunkenness and coma; (2) *withdrawal effects resulting from abstinence*, which may include hallucinatory experiences, withdrawal seizures and delirium tremens; (3) *diseases of the nervous system* associated with alcoholism that are basically due to malnutrition, including the Wernicke-Korsakoff syndrome, optic neuropathy, pellagra, and peripheral neuropathy; (4) *diseases or conditions frequently associated with alcoholism in which the etiology is uncertain*, including cerebral atrophy, cerebellar atrophy, central pontine myelinolysis, Marchiafava-Bignami disease, peripheral neuropathy, and myopathy; (5) *neurological disorders secondary to alcohol-induced cirrhosis of the liver*; and (6) *teratogenic abnormalities* which affect the fetus in women who use alcohol excessively during pregnancy (fetal alcohol syndrome).

The acute effects of alcohol ingestion range from minimal changes to coma. Intervening manifestations may include impaired judgment, a carefree attitude, conviviality, slowing of response time, and more severe symptoms, including disorientation, ataxia, slurred speech, and amnesia for events that occurred during the period of acute intoxication. Neuropathological findings in brains of patients who have died from acute alcoholic intoxication are probably the result of a combination of oxygen deficiency and impaired cerebral blood flow. Autopsy findings include cerebral congestion, edema, and discrete punctate hemorrhages.

Withdrawal signs and symptoms are not uncommon in people who have gone through periods of consistent heavy drinking and then sharply reduce or stop their alcohol intake. The most common manifestations are coarse tremors or shaking of the limbs, irritability, sleeplessness, difficulty concentrating and impaired or inappropriate affective responses.

**Delirium tremens** (DTs) occur in chronic alcoholics who have a long history of heavy alcohol intake. This condition usually begins with severe tremor and irritability, disorientation, hallucinations, delirium and autonomic instability. In addition, the subject may have one or more major motor seizures which usually occur during the first or second day of the withdrawal period. Autonomic nervous system manifestations include rapid pulse, lowered blood pressure, fever, dilated pupils, sweating, nausea and vomiting and may progress to coma. Without treatment, fatalities may occur in up to 10% of persons with delirium tremens. Despite these severe reactions, there are no characteristic pathological changes in the brain except for some instances of cerebral congestion and edema, even in patients who have experienced withdrawal symptoms and seizures.

Nutritional deficiencies frequently associated with alcoholism include optic and peripheral neuropathies as well as brain disorders (Wernicke-Korsakoff syndrome and alcoholic pellagra).

**Wernicke's disease** and **Korsakoff's psychosis**

are not separate diseases but essentially represent a sequential process of a single disease (Victor & Banker, 1978). Wernicke's disease results from thiamine (vitamin $B_1$) deficiency. Thiamine is found in many foods and is absorbed through the small intestine, but only small quantities are stored in the body. Thus, malnutrition among chronic alcoholics may cause Wernicke's disease, a condition characterized by confusion, ocular disturbances, and ataxia. Mortality is as high as 40% during the acute phase of Wernicke disease.

Among survivors, the Korsakoff syndrome becomes manifest in 80% of the patients during recovery from Wernicke disease. Korsakoff's psychosis is a state characterized by a profound amnesic syndrome. Even though the ocular abnormalities, including nystagmus and other indications of impaired functions of extrinsic eye muscles, often improve in the course of recovery from Wernicke's diseases, many patients continue to show these symptoms and, having also developed the amnesia of Korsakoff's psychosis, are referred to as manifesting the Wernicke-Korsakoff syndrome. Although the outstanding deficit in patients with Korsakoff's psychosis involves memory (long-term memory of past events as well as ability to acquire new information), these patients also frequently demonstrate severe impairment of other cognitive functions. In fact, patients with this condition seem to have little insight into their disability, are generally apathetic, and show minimal response to their surroundings. The external surface of the brains of these patients usually appears to be essentially normal unless the types of lesions frequently seen in chronic alcoholics (subdural hematoma, cortical contusion, and cerebral atrophy) are present. However, lesions are consistently found in the thalamus, hypothalamus, midbrain, pons, and medulla and these have been described in detail (Victor, Adams, & Collins, 1971). Only slight or no improvement is seen in nearly one-half of the patients with Korsakoff syndrome.

**Pellagra** is a nutritional disease that is caused by a dietary deficiency of niacin and its precursor, the essential amino acid tryptophan. This condition was very common at one time, particularly in the southern United States and among malnourished chronic alcoholics. Since about 1940 there has been a striking decrease in the incidence of pellagra due to the fortification of bread and cereals with niacin. Symptoms in the early stages of this disease include insomnia, fatigue, nervousness, irritability, and feelings of depression. As the disease progresses the patient may show apathy, impairment of memory, lack of interest in the environment, loss of alertness, and sometimes an acute confusional psychotic state. The pathological changes have been described (Adams & Banker, 1978; Krigman & Bouldin, 1983) and include a swollen and rounded appearance of affected cells with eccentric nuclei and loss of Nissl particles in the motor cortex and nuclei of the brainstem, cerebellum, and the anterior horn cells of the spinal cord.

As noted above, there are several conditions and diseases of unknown etiology that are frequently associated with alcoholism. **Cerebral atrophy** is not necessarily due to alcoholism, but Courville (1967), who had extensive experience in examining the brains of alcoholics, felt that atrophy of the cerebral cortex before the age of 50 years was usually the result of chronic alcoholism. Initially the cerebral atrophy involves the dorsolateral aspects of the frontal lobes; later it extends to involve the precentral gyrus, the postcentral gyrus, and the superior parietal lobule. This atrophy results in dilatation of the lateral and third ventricles. It is apparent that cerebral atrophy, distinct from the Wernicke-Korsakoff syndrome, may occur in chronic alcoholics. It seems likely that these changes in the cerebral cortex may be the basis for consistent findings of neuropsychological deficits in chronic alcoholics who still have relatively normal general intelligence as measured by the Wechsler Scales.

**Cerebellar atrophy** is also frequently seen in chronic alcoholics. Grossly, cerebellar atrophy consistently seems to be most pronounced in the anterior and superior lobules of the vermis and paramedian portions of the anterior lobes. However, other areas of the cerebellar cortex may also be involved and atrophy is apparent either grossly or, in less severe cases, on microscopic examination. Cerebellar atrophy is found in patients who show no clinical symptomatology although it is often associated with abnormal stance, gait, and ataxia of the limbs.

**Central pontine myelinolysis** (CPM) is a relatively uncommon condition in which there is primarily demyelination of the central portion of the pons. Although this condition was first described in patients suffering from severe malnutrition or chronic alcoholism, it also has been reported in instances of renal disease, hepatic disease and infectious illness. Patients with central pontine myelinolysis often show clinical signs of confusion, weakness, and lack of control of muscular movements. This is a rapidly progressive condition that usually results in death within two to four weeks after onset.

Another rare condition, usually seen only among severe chronic alcoholics, is **Marchiafava-Bignami disease.** It is frequently associated with ingestion of crude red wine. This disease has variable clinical symptoms, often with an acute onset and sudden development of stupor and coma. This condition is often fatal; surviving patients often develop a chronic form of the disease and show evidence of definite dysphasia, dyspraxia and other neurological deficits. The pathological characteristics of the disease are more invariable than the clinical manifestations. On gross examination the middle part of the corpus callosum shows evidence of definite degeneration consisting principally of a loss of myelin with relative preservation of the axis cylinders. Although this disease is usually found in chronic alcoholics, cases have been described in nonalcoholic subjects and a nutritional etiology has been postulated but not confirmed.

Brain damage and dysfunction occurs as a result of alcohol-induced cirrhosis of the liver and portal-systemic shunts (shunting of blood around the liver). Victor and Banker (1978) point out that cerebral lesions induced by hepatic failure are the most common among those due to excessive alcohol intake and nutritional deficiencies.

There is considerable evidence that changes in cell structure and composition within the liver may occur after only a relatively short period of heavy drinking. Among long-term heavy drinkers there appear to be repeated episodes of liver dysfunction manifested by gastrointestinal complaints, general malaise, tenderness of the liver, and liver enlargement. Heavy drinking for 5 to 15 years appears to cause death of some liver cells with inflammation, a tendency toward development of fibrous tissue, and some cellular regeneration. At this point the pathological changes appear to be only partly reversible.

Cirrhosis of the liver usually does not occur until at least 15 years after onset of heavy drinking, at which time the liver is usually enlarged and nodular and microscopic examination shows evidence of destruction of liver cells, the development of fibrous tissue, and some evidence of hepatocellular regeneration. The cerebral deficits that are induced by hepatic failure have been described in detail (Victor & Banker, 1978) and are classified as acute hepatic encephalopathy (or hepatic coma) and chronic hepatic encephalopathy.

**Acute hepatic encephalopathy** is accompanied by a confusional state, changes in psychomotor activity (either decreased or increased), followed by drowsiness, stupor and coma. A number of positive neurological findings and EEG changes are present. The condition often terminates fatally but, in some cases, the symptoms regress completely.

**Chronic hepatic encephalopathy** refers to a condition in which the patient may show changes in mood, personality, and some degree of intellectual impairment which may extend over a period of months or even years. In addition, a number of motor abnormalities may be present. The deficits in chronic hepatic encephalopathy are chronic and irreversible and, in some cases, may be gradually progressive. Evidence exists that the basic problem in hepatic encephalopathy stems from a failure by the liver to metabolize ammonium, which results from hepatocellular disease as well as shunting around the liver. According to this view, the clinical symptoms would be a result of a metabolic disorder with rapid accumulation of ammonium in the blood. Continuation of this condition would lead to lesions of the brain tissue and result in a chronic and essentially irreversible condition of deficit.

Victor and Banker (1978) identify only four pathological conditions in which dementia occurs in association with excessive ingestion of alcohol. These are Wernicke-Korsakoff syndrome, alcoholic pellagra, Marchiafava-Bignami disease, and hepatic encephalopathy. The mechanisms of brain pathology and dysfunction in each of these conditions is presumably related to secondary influences on the brain rather than a direct adverse effect on neural tissue. Victor and Banker argue against the notion that ingestion of alcohol directly damages the brain. They believe that "alcoholic deterioration" can nearly always be explained by the presence of Wernicke-Korsakoff disease, trauma to the brain, anoxic encephalopathy as a result of repeated seizures, communicating hydrocephalus, or some other lesion. They do not believe that there is any need to appeal to a possible chronic toxic effect of alcohol on the brain.

Admittedly, the problem of differentiating secondary effects on brain tissues from direct and primary adverse effects is extremely difficult. It is entirely possible that autopsy studies of brain tissue will be insufficient to answer this type of question. In fact, the neuropsychological evidence of slowly progressive neuropsychological deterioration can hardly be ignored, despite the fact that subjects may never reach criteria for diagnosis in any of the four categories of alcoholic dementia identified by Victor and Banker. Although the neuropsychological deficits among chronic alcoholics are not perfectly exclusive to this condition (since they may also be shown by patients in other categories), the changes are fairly characteristic and show few indications of focal involvement, as might be expected from the characteristic autopsy findings in alcoholic dementia. Thus, neuropsychological data suggest that a slowly developing process of deterioration of cerebral functions occurs at a state much earlier than that of patients who are subject to neurological diagnosis of alcohol-related conditions. In fact, neuropsychological studies strongly suggest

that brain functions deteriorate in many chronic alcoholics, including many who have not experienced nutritional deficiencies (Parsons & Farr, 1981; Reitan & Wolfson, 1985).

Finally, we should mention at least briefly the **fetal alcohol syndrome**. Recent evidence has indicated quite clearly that a distinct syndrome of malformations can occur in the offspring of women who abuse alcohol during pregnancy. The abnormalities shown by the offspring include disorders of brain structure and function, intrauterine and postnatal retardation of growth, facial abnormalities, and a number of other malformations. The available data strongly suggest that alcohol ingestion is responsible for the teratogenic effects rather than the use of other drugs or the effects of malnutrition. Mental retardation, poor coordination, diminished muscle tonus, irritability in infancy and hyperactivity in childhood are characteristic of children with fetal alcohol syndrome. Only a limited number of reports have appeared in which detailed examination of the brains of these children have been done, but a wide range of brain malformations have been reported. Thus, it certainly appears that ingestion of alcohol by the mother may have a direct and pronounced adverse effect on the development of the fetus.

## Neuropsychology of Alcoholism

Over the past 25 years, neuropsychological studies of chronic alcoholics have clearly indicated the presence of deterioration of brain-related abilities. As noted above, the medical literature indicates that the pathological changes of the brain frequently seen among alcoholics are due to factors other than alcohol, such as nutritional deficits and head trauma. However, neuropsychological studies suggest that continued ingestion of ethanol may have direct adverse effect on neural tissue.

The characteristic neuropsychological picture in alcoholism is one of relative retention of both Verbal and Performance intelligence levels, adequate ability in dealing with simple tasks that are well-defined and in which the subject is required only to pay continued attention, and relative intactness of measures of primary motor functions. When the task increases in complexity and involves several elements that must be considered simultaneously, alcoholics show a striking deficit. Fitzhugh, Fitzhugh, & Reitan (1960) found that alcoholic subjects were essentially similar to controls with respect to I.Q. scores; however, alcoholics performed more poorly than a comparison group of brain-damaged subjects on a measure of reasoning, abstraction, and logical analysis (Category Test). These results were confirmed by the same authors in 1965 and numerous additional studies have shown similar results (Parsons & Farr, 1981). Thus, there seems to be no doubt that chronic alcoholics show significant brain-related neuropsychological deficits.

Some research findings suggest that young alcoholics do not show these deficits and that it requires a number of years of excessive ingestion of ethanol to produce neuropsychological deficits. There are also clinical observations which suggest that these adverse neuropsychological consequences of chronic alcoholism may be reversible in persons who discontinue consumption of ethanol; however, much remains to be learned in this regard.

# AGING

There is little doubt that as the majority of human beings age they show decremental biological changes that involve essentially all of the bodily systems. Clinical examination indicates that visual and auditory acuity as well as other sensory functions are impaired. Even healthy old people have postural changes resulting in stooped gait and impaired muscular function demonstrated in movement of the extremities. Steadiness of movement is impaired, tremor is often present, and some deficit in coordination and balance occur. Excessive fatigue is also common. Clinical neurological examination shows impairment of light touch perception and vibratory sensitivity. Deep tendon reflexes are changed. Ability to stand on one leg with eyes closed is impaired in more than 60% of healthy subjects beyond the age of 70 years. Muscle strength and bulk are frequently reduced and peripheral nerve conduction speeds are lowered.

Considering the general impairment frequently shown by the aged, one might wonder why debate still continues regarding the possibility of brain changes. This debate centers around a differentiation between aging as the passage of time and its effects on bodily processes and aged individuals in whom age-related biological changes may be classified as disease. Thus, an answer to the question of deterioration of brain functions in association with aging depends, at least in part, on the question being asked. If one is interested in aging as an abstract concept, unrelated to the majority of aged people, the answer might be that the effects are much less than shown by most aged people who are not fortunate enough to escape many of the degenerative changes that have been associated with disease processes. This question will be considered in additional detail at a later point.

Structural, physiological, neurochemical, and psychological deficits of a brain-related nature have been shown to occur in the aging process. Dekaban and Sadowsky (1978) have reported a reduction in brain weight and size among elderly persons, generally averaging a 7%-8% loss from the peak adult weight. Atrophy of brain tissue, shown by shrinkage of the gyri and widening of cortical sulci, occurs especially on the lateral frontal and parietal surfaces (Tomlinson, Blessed, & Roth, 1968). The amount of gray matter with relation to white matter shows a gradual decrease at least up until about middle age (Miller, Alston, & Corsellis, 1980). Both supratentorial and infratentorial structures are reduced in weight. As a result of cortical atrophy, the ventricles also tend to be dilated among elderly persons, including those who show no clinical manifestations of dementia (Tomlinson, Blessed, & Roth, 1968). Brain structure in accordance with aging has also been evaluated using computed tomography of the head. The results generally demonstrate a loss of both white and gray matter, but with the latter showing a more substantial decrement in both cortical and subcortical areas. In addition, there is an increase in the size of the ventricular system (Schwartz, Creasey, Grady, et al., 1985).

Besides these indications of gross (macroscopic) changes that occur in the aging brain, there is also abundant evidence of histological change. Brody (1955; 1970; 1978) has shown that a striking decrease in the number of neurons in the cerebral cortex occurs particularly in the superior frontal gyrus, the superior temporal gyrus, the precentral gyrus, and the visual cortex. He found that the neuronal decrease is a progressive phenomenon in the frontal and temporal areas, with about a 40% reduction by the ninth decade. Other investigators have reported somewhat similar results (Colon, 1972; Shefer, 1973; and Tomlinson & Henderson, 1976). In contrast, glial cells seem to show no reduction in number with advancing age (Henderson, Tomlinson, & Gibson, 1980). Scheibel (1977) has presented a detailed statement of his studies of dendritic tissue with relation to aging. He points out that dendrites constitute 70%-90% of the total membrane area of the neuron and must play a significant role in the information processing capabilities of the individual. In turn, he finds evidence of a definite reduction in the spine systems and dendritic arborization, especially among persons with clinical indications of dementia. Many years ago Ellis (1920) reported that a striking reduction in the number of Purkinje cells in the cerebellum occurred with advancing age.

In addition to these types of changes that occur in the course of normal aging, a number of other histological abnormalities are present that are much more prominent in conditions such as Alzheimer's disease. These include neuritic or senile plaques, neurofibrillary tangles, and granulovacuolar degeneration, all occurring with an increasing frequency in the brains of non-demented persons beginning with the fifth decade in life (Mountjoy, Roth, Evans, & Evans, 1983; Tomlinson, Blessed, & Roth, 1968; and Peress, Kane, & Aronson, 1973). Many other histological abnormalities have been reported to occur in the brains of older persons.

It may be interesting to note that on autopsy presumably normal persons show changes of the type seen in Alzheimer's disease, not only among subjects in North American, Great Britain, and European countries, but also in Japan. Matsuyama and Nakamura (1977) have reported on their examination of 617 brains in Tokyo. They deliberately excluded brains of patients who had evidence of psychosis or any conditions known to be predisposed to the types of pathological changes seen in Alzheimer's disease. Thus, these patients presumably represented a sample of subjects who might manifest the effects of normal aging but not brain disease. Their results indicated a strong association between advancing age and the occurrence of neuropathological changes, including neurofibrillary tangles and senile plaques. Such changes were present in approximately 50% of cases aged from 50-59, in more than 80% of cases aged 60-69, and in almost every patient over age 70. Changes of this kind represent a difference in *degree* regarding pathology in aging and Alzheimer's disease but no apparent difference in *kind*. Besides establishing the fact that neuropathological changes occur in the brains of Japanese as well as other ethnic groups, the results add to the validity of the question of whether

Alzheimer's disease is only an extreme and early form of normal aging.

In recent years many studies concerned with neurochemical changes in association with aging have been done. McGeer and McGeer (1981) have studied neurotransmitter agents and the enzymes concerned in synthesis and metabolism of these agents. They have found evidence of a considerable degree of neurochemical pathology in association with age, and high correlations in many areas between enzyme activity and age. Adolfsson, Gottfries, Oreland, Roos, and Windblad (1977) have also reported relationships between monamines and metabolites and age. They found significant correlations in examination of tissues from the caudate nucleus, globus pallidus, the mesencephalon and the hippocampus, as well as 5-hydroxyindoleacetic acid in the hippocampus and cingulate gyrus. Finch (1978) has developed rodent models for studying neurochemical and neuroendocrine changes with relation to aging. He has found that levels of dopamine are substantially reduced in older as compared with younger mice. Bapna, Neff, and Costa (1971) found that catecholamine metabolism in rat brains is also significantly reduced in older animals. A number of other neurotransmitter systems have been studied with relationship to age and have been shown to have significant relationships (Finch, 1977). McGeer and McGeer (1981) and Perry, Blessed, Tomlinson, et al. (1981) have also provided reviews of research findings in this area.

Electroencephalographic changes have been reported among normal subjects in accordance with advancing age. One of the best sources for information concerning EEG changes is the longitudinal study conducted at Duke University. In this study a large number of normally functioning persons were enrolled with the intent to continue the evaluations until the time of death. Busse (1978) has reported on the EEG findings as well as other results. After the age of 65 there is a progressive slowing of the dominant frequency of alpha activity and the appearance of slow waves in the theta or delta range. Elderly subjects in good health have a mean occipital frequency which is almost a full cycle slower than that found in comparable young adults. This slowing of the dominant EEG frequency is probably related to some degree of decrease in cerebral metabolic functions. The slowing among elderly normal subjects was not closely related to other measures of psychological impairment. It is possible that an insufficient range of EEG variation was represented among these normal subjects or that the selection process did not represent a sufficient range of intellectual deficit.

Probably the most unusual finding was the occurrence of focal EEG abnormalities, consisting of slow waves and sharp waves over the temporal areas of the brain. These findings were observed in 30%-40% of the apparently healthy elderly sample. The left anterior temporal area was involved much more frequently than the right (75%-80%); bilateral focal patterns were found in 18%-20% and 4%-5% of the subjects showed the disturbance on the right side. Comparisons with a similar sample of normal adults under the age of 40 revealed that only 3% have this type of EEG abnormality. An increasing number of subjects show the abnormality as age increases, with the frequency being about 20% at the age of 60. Efforts were made to relate this type of focal EEG abnormality to other factors, but no consistent relationships were established. However, Obrist (1976) observed that more generalized impairment of brain functions was likely to be found when adjacent areas were involved or the patient showed evidence of a more diffuse disturbance.

Using the xenon-133 inhalation method, Obrist, Thompson, Wang, and Wilkinson (1975) compared cerebral blood flow in a group of elderly demented patients and healthy young adults. As might be expected, the demented patients showed a substantial reduction in cerebral blood flow. Other investigators (O'Brien & Mallett, 1970; Hachinski, Iliff, Zhilka, duBoulay, McAllister, Marshall, Russell, & Symon, 1975) compared patients with Alzheimer's disease with a group of patients having definite evidence of cerebral vascular disease. These investigators found that cerebral blood flow was essentially normal among the Alzheimer patients but reduced

among patients with cerebral vascular disorder. Obrist, et al. (1975) combined their data with that of Wang and Busse (1975) and performed a comparison of cerebral blood flow in normal young persons, a group of normal aged persons, and a group of aged persons with dementia. The results indicated a definite stepwise decrease in cerebral blood flow values, with the normal aged group (averaging 80 years) having a 28% reduction compared to the 38% reduction shown by the demented patients (who averaged 60 years of age). Obrist (1977) postulates that the finding by O'Brien and Mallett as well as Hachinski et al. may have related to the fact that they used patients with early Alzheimer's disease and therefore found essentially normal blood flow values. It would appear from these results, however, that there is a definite reduction in cerebral blood flow involving the gray matter in association with normal aging with an additional reduction occurring in older demented patients.

As early as 1956 Kety reported a reduction in cerebral blood flow, the rate of cerebral metabolism of oxygen, and cortical neuron density in aging. His results indicated a gradual decrease in these variables with advancing age and suggested that decrease in brain oxidative metabolism as well as cerebral blood flow were secondary to cell loss. In a study based on subjects who were very carefully examined to exclude all findings related to physiological deterioration (a super-healthy group), Dastur, Lane, Hanson et al. (1963) failed to find any age-related change in cerebral blood flow or cerebral oxygen metabolism. They felt that these results suggested that Kety's conclusions were related to possible deterioration of the cerebral vasculature even though clinical manifestations may not have been evident.

Frackowiak, Lenzi, Jones and Heather (1980) studied regional cerebral blood flow and oxygen metabolism using positron emission tomography; Kuhl, Metter, Riege, and Phelps (1982) conducted a similar study. Both of these reports indicated that glucose and oxygen metabolism, as well as cerebral blood flow, were reduced in the elderly. A recent study by Duara, Margolin, Robertson-Tchabo, et al. (1983), based on carefully selected healthy males, failed to show any age relationship to measures of glucose metabolism even though another study of cerebral structure using computed tomography (Schwartz, Creasey & Rapoport, in press) demonstrated atrophy of the gray matter and ventricular dilatation that was age-related in most of these same subjects.

Creasey and Rapoport conclude that health factors are significant in determining results which suggest that cerebral metabolism and blood flow decrease among older subjects. However, if one screens older subjects to exclude all of the structural, physiological, and neurochemical changes that usually occur among older people, one can hardly expect not to find a reduced incidence of biological deviations from those shown by younger groups. However, such findings would be of little relevance with regard to the customary effects of aging and would be subject to generalization regarding such a highly selected group that they would have little meaning for the majority of the population.

A controversy exists regarding psychological decrements with advancing age. Creasey and Rapoport (1985) note that "crystallized" intelligence, as represented by stored verbal intelligence, is relatively unaffected by aging. On the other hand, "fluid" intelligence, represented by the Performance subtests of the Wechsler Adult Intelligence Scale, decreases with advancing age. They interpret such results as suggesting that a "large part of cognitive processing, related to ability to cope with the environment, remains intact in the elderly" whereas the deficiency in "fluid" intelligence is due to a slower rate of processing associated with a reduction in reaction time and possible slowing of the dominant EEG frequency.

This analysis of impairment of intellectual and cognitive functions in accordance with aging is hardly complete. Reitan (1967) and Reitan and Wolfson (1985, in press) have reported that many of the age-related losses are characterized by striking and significant deterioration of a wide range of abilities related to reasoning, abstraction, logical analysis, adaptation to unusual and novel types of tasks, and a pro-

gressive deficiency as the overall complexity of the task increases. Schaie (1977) has validly criticized cross-sectional research efforts in the assessment of intellectual and cognitive losses resulting from aging, but the differential degree of deficit on certain tasks as compared with others in an age-related context, in the same group of subjects, rather clearly indicates that certain psychological deficits do occur (Reitan, 1973). In fact, the neuropsychological measures that are most closely related to the general biological condition of the brain are also the measures that most strikingly reflect intellectual and cognitive impairment among the aged (Reed & Reitan, 1963).

The preponderance of evidence seems to indicate without doubt that the average normally-functioning person develops many biological and psychological brain-related decremental changes with advancing age. Identification of these changes is important because of the prospect that many of them may be controlled or even reversed (Reitan & Shipley, 1963). A significant problem in this respect, however, concerns the differentiation of aging factors which may be beyond manipulation and those factors which can be controlled. The approach to aging research which emphasizes extremely careful screening of older subjects in order to rule out any possibilty of underlying biological deterioration will scarcely be of significant value in this regard. The approach that must be followed will be to identify the types of changes that characterize aging in the normally functioning population and determine the prospect of arresting or reversing these adverse changes. For example, if atherosclerosis is a factor contributing to intellectual decline in advancing age, the pertinent research must investigate the possibility of limiting the development of atherosclerotic changes and use of pertinent measures to identify the effects (Reitan & Shipley, 1963). If the development of neuritic plaques and neurofibrillary tangles is of critical importance in limiting intellectual and cognitive capabilities and the quality of life experienced by the subject, research showing this must be done and attempts must be made to discover methods for limiting or preventing the development of such neuropathological features within the brain. If cerebral blood flow is reduced in the average aging person (as it certainly seems to be), studies of elderly individuals in whom blood flow is not impaired must be done and the factors that contribute to limitation of cerebral blood flow, as well as cerebral metabolism of oxygen and glucose, should be determined.

It would seem to be possible to make progress in identifying the biological factors that contribute to brain aging and to focus research on further understanding (and perhaps remediation) of such factors. Certainly such an approach would be preferable to the rather circular procedure in which every effort is made initially to rule out the biological correlates of aging, to then study such a select and non-representative group in detail, and to prove that such a group fails to show significant impairment in comparison with younger subjects. Such a tendency appears to have been fostered by the initial efforts of the National Institutes of Health to study the effects of aging without the complicating factors of the biological and psychological changes that customarily accompany aging (Birren, Butler, Greenhouse, et al., 1963) and the continuing efforts to establish the fact that once the normally accompanying adverse components have been screened out, aging has essentially no adverse effects (Creasey & Rapoport, 1985).

In this regard it may be helpful to refer to a suggestion made by Busse (1977), a person who spent most of his professional career contemplating and studying the aging process. Busse indicated that for operational purposes he had learned to differentially define primary aging, or senescence, and secondary aging or dementia. He felt that primary aging is represented by inborn and inevitable detrimental time-related changes, rooted in heredity, but independent of stress, trauma, or acquired disease. He felt that secondary aging was caused by an inherent biological defect that is initiated or exacerbated when the person is in a vulnerable physiological condition which has been produced by insults or disease, including trauma, infection, toxins, or psychosocial stress. Busse recognized that this differentiation did not provide for a perfect separation of the aging process and conditions of insult or disease, but did postulate that it was relevant to the ultimate question of whether medical science can provide the diagnostic skills and techniques for prevention and intervention that control the aging process.

Clinical neuropsychological evaluation as well as many research studies (Reitan & Wolfson, in press) indicate that significant impairment of brain-related adaptive abilities gradually accrue with advancing age among healthy human beings (Reitan & Shipley, 1963). Neuropsychological deficits, even of a pronounced nature, can often be measured in persons who show no gross neurological evidence of brain deterioration (Reitan & Wolfson, 1985). These deficits, however, have profound significance in the overall adjustment of many older persons. Clinical neuropsychology is a discipline that is growing in significance within the field of gerontology, in terms of its clinical contributions as well as research potential.

# EPILEPSY

Epilepsy is an excessive, uncontrolled discharge of electrical impulses from neurons in the brain causing involuntary movements, usually a loss of consciousness, occasional abnormal sensations, and an increase in autonomic activity. Epilepsy is not a disease; it is a symptom that may be caused by a large number of factors. Although the cause of epilepsy may be identified in many cases, most epileptics are said to have "idiopathic" epilepsy, meaning that the cause is unknown. In fact, the etiology is unknown in more than 50% of children with epilepsy and among adults the percentage is only somewhat smaller. Careful studies of the brain have been done in many cases and although electrical activity is periodically abnormal, the brain has been shown to be normal, either grossly or microscopically, in a morphological sense. There appears to be little doubt that biochemical or metabolic causes may be responsible for epilepsy in many cases.

Despite the fact that epilepsy is only a symptom of some type of brain disorder, steady progress has been made in treating this symptom. Using a non-impairing level of antiepileptic medication, effective seizure control can be achieved in over 85% of patients. Therefore, even though the cause may not have been discerned, most patients with epilepsy can effectively control their seizures with medication and function normally. Despite this progress, epilepsy remains an important public health problem. It is difficult to determine the exact incidence of epilepsy, but estimates have been made that 4-7 people per 1,000 members of the population are affected. This means that there are 0.8-1.4 million epileptics in the United States. Although seizures can occur at any age, an adult having an epileptic seizure for the first time must be evaluated carefully in order to identify the type of brain disorder responsible for the seizure. Thirty percent of epileptics have their first seizure before the age of 4 years, 50% by the age of 10 years, and 75% by the age of 20 years. Initial seizures are very rare beyond the age of 50 years. Thus, the onset of epilepsy occurs particularly among children and adolescents.

Certain types of seizures seem to run in families, particularly absence (or petit mal) epilepsy in children and partial complex epilepsy. Studies of parents and siblings of children who have these types of seizures show a higher-than-normal incidence of EEG abnormalities, even though the relatives have shown no overt indications of epileptic seizures. In addition, epilepsy is a symptom manifestation of a number of hereditary degenerative diseases of the nervous system, and this factor increases the hereditary influence.

Developmental defects may also cause epilepsy. Diseases such as *tuberous sclerosis* and *Sturge-Weber disease* may cause epilepsy. Viral infections of the fetus, maternal infection with toxoplasmosis, irradiation of the uterus, and drugs or toxic substances ingested particularly during the first months of pregnancy may cause the eventual development of epilepsy. Birth trauma is another factor that may result in cerebral anoxia or contusion and sometimes cerebral thrombosis or embolism.

Herniation of the medial aspect of the temporal lobe over the free edge of the tentortium during the birth process may also occur. Damage of this kind gives rise to proliferation of glial tissues and may cause epilepsy later in life. Anoxic episodes in infancy or childhood may also have a similar effect. In fact, anoxia during an epileptic attack seems to produce additional cerebral damage in some cases which, in turn, increases the probability of further seizures.

Brain injury due to head trauma causes epilepsy in many persons. Head injury is probably the single most common cause of epilepsy, adding 190,000 new epileptics to the pool each year. An initial seizure occurring during the first week as an acute effect of the head injury is unlikely to be followed by further seizures. However, if the first seizure occurs 2-7 weeks after the head injury, after the brain has had some opportunity to reorganize and stabilize, the probability of another seizure increases to 20%. The development of epilepsy following a head injury is more common when there has been penetration of the dura and direct damage of the brain tissue. Gliosis and scar-tissue formation, which occurs in such instances, seems to produce an epileptic focus. Post-traumatic seizures are much less common in persons who have sustained closed head injuries even though the damage to the brain may be substantial. Early seizures following head injuries are usually of the focal motor type; seizures that develop later are often of the psychomotor type.

Infectious involvement of the brain is frequently a cause of seizures. Brain abscess and neurosyphilis were common causes in the past but the frequency has been reduced because of treatment available to control these types of brain lesions. Viral encephalitis, particularly among children, is a common cause of seizures. Although occurring less frequently, bacterial, fungal, and yeast infections leading to meningo-encephalitis may also cause epilepsy.

Both primary and metastatic tumors of the brain may cause seizures. Slowly growing tumors and those which involve cerebrocortical tissue directly are more frequently associated with epilepsy. As noted above, neurologists and neurosurgeons feel that any onset of focal seizures in adulthood requires an aggressive diagnostic approach to rule out the possibility of brain tumor. Nutritional and metabolic disorders have also been related to the development of epilepsy, particularly in children. Heavy metal poisoning is also a factor, with lead poisoning being more common in children. A considerable number of drugs may cause seizures in susceptible persons and sometimes sudden withdrawal of drugs (such as barbiturates) after prolonged use may precipitate seizures. Chronic alcoholic adults frequently have epileptic seizure disorders, although it is often difficult to differentiate between the effects of alcohol ingestion and head injuries that may have been sustained. Seizures are not usually associated with cerebral infarction, although seizures may occur if there is cerebral bleeding. Vascular malformations, particularly arteriovenous malformations, may cause seizures with or without evidence of bleeding. Seizures are uncommon in patients with multiple sclerosis and in primary neuronal degenerative diseases such as Alzheimer's,

Pick's, Huntington's chorea, and Jakob-Creutzfeldt disease. However, seizures may occur in perhaps 10%-20% of patients with these conditions.

As noted above, epileptic seizures are caused by abnormal, synchronous discharges of neurons. The "epileptic" neuron has been studied in considerable detail and it appears that a number of factors may contribute to electrical instability or irritability of affected neurons. These factors may include disorders of metabolism within the neuron, instability of the neuronal membrane, or other factors that affect the excitability of the cell body or synapses. Neurotransmitters may play a role either in the inhibition or spread of seizure activity. In any case, the seizure may begin with a small population of electrically unstable neurons whose electrical discharges are transmitted to other neurons resulting in synchronous discharges of increasing numbers of neurons. As this process develops, EEG recordings show high-voltage brief discharges (spikes) and slow wave discharges. This process continues as the basis for the clinical manifestations of the epileptic seizure. Finally, the frequency of synchronous discharges decreases, there is a lengthening of the refractory period, and the synchronous discharges finally cease. The termination of the seizure is apparently due to a number of factors, including depletion of energy reserves, anoxia, changes in electrolyte concentrations, and accumulation of toxic end-results of metabolism.

Although seizures may occur suddenly and without warning, many patients report that they know in advance that a seizure is imminent; in other persons with epilepsy strange sensations may occur for a brief period of time before the seizure begins. The warning symptoms, which may be present for hours or days before the seizure, often consist of mood changes, irritability, difficulty in thinking and organizing thoughts, and feelings of depression. Signs and symptoms of changes in autonomic function may also precede a seizure, including either pallor or flushing of the skin, pupillary dilatation, increase in heart rate, urinary frequency, and the desire to defecate. Many patients report specific changes, known as the *aura*, only seconds or minutes before the seizure. These may consist of automatic contraction of small muscle groups, perception of strange smells, etc. The aura may be of importance in identifying the neuronal population that gives rise to the seizure. For example, perception of strange odors suggests that the neuronal discharge begins in the uncinate gyrus and then spreads into the temporal lobe. The rapid spread throughout the brain may result in a generalized seizure.

Usually epilepsy is clinically classified according to description of the nature of the seizure. The major classifications are: (1) **generalized seizures** (with or without convulsions); (2) **partial seizures**; (3) **reflex seizures**; and (4) **status epilepticus**. The most common generalized convulsive seizure is the tonic-clonic seizure often referred to as "grand mal." Generalized convulsive seizures that occur particularly among children are infantile spasms (resulting from perinatal infections, developmental abnormalities, severe trauma, or degenerative disorders of the brain and associated with severe mental retardation in about 90% of patients) and *akinetic seizures* or *drop attacks* (represented by a sudden loss of muscle tone and a precipitous fall to the ground. They are often precipitated by sudden noises.)

Gilroy and Meyer (1979) differentiate tonic-clonic seizures into those that occur without warning and those that are preceded by warning symptoms or a specific aura. The latter are called *secondary generalized seizures with focal onset*, and the differentiation is made because of the value of the aura in identifying the locus of the initial epileptic discharge.

Tonic-clonic seizures customarily go through three phases. The first phase is *tonic seizure*, in which all muscles contract, the limbs and the trunk extend and may be so pronounced as to resemble decerebrate rigidity, and marked cyanosis occurs. The patient usually remains in this condition for 20-60 seconds. As the rate of neuronal discharge slows, the second, or *clonic phase*, of the seizure begins and all muscles are involved in contractile movements. In this phase it is important to maintain the airway in order to avoid possibly fatal asphyxia and to protect the tongue from damage that may occur by contraction of the jaw muscles. The clonic phase usually lasts about 40 seconds but in many instances may be considerably more prolonged. The patient then enters the third stage, *coma*, characterized by general flaccidity of muscles and a number of abnormal or diminished reflexes, including absence of response to painful stimuli. This stage usually lasts for about one minute.

Following the three stages of the epileptic seizure the patient lapses into deep sleep which may last for several hours. If aroused during this sleep the patient often complains of severe headache, is confused and disoriented and unaware that the seizure has occurred. After the patient awakens, post-ictal manifestations may be present, including persistence of headache and confusion, muscle pain, and feelings of extreme fatigue. These symptoms may last for only a brief period or several days.

Seizures that include the tonic phase but not the clonic contractions are relatively rare but sometimes occur. This type of seizure rarely lasts more than a few seconds.

**Generalized non-convulsive seizures**, which occur particularly in children, consist of absence (or petit mal) seizures or unilateral seizures that involve the whole side of the body. **Absence** or **petit mal attacks** in children are characterized by brief episodes of loss of consciousness lasting approximately 5-15 seconds. During this period the child seems to be unaware of his/her surroundings and stares with a vacant expression. This type of seizure is not totally devoid of motor activity. Automatisms have been identified through careful observation that may include blinking of the eyelids in a standard rhythm, swallowing, or movement of an arm. Most children do not continue to have these seizures into adulthood; about one-third have a change in their seizure pattern and may develop generalized seizures. Continuing absence attacks (or petit mal status) tends to occur in young adults rather than children and consists of attacks that may last for several hours to several days. The patient does not lose consciousness but is in a state of reduced alertness and awareness.

**Unilateral seizures** of a clonic (contractile) nature, not uncommon in children, are infrequent in adults. When present in an adult they may suggest the presence of a brain tumor. One part of the body may be especially involved but careful observation shows that the whole side is affected and, as a result, these seizures are referred to as "generalized." These seizures may last from several minutes to several hours and the degree of clonic movement may be variable. These seizures often are followed by **postictal paralysis** (Todd's paralysis) which may last on the affected side for an hour or more after the clonic movements have ceased. In some children the seizure may involve one side of the body or the other in successive attacks or even alternate from one side to the other during the same episode.

**Partial seizures** frequently center on one site or one type of behavior as the principal manifestation. Partial seizures may be motor, sensory, or complex (psychomotor) in nature. *Partial motor seizures* may involve one muscle or a small group of muscles and not spread to involve other parts of the body. For example, the seizure may involve a thumb, a thumb and index finger, the whole hand, the face, or a foot. This type of seizure usually lasts for a few seconds to a few minutes.

A second type of a partial motor seizure is often referred to as **Jacksonian epilepsy**. This seizure begins with a rhythmic clonic jerking of the particular muscles initially involved and then spreads to include adjacent muscles. This spread of muscular involvement is frequently referred to as the *"Jacksonian march"* and many neurologists require this type of manifestation before referring to the epilepsy as Jacksonian in type. The spread may be rather delimited or may progress to involve the entire side of the body and spread to the opposite side and develop into a generalized tonic-clonic seizure. Partial motor seizures have been identified by additional terms, depending upon their particular characteristics. Some patients, for example, have a temporary loss of speech and language abilities

during the seizure; other patients have abnormal postures of an affected limb. Sometimes the clonic movements, even though involving just one part of the body, may continue for many hours.

*Partial sensory seizures* may also occur. They may be quite localized, spread in a systematic fashion, and may persist for variable periods of time. The sensations may be described as numbness, tingling, loss of feeling, electrical sensations, or as if an insect is crawling on the skin. These seizures are also known as *sensory Jacksonian seizures* or *sensory fits*. Seizures of this type are fairly often associated with developing brain tumors.

*Partial complex seizures* have previously been referred to as psychomotor seizures or temporal lobe seizures. However, the range of variations in manifestations of these seizures extends beyond the descriptive characteristics of the word "psychomotor" and their origin or limitation to temporal lobe involvement is far from exact. These seizures are classified according to the initial symptom or the predominant symptom. In many instances the initial symptom predominates but in others they may develop into a much more complex seizure pattern with a variety of complex behaviors or develop into a secondary generalized tonic-clonic seizure.

Many of these seizures involve complex motor behavior involving rapid chewing, blinking, swallowing, incoherent mumbling, repetitive movements of extremities, wandering around a room or office usually inspecting things with a blank look, etc. The patient resists any attempt at restraint and is amnesic for the episode. In some instances patients with seizures of this type may engage in complex behaviors during the seizure, performing difficult tasks that appear to be relatively normally done, but the patient essentially is in a fugue state. Disturbances of language use may also be seen, either with unintelligible automatic speech utterances or dysphasic types of manifestations.

A variety of sensory symptoms is reported by these patients, including auditory perceptions such as a shrill whistle or sounding of bells, olfactory symptoms such as experiencing adverse chemical smells, visual hallucinations of flashing lights or floating objects, sensations of spinning, reports of a bitter taste, a feeling of extreme nervousness in the stomach area followed by a urgent need to defecate, a feeling of fluttering in the left chest area with tachycardia, instances of fear and withdrawal followed by agitated behavior and disorganized thought processes, and a "dreamy" type of re-experiencing of events of the past, often in childhood, with vivid detail, and even hallucinatory experiences of the voices of persons who have died.

Many patients with partial complex seizures have definite personality problems in the interictal period that do not reflect the acute seizure episodes. Attempts have been made to characterize these patients (Bear & Fedio, 1977; Geschwind, 1977). In fact, these personality characteristics differ according to which temporal lobe is affected. With a right temporal lobe focus the patient is described as being emotionally labile, alternately aggressive and depressed and somewhat irresponsible. Patients with left temporal lobe foci are supposedly obsessed with considerations regarding personal destiny and religion, emphasize negative features of experiences, and need to write things out in obsessive detail. These patients also have great difficulty maintaining composure under stress. However, careful review of the evidence supporting these personality and behavioral differences in patients with right and left temporal lobe foci suggests that they represent generalizations that fall far short of applying to all patients.

A great number of antiepileptic drugs have been developed, some of which are more effective for patients with certain symptoms than others. Partial complex seizures are by far the most difficult to treat effectively. In most seizure types the first drug tried is diphenylhydantoin (Dilantin), followed by another drug if adequate control is not achieved. As noted in the early part of this section, complete control or great improvement of seizure frequency and intensity can be achieved in over 85% of epileptic patients. Surgical treatment is definitely indicated if the patient has a lesion such as an abscess, cyst, arteriovenous malformation, or tumor. In such cases surgery may result in improved control of epilepsy only as a secondary factor; the surgery is performed essentially for treatment of the lesion. Excision of epileptogenic foci that cause intractable seizures is also useful in patients who meet criteria related to inadequate response to drug treatment, unilateral and stable location of the focus, careful study to rule out multiple foci, and at least sufficient intellectual competence to be able to benefit from seizure control. Often surgical excision of the focus will be of definite assistance in limiting the epilepsy, particularly when complemented by post-surgical drug treatment.

It is not possible to describe the neuropsychological correlates of epilepsy briefly because the nature of deficits is variable from one person to another and heavily dependent on the underlying brain disorders. However, the neuropsychology of epilepsy has been studied in detail and the reader is referred to available sources (Dodrill, 1981; Reitan, 1976; Reitan & Wolfson, 1985).

# Glossary

# GLOSSARY

## A

**Abscess.** A localized collection of pus in a cavity, formed by the disintegration of tissues.

**Absence epilepsy.** A type of epilepsy that occurs especially in children and is manifested by a sudden momentary loss of consciousness with minimal motor manifestations.

**Acoustic neuroma.** A tumor or new growth which involves the acoustic division of the eighth cranial nerve, largely made up of nerve cells and nerve fibers.

**Adipose tissue.** Fatty tissue.

**Afferent.** Conducting inward to a part or organ. In neurophysiology, a nerve impulse carried from sensory receptors in toward a synapse en route to the brain.

**Agnosia.** Denoting an absence of knowledge. In aphasia, impairment of ability to recognize the symbolic meaning of stimulus material.

**Akinetic mutism.** Inability to speak, usually accompanied by a more general failure of ability to respond. It is frequently associated with lesions of the anterior brainstem.

**Alpha rhythm.** A uniform rhythm of brain waves in the normal electroencephalogram, with an average frequency of about 8 to 13 cps.

**Alzheimer's disease.** Pre-senile or senile dementia with progressive mental impairment. Characterized pathologically by the presence of excessive neurofibrillary tangles and senile plaques.

**Amaurosis fugax.** Temporary impairment or loss of vision (blindness) in one eye due to impairment of blood supply through the internal carotid artery or the ophthalmic artery.

**Amygdaloid body.** A small gray mass of several small nuclei located in the roof of the terminal part of the inferior horn of the lateral ventricle.

**Anaplasia.** A characteristic of tumor tissue in which there is a loss of differentiation of cells (dedifferentiation), of their orientation to one another, and to their axial framework and relationship to blood vessels. The degree of anaplasia is related to the malignancy of the tumor.

**Anterior.** Before or toward the front.

**Aneurysm.** A sac (or bulging) of an artery or vein caused by dilatation of the walls of the vessel.

**Anterior cerebral artery.** An artery originating from the internal carotid artery serving principally the frontal lobe, corpus collosum, olfactory and optic tracts. Branches include the anterior communicating, ganglionic, commissural, and hemispheral arteries.

**Anterior commissure.** A band of fibers that passes transversly through the lamina terminalis and connects the basal portions of the two cerebral hemispheres.

**Anterior communicating artery.** An artery that originates from the anterior cerebral artery, supplies the caudate nucleus, and helps form the anterior part of the circle of Willis.

**Anticholinergic drugs.** Drugs which block the passage of nerve impulses through the parasympathetic nerves.

**Aphasia.** Impairment, due to cerebral damage, of receptive or expressive abilities in use of language symbols for communicational purposes.

**Apraxia.** Impaired ability, due to brain damage, to perform functional or purposeful acts.

**Aqueduct of Sylvius (Cerebral aqueduct).** A narrow canal, about three-quarters of an inch long, that connects the third and fourth ventricles.

**Arachnoid.** The middle layer of the meninges of the brain; so-named ("like a cobweb") because of its delicate network of tissue.

**Arachnoid villus.** A microscopic projection of the arachnoid tissue into the venous sinuses. Arachnoid villi absorb CSF.

**Arcuate fasciculus.** A bundle of fibers which connects the superior and middle frontal convolutions with the temporal lobe and temporal pole.

**Arteriosclerosis.** A condition marked by loss of elasticity, thickening, and hardening of the arteries.

**Arteriovenous malformation.** An abnormal formation of arteries and veins. It may be only a small tangle of vessels or a large collection of abnormal vessels occupying a large area.

**Artery.** A blood vessel that carries oxygenated blood.

**Association fibers.** Fibers which connect various cortical portions of the same cerebral hemisphere.

**Astereognosis.** Inability to identify objects through the sense of touch.

**Astrocytoma.** An intrinsic tumor of the brain that arises from star-shaped cells (astrocytes) of the neuroglia.

**Ataxia.** Disordered movements due to irregularity of muscular action and failure of muscular coordination.

**Atherosclerosis.** A degenerative process of arteries in which there are fatty deposits and degeneration of the inner lining of the vessel which, in turn, may lead to narrowing of the lumen of the vessel.

**Athetosis.** Involuntary, purposeless, disordered movements, caused by a brain lesion, in which there is a constant recurrence of slow writhing movements of the hands and feet.

**Atrophy.** A wasting away or decrease in size of a cell, tissue, organ, or part of the body due to lack of nourishment.

**Autonomic nervous system.** That part of the nervous system concerned with visceral and involuntary functions.

**Auditory verbal dysgnosia.** An aphasic deficit characterized by impairment of ability to understand the symbolic significance of verbal communication through the auditory avenue (loss of auditory-verbal comprehension).

**Autoimmune disorders.** Impairment of bodily processes by which immunization is effected.

**Axon.** A long, slender, and relatively unbranched process of a nerve cell which conducts impulses away from the cell body.

# B

**Babinski response.** Extension (instead of flexion) of the toes on stimulation of the sole of the foot, occurring in persons with lesions of the pyramidal tract.

**Bacterial infection.** Infection by minute, one-celled organisms which multiply by dividing in one or more directions.

**Basal ganglia.** A group of forebrain nuclei located within the diencephalon. Most anatomists include all or at least parts of the thalamus, caudate nucleus, and lentiform nucleus.

**Basilar artery.** An artery formed by the right and left vertebral arteries which supplies blood to parts of the cerebrum and cerebellum. It supplies blood to many brainstem structures and leads to the right and left posterior cerebral arteries.

**Basophil.** A granular leukocyte with an irregularly shaped, relatively pale-staining nucleus with cytoplasm that contains coarse bluish-black granules of variable size. Basophils contain vasoactive amines, such as histamine and serotonin, which are released on appropriate stimulation.

**Bell's palsy.** Unilateral facial paralysis of sudden onset, caused by a lesion of the facial nerve.

**Beta rhythm.** Rhythmic waves in the electroencephalogram that have a smaller amplitude than alpha waves and have an average frequency of about 25 cps.

**Bilateral sensory stimulation.** Stimulation of both sides of the body simultaneously, using touch, hearing, or vision, in order to determine whether an individual imperceives the stimulus on one side or the other.

**Bilateral transfer.** Facilitation of performance of a task by one hand as a result of having practiced the task with the other hand.

**Blepharospasm.** Spasmodic and frequent blinking of the eyes (tonic spasm of the orbicularis oculi muscle).

**Blood-brain barrier.** A process whereby certain substances fail to leave the blood circulation and enter the gray and white matter of the brain. The "barrier" is more of a physiological concept than a defined anatomic structure. In addition, the barrier does not exist at certain sites in the brain, including the pituitary gland, the pineal gland, and choroid plexus.

**Blood dyscrasia.** A disorder characterized by an abnormal composition of the blood.

**Body dysgnosia.** A deficit, associated with aphasia, in which the subject is impaired in ability to identify body parts.

**Brachia pontis.** A pair of peduncles which attach the pons to the overlying cerebellum.

**Bradykinesis.** A motor disorder, frequently seen in Parkinson's disease, resulting from rigidity of muscles and manifested by slow finger movements and difficulty in fine motor performances, such as writing.

**Brain abscess.** A localized collection of pus in a cavity in the brain, formed by the disintegration of tissues.

**Brain contusion.** A bruise of brain tissue in which there is capillary bleeding.

**Brain infection.** An invasion of brain tissues by pathogenic organisms in such a way that injury of brain tissue follows with symptoms of illness.

**Brain lesion.** Any pathological or traumatic damage of brain tissue.

**Bruit.** A sound or murmur, especially of an abnormal nature, that is heard in auscultation.

# C

**Calvarium.** The cranium, or more specifically, the skull cap.

**Capillary.** A minute blood vessel which connects an arteriole and a venule, forming a network in nearly all parts of the body and effecting a transition from arterial to venous blood flow.

**Carcinogen.** Any substance which produces cancer.

**Carcinoma.** A malignant new growth (cancer) that tends to infiltrate surrounding tissue and give rise to metastases.

**Carotid system.** A system of blood circulation to certain parts of the brain deriving from the internal carotid arteries.

**Caudate nucleus.** An elongated, arched mass of gray matter that is adjacent to the lateral ventricle of the brain throughout its entire extent and consists of a head, body, and tail. The caudate nucleus, lentiform nucleus, and putamen compose the corpus striatum, which is located in front of the thalamus.

**Cellular pleomorphism.** Assumption by cells of various distinct forms. Also, the property of crystalizing in two or more forms.

**Central dysarthria.** Impairment of ability to enunciate words, characterized by an omission, addition, or transposition of syllables.

**Central fissure (Rolandic fissure).** A fissure is a deep fold in the cerebral cortex which involves the entire thickness of the brain wall. The central fissure is the deep fold between the frontal and parietal lobes.

**Central nervous system.** The part of the nervous system made up of the brain and spinal cord.

**Cerebellar fits.** Episodes of decerebrate rigidity usually associated with large midline cerebellar masses.

**Cerebellum.** The portion of the brain that lies behind the cerebrum and above the pons and fourth ventricle. The cerebellum is concerned particularly with coordination of voluntary movements.

**Cerebral angiogram.** A procedure of visualization of blood vessels of the brain, using x-rays taken after injection of radiopaque material into the arterial blood stream.

**Cerebral anoxia.** A condition in which the cells of the brain do not have (or cannot utilize) sufficient oxygen to perform normal functions.

**Cerebral aqueduct.** See Aqueduct of Sylvius.

**Cerebral atrophy.** A wasting away or diminution in the size of cells or tissue structures of the brain.

**Cerebral blood flow.** The rate of blood flow through the brain, which may be measured by various techniques and determined for various regions of the brain.

**Cerebral cortex.** The thin surface layer of gray matter (nerve cell bodies) that forms the outer surface of the cerebrum.

**Cerebral embolism.** A sudden blocking or obstruction of an artery or vein by a clot which has been brought to the position of blockage by the current of blood flow.

**Cerebral hemisphere.** The large structure representing either half of the cerebrum.

**Cerebral hemorrhage.** Bleeding of a blood vessel within the cerebrum.

**Cerebral infarct.** An area of coagulation necrosis in a cerebral vessel which obstructs circulation and results in pathological changes in the area deprived of blood supply.

**Cerebral vascular accident (CVA or stroke).** An embolism, infarct, or hemorrhage of a cerebral vessel.

**Cerebral vascular insufficiency.** Lack of a sufficient supply of blood (which can be due to many factors) for the brain to perform its normal functions.

**Cerebrospinal fluid.** The fluid contained within the cerebral ventricles, subarachnoid sinus, and the central canal of the spinal cord. It acts as a water cushion to protect the brain and spinal cord from shock.

**Cerebrum.** The main portion of the brain which occupies the upper portion of the cranium and consists principally of the two cerebral hemispheres which are united by large masses of tissue fibers (white matter) called the anterior commissure, the corpus callosum, and the posterior commissure. Some anatomists also include the anterior part of the brainstem in the cerebrum.

**Chiasm.** A crossing or decussation of parts. The *optic chiasm* refers to the crossing of fibers of the optic nerve, forming the optic tract, that lies on the ventral surface of the brain.

**Chordoma.** A malignant tumor which arises from the embryonic remains of the notochord.

**Choreiform movements.** Movements that occur in the various forms of chorea which consist of rapid, highly complex, jerky movements that appear to be well coordinated but are performed involuntary and go on continuously in a variety of expressions.

**Choreoathetotic movements.** Movements of both a choreic and athetoid nature. *Athetosis* is marked by ceaseless occurrence of slow, sinuous, writhing movements that are involuntary and may be particularly severe in the hands.

**Choroid plexus.** A highly vascularized fold of the pia matter in the third, fourth, and lateral ventricles that secretes the cerebrospinal fluid.

**Cingulate gyrus.** A convolution (gyrus) which is arch-shaped and closely adjacent to the surface of the corpus collosum, from which it is separated by the callosal sulcus.

**Circle of Willis.** A circular system of cerebral arteries formed principally by the internal carotid, the anterior and posterior cerebral arteries, and the posterior communicating arteries.

**Cisternography.** Radiographic visualization of the basal cisterns of the brain after injection of a contrast substance.

**Cogwheeling.** A phenomenon that occurs among patients with Parkinson's disease in which a muscle, when passively stretched, develops a degree of hypertonicity and resistance, occurring in the form of irregular jerkiness of movement.

**Collagen.** The protein substance of white (collagenous) fibers of connective tissue.

**Colloid cyst.** A cyst that occurs particularly in the third ventricle and contains jelly-like material.

**Commissural fibers.** See Transverse fibers.

**Communicating hydrocephalus.** Hydrocephalus is a condition in which there is an abnormal accumulation of cerebral spinal fluid within the skull. Communicating hydrocephalus is a condition in which there is no obstruction in the ventricular system and cerebrospinal fluid is able to pass out of the brain but is not re-absorbed.

**Computed tomography (CT or CAT scan).** An x-ray procedure in which images or "slices," taken by scanners which rotate around the head, are reconstructed through computer-assisted methods. Computed tomography scanning permits identification and differentiation of many soft tissues in the body because of their absorption differences and the thin sections represented by the images in CT scanning.

**Concussion.** A condition caused by a physical blow to the head or extreme airblast, often resulting in loss of consciousness, vertigo, nausea, weak pulse, and slow respiration.

**Congenital lesions.** Lesions present at or dating from birth.

**Constructional dyspraxia.** Impaired ability to deal with spatial relationships either in a two- or three-dimensional framework. This symptom is commonly manifested by impaired ability to copy simple shapes, such as a cross.

**Contrecoup damage.** Damage to the opposite side of the brain from the point of injury.

**Contrast radiography.** X-ray procedures in which a contrast substance is injected in order to enhance visualization of particular structures. Customarily a contrast substance is injected into the blood circulation of the organ before x-rays are taken.

**Convolution.** A rounded, elevated part of the cerebral cortex (gyrus) that is generally fairly well demarcated by fissures (sulci).

**Cornea.** A transparent tissue that forms the outer anterior tissue of the eye.

**Corneal reflex.** Reflex closure of the eyelid as a result of irritation of the cornea.

**Corpus callosum.** An arched mass of white matter (nerve fibers), located at the bottom of the longitudinal fissure, made up of transverse fibers which connect the cerebral hemispheres.

**Corpus striatum.** A subcortical mass of gray and white matter that lies in front of and lateral to the thalamus in each cerebral hemisphere, forming one of the components of the basal ganglia.

**Cortex (pallium).** The surface layer (gray matter) of the cerebral and cerebellar hemispheres.

**Cortical atrophy.** Wasting, diminution or shrinkage of the cerebral cortex.

**Corticosteriods.** Any of the steroids elaborated by the adrenal cortex in response to the release of adrenocorticotropic hormone by the pituitary gland. Corticosteroids also refer to the synthetic equivalents of these steroids.

**Craniectomy.** Surgical removal (excision) of a part of the skull.

**Craniopharyngioma.** A tumor that arises from cells derived from the hypophyseal stalk.

**Cranium.** The skull.

**Cremasteric reflex.** A retraction of the testis on the same side and following stimulation of the skin on the front and inner side of the thigh. Presence of this reflex demonstrates integrity of the first lumbar nerve segment of the spinal cord.

**Creutzfeldt-Jakob disease.** A viral infection of the brain which usually occurs in middle life and causes partial degeneration of the pyramidal and extrapyramidal systems, accompanied by tremor, athetosis, spastic dysarthria, sometimes wasting of the muscles, and progressive dementia.

**Cyst.** A closed cavity or sack, lined by epithelium, and usually containing semisolid material.

**Cytology.** Study of the origin, structure, function, and pathology of cells.

# D

**Deep tendon reflexes (also called tendon reflexes and muscle stretch reflexes).** Tendon reflexes or muscle stretch reflexes are contrasted with reflexes of a superficial type. In muscle stretch reflexes the tendon or insertion of a muscle is briskly tapped with a reflex hammer and the resulting contraction of the muscle is graded from 0 (no response) to 4 + (maximal response or clonus).

**Delta waves (electroencephalography or EEG).** Random slow waves of 1 to 3 cps on EEG tracings.

**Dementia.** Significant deterioration of intellectual and cognitive functions.

**Demyelinating diseases.** Diseases characterized by destruction or removal of the myelin of nerve tissue.

**Dendrite.** A tree-shaped protoplasmic process from a nerve cell which receives impulses and conducts them toward the cell body.

**Dentate nucleus.** A major nucleus lying in the white matter of the cerebellum.

**Diabetes insipidus.** A metabolic disorder due to injury of the neurohypophyseal system, which results in a deficient quantity of antidiuretic hormone being released or produced. It is characterized by passage of large amounts of urine of low specific gravity and a great thirst.

**Diabetes mellitus.** A metabolic disorder in which there is a severe deficiency in ability to oxidize carbohydrates due to faulty pancreatic activity and consequent disturbance of normal insulin mechanism. This produces hyperglycemia with a variety of symptoms, including thirst, hunger, emaciation and weakness.

**Diaphragma sellae.** The membrane which forms the roof of the sella turcica and separates the pituitary gland from the hypothalamus and the optic chiasm.

**Diencephalon.** An ovoid mass of gray matter which forms the central core of the cerebrum, composed of the epithalamus, thalamus, hypothalamus and subthalamus.

**Diplopia.** Double vision, or seeing one object as if it were two.

**Dissecting aneurysm.** An aneurysm resulting from hemorrhage that causes longitudinal splitting of the arterial wall.

**Distal.** Toward the periphery or away from the center of the body.

**Dopamine.** A neurotransmitter, produced in the neurons of the pars compacta of the substantia nigra which reaches the corpus striatum by way of the axons of the nigrostriatal pathway, and is necessary for the normal functioning of the excitatory pathways to the gamma motor neurons.

**Dorsal.** Pertaining to or situated toward the back of the structure.

**Dura mater.** The tough and mostly fibrous outer layer of the meninges or membranes surrounding the brain.

**Dysarthria.** Imperfect articulation of speech due to disturbances of muscular control which result from damage to the central or peripheral nervous system.

Dyscalculia. An aphasic symptom characterized by impairment in the ability to appreciate the symbolic significance of numbers and the nature of arithmetical processes.

Dysdiadochokinesis. The ability to arrest one motor impulse and substitute one that is exactly the opposite. The clinical test for this condition is to have the patient hold out both hands and pronate and supinate them as rapidly as possible.

Dysgnosia. In contrast to agnosia, dysgnosia represents a partial rather than complete loss of the symbolic significance of information reaching the brain.

Dysgraphia. A loss of ability to form letters when writing, resulting from a brain lesion. A symptom of dysphasia.

Dyskinesia. A general term referring to impairment of voluntary movement which may be expressed in a number of specific ways.

Dyslexia. Impairment (due to a brain lesion) of reading ability and the understanding of the symbolic significance of words. A symptom of dysphasia.

Dysmetropsia. A defect in the visual appreciation of the measure of the size of objects. Also known as "past-pointing phenomenon."

Dysnomia. Impairment of the ability to name objects, resulting from a brain lesion. A symptom of dysphasia.

Dysphagia. Difficulty in swallowing.

Dyspraxia. Impairment of ability to perform coordinated and purposeful movements, resulting from a brain lesion.

Dysrhythmia. A disturbance or irregularity in the rhythm of EEG tracings.

Dysstereognosis. Impairment of ability to recognize objects through touch.

# E

Echoencephalography. A procedure in which ultrasonic waves are beamed through the head from both sides and echos from the midline structures as well as from other tissues are recorded as graphic tracings. The tracings may indicate the presence of a mass lesion on one side or the other.

Edema. Accumulation of abnormally large amounts of fluid in the intercellular tissue spaces of the body.

Efferent. In reference to nerve impulses, conveying impulses outward or toward an effector organ.

Electromyography. Recording of the electrical properties of skeletal muscles to determine whether or not the muscle is contracting, detecting the nature and location of motor unit lesions, and providing information regarding neuromuscular function, neuromuscular conduction, extent of nerve lesion, reflex responses, etc.

Electronystagmography. Caloric (both heat and cold) stimulation of the vestibular nerve with recording of nystagmus (or rhythmic contractions of extrinsic eye muscles resulting in patterns of eye movements).

Encephalitis. Infection and resulting inflammation of the brain.

Encephalon. A general term referring to the brain.

Endarterectomy. Surgical removal of deposits along the inner lining of arteries, intended to improve patency of the vessel.

Endocrinological disorders. Any disease or disorder due to malfunction of the organs of internal secretions (endocrine glands).

Eosinophil. A cell that is readily stained by eosin. The cell is usually a granular leukocyte with a nucleus that usually has two lobes and cytoplasm that contains coarse, round granules that are uniform in size.

Ependymoma. A tumor of the brain, classified as a glioma, which arises from adult ependymal cells.

Epidermoid. A tumor that includes epidermoid elements but occurs in a noncutaneous site such as the skull, brain, or meninges.

**Epidermoid cyst.** An epidermoid that is cystic in nature.

**Epidural hematoma.** An area of bleeding or accumulation of blood outside of the dura mater and in the epidural space. These lesions are usually due to damage of the middle meningeal artery and may produce compression of the dura mater and thus compression of the underlying brain tissue.

**Epilepsy.** A disorder characterized by seizures of a number of different types. It may be due to one of many known causes but frequently is of unknown etiology.

**Epithalamus.** The part of the diencephalon superior and posterior to the thalamus, comprising the pineal body, the habenula and habenular trigone.

**Epithelium.** The tissue that covers the internal and external surfaces of the body, including the lining of blood vessels and other small cavities.

**Erythrocyte.** A red blood cell or red blood corpuscle that is adapted by virtue of its form and hemoglobin content to transport oxygen.

**Essential hypertension.** Elevated blood pressure due to unknown etiology.

**Exophthalmos.** Abnormal protrusion of the eyeball.

**External capsule.** A thin lamina of white matter which separates the claustrum from the median putamen.

**Extraneuronal neuritic plaques (senile plaques).** Areas of incomplete necrosis in the brains of patients with Alzheimer's disease and in older persons.

**Extreme capsule.** A thin layer of white matter which separates the claustrum and the insula.

**Extrinsic brain tumor.** A tumor that arises from tissue surrounding the brain and produces brain-related symptoms through compression of brain tissue.

# F

**Facial paresis.** Weakness or partial paralysis of facial muscles.

**Falx.** The dural tissue which separates the cerebral hemispheres.

**Falx cerebelli.** The partition between the cerebellar hemispheres.

**Falx cerebri.** The partition between the cerebral hemispheres in the midline.

**Fasciculation.** A small local contraction of muscles caused by a spontaneous discharge of a number of nerve fibers innervated by a single motor nerve filament. A fasciculation is often visible through the skin.

**Finger dysgnosia.** Impaired ability to identify individual fingers following tactile stimulation.

**Fissure (sulcus).** A deep fold in the cerebral cortex which involves the entire thickness of the brain wall and tends to define the limits of a gyrus or convolution.

**Fistula.** An abnormal passage or communication, usually between two internal organs. It may also lead from an internal organ to the surface of the body. Fistulae may be created for purposes of experimental study.

**Flaccid.** Relaxed, flabby or absent muscular tone.

**Folia (of cerebellum).** The numerous long narrow folds of the cerebellar cortex, separated by sulci and supported by white laminae.

**Foramen.** A natural opening or passage from one area to another.

**Foramen of Magendie.** The aperture in the fourth ventricle through which CSF escapes into the subarachnoid space.

**Foramen of Monro (interventricular foramen).** A passage connecting the lateral with the third ventricle.

**Foramina of Luschka.** Two lateral apertures in the fourth ventricle which permit escape of CSF into the subarachnoid space and its various cisterns.

**Formication.** A sensation of small insects crawling over the skin.

**Fornix.** A large tract which is a major connection between the forebrain and midbrain.

**Fovea.** A term used to describe a small pit or depression in the surface of a structure. The term is often used to indicate the central area of the retina which consists of slim, elongated cones and subserves the area of clearest form vision.

**Frontal lobe.** The anterior lobe in each cerebral hemisphere, bound posteriorly by the central fissure.

**Fundus (of the eye).** The posterior aspect of the internal coat of the eye.

**Fungal infections.** Infections caused by any one of a class of vegetable organisms of a low order of development, including molds.

## G

**Galvonometer.** An instrument for measuring current by electromagnetic action.

**Ganglioneuroma.** A benign neoplasm composed of nerve fibers and mature ganglion cells.

**General dyspraxia.** A general impairment in the ability to perform coordinated and purposeful acts.

**General paresis (dementia paralytica).** A chronic syphilitic meningoencephalitis, characterized by progressive dementia and a generalized paralysis.

**Geniculostriate tract.** A tract of nerve fibers in the visual system extending from the lateral geniculate body of the thalamus to the striate cortex of the occipital lobe.

**Glabellar tap sign.** Failure to discontinue eye-blinking after several taps have been delivered to the glabella (the smooth area on the frontal bone between the eyebrows).

**Glasgow Coma Scale.** A scale used to assess potential outcome in cases of head injury.

**Glia.** Neuroglia cells are part of the supporting structure of nervous tissue in the brain. This structure consists of a fine web of tissue made up of ectodermic elements in which are enclosed odd-shape branched cells known as neuroglia or glial cells. These cells are of three types: macroglia or astroglia, oligodendroglia, and microglia.

**Glioblastoma multiforme (astrocytoma grades III or IV).** A rapidly growing glioma originating from astrocytes (star-shaped cells) of the neuroglia.

**Glioma.** A brain tumor composed of tissue which represents neuroglia in any of its stages of development.

**Granuloma.** A tumor-like mass or nodule of granulation tissue associated with an infectious disease.

**Granulovacuolar degeneration.** A degenerative change in neurons that occurs particularly in the hippocampal regions and a prominent finding in Alzheimer's disease.

**Gray matter.** Cell bodies of neurons in the central nervous system composed of the cerebral cortex and various nuclei.

**Gyrus (convolution).** On the surface of the brain, a convoluted ridge of cerebral cortex between fissures or sulci.

## H

**Haptic sensitivity.** Sensitivity to stimuli through touch.

**Hemangioblastoma.** A hemangioma (a benign tumor made up of newly formed blood vessels) that consists of capillaries.

**Hemangioma.** A benign tumor made up of newly formed blood vessels.

**Hemangiopericytoma.** A tumor composed of spindle cells with a rich vascular network which apparently arises from pericytes.

**Hemianopia.** Loss of vision in half of each eye.

**Hemiballismus.** A violent form of motor restlessness involving only one side of the body and most marked in the upper extremity. It results from a lesion of the hypothalamic nucleus.

**Hemihypalgesia.** Diminished sensitivity to pain affecting one lateral half of the body.

**Hemiparesis.** Partial paralysis or weakness of one side of the body.

**Hemiplegia.** Paralysis of half of the body.

**Hemisensory deficit.** Sensory losses, usually including tactile impairment, on half of the body.

**Hepatic encephalopathy.** A brain disorder or dysfunction caused by liver disease or damage.

**Herpes simplex encephalitis.** An infectious invasion of the brain by the virus causing herpes simplex.

**Hippocampus.** A curved structure that forms an elevation in the floor of the inferior horn of the lateral ventricle. It is an important functional component of the limbic system. The hippocampus has been identified as being especially important in memory.

**Histological examination (histology).** An examination or study of the fine (microscopic) structure of tissues of the body.

**Hodgkin's disease.** A disease of unknown etiology producing painless, progressive enlargement of the lymph nodes, spleen, and general lymphoid tissues. It often begins in the neck and spreads to other parts of the body.

**Homonymous hemianopia.** A loss of half of the visual field for each eye with the loss being on the same side (left or right) for each eye.

**Homonymous quadrantanopia.** A loss of one quadrant of the visual field (either upper or lower) on the same side (either right or left) for each eye.

**Huntington's disease (Huntington's chorea).** A hereditary disease, resulting in dementia, and characterized by chronic, progressive choreic movements and mental deterioration.

**Hydrocephalus.** An abnormal accumulation of cerebrospinal fluid within the skull, usually with dilatation of the cerebral ventricles, caused most often by obstruction of normal cerebrospinal fluid circulation.

**Hydrocephalus ex vacuo.** Replacement of the space lost by cerebral tissue (in atrophy) by cerebrospinal fluid.

**Hypalgesia.** Diminished sensitivity to pain.

**Hyperostosis.** Hypertrophy or excessive growth of bone tissue.

**Hypertension.** Abnormally high blood pressure.

**Hypertensive encephalopathy.** Brain dysfunction or disease due to elevated blood pressure.

**Hypesthesia.** Impairment or lessening of tactile sensitivity.

**Hypoglycemia.** A below-normal concentration of glucose in the blood.

**Hypothalamus.** A region of the diencephalon below the thalamus which forms the floor and part of the lateral wall of the third ventricle.

**Hypotonia.** A condition of diminished tone of the skeletal muscles.

**Hypoxic encephalopathy.** Disease or damage of the brain due to a diminished supply of oxygen.

# I

**Ictal.** The symptoms and manifestations characterized by a stroke or an acute epileptic seizure.

**Idiopathic.** A term referring to conditions of unknown cause.

**Idiopathic epilepsy.** Epilepsy of unknown cause.

**Imperception (tactile, auditory, visual).** Failure to perceive a sensory stimulus on one side when stimuli are delivered to both sides simultaneously, even though unilateral stimuli on both sides can be perceived correctly.

**Inclusion bodies.** Anything that is enclosed; often used to refer to inclusion of substances in cells which may be lifeless, often temporary (such as an accumulation of proteins, fats, carbohydrates, pigments, secretory granules, crystals, or other insoluble components) contained within the cytoplasm of a cell.

**Insula.** The lateral part of the cerebral hemisphere covered by the frontal, parietal and temporal lobes.

**Intracranial hypertension.** Elevated pressure within the cranium or skull.

**Intraneuronal deterioration.** Deterioration of structures within the neuron.

**Intracranial tumor.** A tumor that occurs within the cranium.

**Intention (Kinetic) tremor.** A tremor which arises or is intensified when a voluntary movement is attempted.

**Internal capsule.** A broad band of white fibers separating the lenticular nucleus from the medial caudate nucleus and thalamus.

**Internal carotid artery.** An artery that originates from the common carotid artery and with its branches supplies blood to a large portion of the brain, the orbit, internal ear, nose, and forehead.

**Interthalamic adhesion.** *See* Massa intermedia.

**Intrinsic tumor.** A tumor arising from tissues within the brain.

**Ipsilateral.** Refering to (situated on or affecting) the same side, as opposed to contralateral.

**Iris.** The circular pigmented membrane behind the cornea that surrounds the open space represented by the pupil of the eye. Circular muscular fibers of the iris (surrounding the pupil) permit constriction of the pupillary space when they contract; a thin layer of radial smooth muscle fibers dilate the pupil when they contract. This mechanism regulates the amount of light entering the eye.

**Ischemia.** A local and temporary deficiency of blood.

## J

**Jacksonian seizures.** Epileptic seizures which begin with a small, localized group of muscles and gradually spread to involve a larger muscle group.

**Jakob-Creutzfeldt disease.** *See* Creutzfeldt-Jakob disease.

## K

**Kinesthesis.** A sense by which muscular motion and degree of muscular contraction permits perception of weight, bodily position, etc.

**Korsakoff's syndrome.** A psychotic state, associated with chronic alcoholism, marked by disturbance of orientation, confusion, delusions, hallucinations, and inaccurate memories. Polyneuritis and wrist drop are also usually present.

## L

**Laminography.** A special radiographic technique to show detailed images of structures lying in a predetermined plane of tissue, while blurring or eliminating detail of structures in other planes.

**Lateral geniculate body.** A prominent nucleus of the thalamus, which receives input from the retinal ganglion cells and projects to the visual cortex.

**Lesion.** Any damage to bodily tissues as a result of disease or injury.

**Levodopa.** A drug that plays an important role in treatment of Parkinsonism. The neurotransmitter dopamine is unable to pass the blood-brain barrier, but levodopa is converted to dopamine in the brain and replenishes depleted dopamine in the brainstem and basal ganglia.

**Leukemia.** A disease of blood-forming organs characterized by an increase in the number of leukocytes and their precursors in the blood. It is accompanied by enlargement and proliferation of the lymphoid tissue of the spleen, lymphatic glands, and bone marrow.

**Leukocyte.** A white blood cell or corpuscle, which may be classified into various types falling within two main groups refered to as *granular* and *nongranular* leukocytes.

**Leukodystrophies.** A group of familial conditions occuring predominantly in infancy and childhood in which there is abnormal formation of myelin.

**Lipid storage diseases.** Diseases which involve neuronal storage of lipid and cerebromacular degeneration (an accumulation of lipid in the ganglion cells of the retina).

**Lipoma.** A benign tumor composed of fat cells.

**Lumbar puncture.** Insertion of a needle into the lumbar subarachnoid space to determine cerebrospinal fluid pressure and to withdraw cerebrospinal fluid for examination.

**Lymphocyte.** A mononuclear leukocyte which is chiefly a product of lymphoid tissue and participates in the immune process.

**Lymphoma.** A tumor made up of lymphoid tissue.

**Lysis.** A term used to refer to (1) destruction of cells by a specific lysin; (2) decomposition of a chemical compound by a specific agent; or (3) the gradual decrease of symptoms of a disease.

# M

**Macrophage.** Large, mononuclear cells occuring in the walls of blood vessels and in loose connective tissue which are highly phagocytic in nature. Phagocytes are cells that ingest microorganisms or other cells and foreign particles.

**Major motor seizures.** Epileptic seizures characterized by loss of consciousness and tonic-clonic muscular activity. Also referred to as *grand mal epilepsy*.

**Malleolus.** A rounded process or protuberance.

**Manual dexterity.** Proficiency in performances using the hands.

**Massa intermedia (interthalamic adhesion).** A mass of gray matter connecting the thalami across the midline of the third ventricle.

**Mastication.** The process of chewing food.

**Medulla oblongata.** The lowest part of the brain, continuous with the spinal cord on the lower end and the pons on the upper end. It lies below the cerebellum. The back of the medulla forms the floor of the fourth ventricle.

**Medullary center.** The white matter of the cerebral hemisphere.

**Medulloblastoma.** A malignant tumor in the region of the fourth ventricle and involving the cerebellum. It is composed of immature neuroglial cells.

**Meninges.** The three membranous tissues (dura mater, arachnoid, and pia mater) that envelop the brain and spinal cord.

**Meningo-cortical scar.** Scar tissue that involves the meninges and the cerebral cortex of the brain.

**Meningioma.** A tumor of the meninges. These tumors are classified as benign and are usually slowly growing.

**Meningitis.** Inflammation of the meninges. When the dura mater is affected the disease is referred to as *pachymeningitis*; when the arachnoid tissue and pia mater are also involved it is called *leptomeningitis*.

**Metabolic brain disorder.** A disorder of the brain tissue involving the physical and chemical processes by which living organized substance is produced and maintained and by which energy is made available.

**Metastatic tumor.** A tumor that is transferred from one organ or part of the body to another organ or part not directly connected with it. In metastatic brain tumors there is a transfer of cells via the lymphatics or blood stream from the initial malignant tumor (carcinoma) to the brain.

**Midbrain (mesencephalon).** A portion of the brain which consists of the corpora quadrigemina, tegmentum, cerebral peduncles, and cerebral aqueduct (Sylvian aqueduct).

**Micrographia.** Small, cramped handwriting.

**Middle cerebral artery.** One of three major arteries that serves the cerebral hemispheres. It arises from the internal carotid artery and distributes blood to the frontal, parietal, part of the temporal lobe, and the basal ganglia.

**Mitosis.** A process of indirect division of a cell by which the body grows and replaces cells. Pathologic mitosis indicates malignancy.

**Monocyte.** A phagocytic leukocyte which is formed in the bone marrow and transported to other tissues where they develop into macrophages.

**Morphology.** The science of the form and structure of organisms or parts of organisms.

**Motor area.** The pre-central gyrus represented in the posterior part of the frontal lobe. This area serves primary motor functions.

**Multi-infarct dementia.** Dementia resulting from small infarcts due to arteriosclerosis, distributed throughout the brain.

**Multiple sclerosis.** A disease characterized by sclerosis (plaques) resulting from degeneration of myelin occurring in patches throughout the brain and spinal cord.

**Myelin sheath.** A sheath that surrounds the axis-cylinder of some nerve fibers. Fibers which have myelin sheaths are referred to as myelinized fibers.

**Myeloma.** A tumor composed of cells originating from the bone marrow.

**Myoclonic epilepsy.** An epileptic seizure in which shock-like contractions occur in a portion of a muscle, an entire muscle, or a group of muscles. These seizures are sometimes restricted to one area of the body or appear either in or out of synchrony in several areas.

**Myxedema.** A condition due to hypoactivity of the thyroid gland. It results in a lowering of basal metabolism and a number of signs and symptoms.

# N

**Necrosis.** The morphological changes occuring as a result of cell death and caused by progessive degradative action of enzymes.

**Nephrectomy.** The excision or removal of a kidney.

**Neuritic (or senile) plaque.** Areas of incomplete necrosis in the cerebral cortex; associated with aging and certain pathological states such as Alzheimer's disease.

**Neuroblastoma.** A tumor composed principally of neuroblasts which occurs principally in infants and children up to about 10 years of age.

**Neurofibrillary tangles.** Tangles of neurofibrilla, which are fibers that form a delicate network among nerve cells. These tangles are observed particularly in patients with Alzheimer's disease but are also seen in the brains of older people generally.

**Neurofibroma.** A connective tissue tumor of the nerve fiber.

**Neuroglia.** The supporting structure of nervous tissue consisting of a fine web of tissue that contains neuroglial cells or glial cells. These glial cells fall in three categories: astrocytes, oligodendrocytes, and microglia.

**Neurolemmoma.** A neurofibroma.

**Neurology.** A branch of medical science that deals with nervous system functions and diseases.

**Neuron.** A nerve cell, or the structural unit of the nervous system, including the cell body and the various processes, collaterals, and terminations of the cell.

**Neuronal degenerative disease.** A disease in which the primary underlying factor is degeneration of neurons.

**Neuronal loss.** A depletion in the number of neurons which occurs with aging and many neurological diseases (e.g., Alzheimer's disease).

**Neuropathology.** A branch of medicine which deals with diseases of the nervous system and pathology of nerves and nerve centers.

**Neuropsychology.** A branch of psychology which deals with brain-behavior relationships and measurement of the manifestations of brain functions.

**Normal-pressure hydrocephalus (also refered to as occult hydrocephalus).** Hydrocephalus occurring in middle-aged and older persons in which cerebrospinal fluid pressure is normal but the ventricles are enlarged. The patient often shows evidence of dementia, ataxia, and urinary incontinence.

**Nuchal rigidity.** Stiffness of the back of the neck.

**Nucleus ambiguus.** A nucleus located in the reticular formation of the medulla. Its fibers innervate cranial nerves IX, X, and XI.

**Nystagmus.** An involuntary rapid movement of the eyeball, which may be lateral, vertical, rotatory, or a mixed combination.

# O

**Obstructive hydrocephalus (also called noncommunicating hydrocephalus).** Hydrocephalus due to a ventricular block that obstructs the normal flow of cerebrospinal fluid.

**Occipital lobe.** The most posterior lobe of each cerebral hemisphere.

**Occlusion.** The process of closure or the state of being closed. Vascular occulsion refers to the closing of a blood vessel.

**Oculogyric crisis.** An episode, usually in patients with Parkinson's disease, in which the eyeballs become fixed in one position for an extended period of time.

**Oculomotor signs.** Signs pertaining to abnormal movements of the eye through impaired control or coordination of the extrinsic eye muscles.

**Oligodendroglioma.** A tumor of the brain that arises from oligodendroglial cells.

**Ophthalmic artery.** An artery that arises from the internal carotid artery and supplies blood to the eye and adjacent parts of the face.

**Ophthalmoplegia.** Paralysis of the eye muscles.

**Optic chiasm.** The point at which there is crossing of the fibers from each optic nerve to form the optic tracts, located on the ventral surface of the brain.

**Optic disc.** The area of the retina where the optic fibers converge to leave the back of the eye as the optic nerve.

**Optic disc pallor.** An appearance of paleness in the vicinity of the optic disc.

**Optic neuritis.** An inflammation of the optic nerve.

**Optic tract.** A tract made up of contributions of fibers from both the right and.left optic nerves and extending from the optic chiasm to the point of synapse in the lateral geniculate body.

**Orbital surface (of the skull or frontal lobes).** The surface adjacent to the eyes.

**Oropharynx.** The part of the pharynx that lies between the soft palate and the upper edge of the epiglottis.

**Osteomyelitis.** An inflammation of bone caused by a pyogenic (pus-producing) organism which may be localized or spread through the bone more generally.

**Osteoporosis.** Abnormal rarefaction (decrease in density and weight, but not in volume) of the bone, most commonly seen in the elderly. Subclassifications of osteoporosis may occur with particular diseases or injuries.

# P

**Pacchionian granulations.** Enlarged arachnoid villi through which cerebrospinal fluid is reabsorbed into the blood of the venous system of the central nervous system.

**Palepbral fissure.** The longitudinal opening between the eyelids.

**Pallium.** *See* Cortex.

**Palsy.** Paralysis or weakness of muscles.

**Papilledema.** Edema or swelling of the optic papilla which gives rise to an elevation of the optic disk ("choked disk"). Papilledema is usually a sign of increased intracranial pressure.

**Paralysis agitans.** Idiopathic Parkinson's disease.

**Paranoid schizophrenia.** Psychosis characterized by suspiciousness, systematized delusions of persecution, and feelings of grandeur, often built up in logical form.

**Paraparesis.** A partial paralysis of the lower extremities.

**Paraplegia.** Paralysis of the legs and lower part of the body with sensation also often being affected.

**Parenchyma.** Referring to the functional elements of an organ as distinguished from the elements representing its framework.

**Paresis.** A partial or incomplete paralysis.

**Paresthesia.** An abnormal tactile sensation such as numbness, burning, prickling, or tickling.

**Parietal lobe.** One of the four lobes of each cerebral hemisphere that is bound by the frontal lobe anteriorly, the occipital lobe posteriorly, and the temporal lobe principally inferiorly.

**Partial complex epilepsy.** Epilepsy in which the seizures include inappropriate complex acts and performances for which the patient is amnesic.

**Pathognomonic signs.** A sign or symptom specifically distinctive or characteristic of a disease or pathological condition and on the appearance of which a diagnosis can be made.

**Peripheral dysarthria.** Impaired enunciatory ability characterized by slurring of speech.

**Petechial hemorrhage.** A hemorrhage characterized by petechiae or small spots of bleeding.

**Petit mal epilepsy.** A type of epilepsy seen particularly in children in which there is a sudden and momentary loss of consciousness with only minor myoclonic jerking. After adolescence it may develop into another form of epilepsy.

**Pick's disease.** Atrophy of the lobes of the brain resulting in a clinical picture that is very similar to Alzheimer's disease.

**Pineal gland (pineal body).** A small, somewhat flattened, cone-shaped structure that lies above the superior colliculi and below the splenium of the corpus callosum.

**Pinealoma.** A tumor of the pineal gland.

**Pituitary adenoma.** A tumor of the pituitary gland.

**Pituitary gland.** A body located at the base of the brain in the sella turcica. It is attached by a stalk to the hypothalamus, from which it receives an important neural outflow. The pituitary gland consists of two main lobes: the anterior pituitary and the posterior pituitary (or neurohypophysis). The pituitary gland secretes several important hormones which regulate the functioning of the thyroid, gonads, adrenal cortex, and other endocrine organs. Thus, it is of great importance in the growth, maturation, and reproduction of the individual.

**Plantar.** Pertaining to the sole of the foot.

**Plantar reflex.** Contraction of the toes with irritation of the middle part of the sole of the foot.

**Plasma cell.** A spherical or ellipsoid cell having certain morphological characteristics that result from differentiation of certain lymphocytes and are the most active cells in secreting antibodies.

**Pleurothotonos.** Bending of the body to one side.

**Pneumoencephalography.** A procedure in which cerebrospinal fluid is replaced with air in order to permit x-ray visualization of structures within the brain.

**Polycythemia.** An excessive number of red corpuscles in the blood.

**Polymorphonuclear cell.** A cell that has a nucleus so deeply lobed or divided that it appears to be multiple. A polymorphonuclear leukocyte, for example, has a nucleus with three to five lobes connected by slender threads of chromatin.

**Pons.** The region of the brain stem between the midbrain and the medulla, lying in front of the cerebellum.

**Porencephaly.** The presence of cavities in the brain which developed in fetal life or early infancy, usually resulting from destructive lesions such as small areas of bleeding. These lesions may be cystic and communicate with the arachnoid space.

**Posterior cerebral artery.** An artery arising from the basilar artery and supplying blood to the occipital area and parts of the temporal area.

**Posterior commissure.** A band of nerve fibers that join nuclei of the thalamus.

**Posterior communicating artery.** An artery that arises from the internal carotid artery, forms part of the circle of Willis, and supplies blood to the uncinate gyrus and part of the thalamus.

**Primary tumor.** A tumor that develops within the affected organ rather than originating in other parts of the body.

**Presenile dementia.** Severe deterioration of mental functions before the age of 65 years.

**Projection fibers.** Fibers which connect the cerebral cortex with the lower portions of the brain and spinal cord.

**Proximal.** Next to or nearest, as in a part of the limb with relation to the body.

**Psychomotor epilepsy.** A condition now referred to as "partial complex epilepsy."

**Ptosis.** Drooping of the upper eyelid as a result of involvement of the third oculomotor cranial nerve or impairment of sympathetic innervation.

# R

**Radicle.** Any one of the smallest branches of a vessel or nerve.

**Radionuclide imaging.** A procedure in which radioactive materials are injected into the blood stream and a quasi-pictorial representation of the distribution of radioactive materials is obtained. In terms of the brain, if there is a breakdown in the blood-brain barrier or an abnormal accumulation of blood in a particular area, the radionuclide image may represent the abnormality.

**Reflex seizure.** An epileptic attack occurring in response to a specific type of stimulus. Reflex epilepsy may be broken down into a number of categories, depending upon the type of stimulus that precipitates the epileptic attack. For example, musicogenic epilepsy is a type of reflex epilepsy that occurs in response to a musical stimulus, in some instances requiring a highly selective musical piece (the music of a particular band or even a particular musical composition).

**Renal insufficiency.** A condition in which the kidneys are unable to remove a sufficient proportion of waste matter from the blood.

**Rest tremor.** Tremor which occurs in the absence of voluntary movements, frequently seen in patients with Parkinsonism.

**Retrobulbar neuritis.** Neuritis (nerve inflammation) of the portion of the optic nerve that is immediately posterior to the eyeball.

**Reye's syndrome.** An acute and severe illness that often occurs as a sequel of influenza and other viral infections of the upper respiratory tract. The syndrome is marked by acute brain swelling associated with hypoglycemia, fatty infiltration of the liver, hepatomegaly (enlargement of the liver), impairment of consciousness and the occurrence of epileptic seizures.

**Right-left confusion.** Confusion of the right and left sides of one's own body or of other persons or objects.

**Rigidity.** Abnormal or pathological stiffness or inflexibility of muscles.

**Rolandic fissure (central fissure).** The fissure between the frontal and parietal lobes.

**Romberg test.** A test used for differentiating between peripheral and cerebellar ataxia. In this test the patient is required to stand in a motionless position with the eyes closed. An increase in movements and uncertainty of physical position with swaying indicates the presence of peripheral ataxia. The test is also used more generally to evaluate clumsiness in movements and the width and uncertainty of gait when the patient's eyes are closed. Absence of difficulties with the eyes closed is characteristic of cerebellar ataxia.

# S

**Sarcoma.** A tumor, often highly malignant, made up of embryonic-like connective tissue or of tissue composed of closely packed cells embedded in a fibrillar or homogenous substance.

**Sagittal.** Pertaining to the sagittal or midline suture of the skull and in any plane that is parallel to this suture.

**Schizophrenia.** A psychotic disorder manifested by a variety of symptoms depending upon the type of schizophrenia. Often characterized by withdrawal, ineffectiveness in behavior, disorientation, delusions, and hallucinations.

**Scotoma.** An area in the visual field that is characterized by lost or depressed vision and surrounded by an area of less depressed or normal vision. In other words, specific areas of decreased vision or blindness within the visual field.

**Sella turcica.** A saddle-shaped depression crossing the midline on the superior surface of the body of the sphenoid bone.

**Senile dementia.** Severe deterioration of mental functions in persons over the age of 65 years.

**Senile plaque (Extraneuronal neuritic plaque).** An area of incomplete necrosis seen in persons with primary neuronal degenerative diseases of the brain and, to a lesser degree, in older persons.

**Septum pellucidium.** A double membrane, triangular in shape, that separates the anterior horns of the lateral ventricles of the brain. It is situated in the median plane and bounded by the corpus callosum and the body and columns of the fornix.

**Sickle-cell anemia.** An inherited disease characterized by anemia and ulcers in which the red blood cells acquire a sickle-like or crescent shape.

**Somatic complaints.** Complaints referring to disorders of bodily functions.

**Spastic paraparesis.** Partial paralysis of the lower extremities characterized by spastic movements.

**Spelling dyspraxia.** Impairment of spelling ability as a result of cerebral damage. A symptom of aphasia.

**Status epilepticus.** A series of rapidly repeating epileptic seizures that continue without any intervening periods of consciousness.

**Stereotaxic surgery.** Surgery in which the purpose is to place a therapeutic lesion in a precise area of the brain. Mechanical equipment and x-rays are used to localize the specific area.

**Sternocleidomastoid muscle.** A muscle originating from the sternum and clavicle, inserting in the mastoid process and a part of the occipital bone. It is used to depress and rotate the head and flex the head and neck.

**Strabismus.** Involuntary deviation of the eye from the normal position.

**Stroke.** A general term referring to a cerebral vascular accident.

**Sturge-Weber disease (syndrome).** A congenital syndrome consisting of an area of the skin that is pink to dark bluish red in color and involves otherwise normal skin (also called *capillary hemangioma* or *port-wine stain*). The angioma may be more extensive and is frequently associated with intracranial calcification, mental retardation, contralateral hemiplegia, and epilepsy.

**Subacute sclerosing panencephalitis.** A rare and devasting form of leukoencephalitis usually affecting children and adolescents. This disease is insidious in onset, characterized by progressive cerebral dysfunction over a course of weeks or months and usually results in death within a year. The disease has been associated with the measles virus.

**Subarachnoid hemorrhage.** Bleeding into the subarachnoid space.

**Subclavian artery.** The artery which arises from the brachiocephalic artery on the right side and the aortic arch on the left side and distributes blood to the brain, meninges, and other parts of the body.

**Subdural hematoma.** Bleeding into the subdural space.

**Substantia nigra.** The layer of gray substance that separates the tegmentum of the midbrain from the crus cerebri. The substantia nigra consists of two zones, a dorsal compact zone with melanin-containing cells and a ventral reticular zone in which melanin is lacking.

**Sulcus (fissure).** An indentation in the cerebral cortex marking the limit of a gyrus or convolution.

**Superior sagittal sinus.** A single venous sinus formed by the walls of the dura mater, beginning in the front at the crista galli and extending in the midline backward to the convex border of the falx cerebri, ending near the occipital protuberance in a confluence with other sinuses.

**Suprasellar tumor.** A tumor above the sella turcica.

**Supratentorial.** Above the tentorium of the cerebellum.

**Sylvian area.** The area of the cerebral cortex in the vicinity of the Sylvian fissure.

**Sylvian fissure.** A fissure that runs along the superior surface of the temporal lobe, dividing it in its anterior portion from the frontal lobe and in the more posterior portion from the parietal lobe.

**Synapse.** The region of contact between processes of two adjacent neurons, forming the place where a nervous impulse is transmitted from one neuron to another.

**Syphilitic gumma.** A soft, gummy tumor that occurs in the tertiary stages of syphilis.

**Syphilitic infection of the brain.** Syphilis is a contagious venereal disease that leads to many lesions throughout the body and, if untreated, eventually will involve the brain.

# T

**Tactile.** Pertaining to touch.

**Tactile form discrimination.** Ability to discriminate form or shape through the sense of touch.

**Tay-Sachs disease.** An inherited lipid storage disease with onset in early life resulting from an enzyme deficiency leading to accumulation of lipids and other material in the neurons of the retina and central nervous system.

**Telencephalon.** The cerebral hemispheres.

**Temporal lobe.** One of the four lobes of the cerebral hemisphere; it lies in an inferior and lateral position.

**Tentorium.** A layer of dura mater which forms a partition between the cerebrum and the cerebellum and covers the upper surface of the cerebellum.

**Teratogenic abnormalities.** Abnormalities that result from physical defects of the offspring in utero.

**Teratoma.** A tumor, or true neoplasm, which is made up of a number of different types of tissue, none of which is appropriate in the area in which the tumor occurs.

**Thalamus.** A structure constituting the middle and larger portion of the diencephalon, which forms part of the lateral wall of the third ventricle and lies between the hypothalamus and the epithalamus. It contains various nuclei and is the main relay center for sensory impulses and cerebellar and basoganglia projections to the cerebral cortex. Thalamic nuclei include the anterior, central, intralaminar, lateral, medial, posterior, and reticular thalamic nuclei. The lateral and medial geniculate bodies are also often considered to be part of the thalamus.

**Thalamotomy.** A stereotaxically imposed surgical lesion in the thalamus (usually placed in the ventrolateral nucleus for relief of dyskinesia on the contralateral side of the body).

**Theta rhythm.** Brain waves in the electroencephalogram that have a frequency of four to seven cycles per second. Theta waves occur principally in children but also in adults during periods of emotional stress.

**Thrombosis.** The formation of a clot (thrombus) in a blood vessel.

**Tinnitus.** A noise in the ears such as ringing, buzzing, roaring, or clicking.

**Tonic-clonic seizure.** A seizure characterized by alternate muscular contraction and relaxation in rapid succession.

**Toxic brain disorder.** Damage or dysfunction of the brain as a result of toxic influences.

**Toxoplasmosis.** A protozoan disease that may be congenital or acquired and infects many organs of the body, including the brain.

**Transient ischemic attack (TIA).** A temporary manifestation of brain disorder which may last from a few minutes for up to 24 hours. It usually represents focal manifestations with a great range of symptoms, due to cerebral circulatory insufficiency.

**Transverse (commissural) fibers.** Fibers which interconnect the two cerebral hemispheres.

**Tremor.** An involuntary trembling or quivering.

**Trigeminal neuralgia (tic douloureux).** A condition resulting from a lesion of the trigeminal nerve, characterized by paroxysms of pain in the distributions of one of the trigeminal divisions.

**Tuberculoma.** A tumor-like mass that results from enlargement of a caseous (resembling cheese or curd) tubercle.

**Tuberous sclerosis.** A congenital familial disease in which tumors occur on the surfaces of the lateral ventricles and sclerotic patches are found on the surface of the brain. The disease is manifested clinically by progressive mental deterioration and epileptic convulsions.

## U

**Uncinate fasciculus.** A bundle of fibers which connects the inferior frontal lobe gyri with the anterior temporal lobe.

**Uncinate fits.** Olfactory hallucinations characterized by sensations of peculiar odors and tastes. Often associated with a dreamy state, uncinate fits may occur as an epileptic aura.

**Uncinate gyrus.** The medially curved anterior end of the parahippocampal gyrus.

## V

**Vascular malformation.** A congenital abnormality of blood vessels represented by a weakness of the vessel wall with focal enlargement (such as a berry aneurysm) or a tangled mass of arteries and veins (arteriovenous malformation).

**Ventral.** Referring to the side that is toward the front, as opposed to dorsal (toward the back).

**Ventricle.** A small cavity, such as the right or left ventricles of the heart or the ventricles of the brain.

**Ventriculography.** A procedure in which burr holes are made in the skull to permit direct access to the cerebral ventricles. Cerebrospinal fluid is removed from the cerebral ventricles, replaced by air or other contrast medium, and the brain structures are visualized by x-ray.

**Ventrolateral nucleus of the thalamus.** One of the nuclei of the thalamus which is often the target in stereotaxic surgery for relief of involuntary movements.

**Vertebral artery.** One of the four major arteries (two internal carotid and two vertebral) which supply blood to the brain. This artery arises from the subclavian artery and supplies blood to the cerebellum, muscles of the neck, vertebrae, the spinal cord and interior portions of the cerebrum.

**Vertebral-basilar system.** A system for supply of arterial blood to the brainstem and posterior part of the brain. The other system of arterial blood supply to the brain is the carotid system.

**Vertigo.** A sensation of external objects revolving around the subject or the subject revolving in space. In common practice, however, this term frequently refers to a feeling of dizziness.

**Viral infections.** Any infection of the body resulting from invasion by a virus.

**Visual agnosia.** Inability to recognize objects through vision.

**Visual form dysgnosia.** Impairment in the ability to recognize forms or shapes through visual observation.

**Visual letter dysgnosia.** Impairment of the ability to recognize the symbolic significance of letters of the alphabet through visual perception.

**Visual imperception.** Impairment of the ability to recognize stimuli presented visually on both sides simultaneously, even though the stimulus can be perceived and reported when given unilaterally. The deficit is usually contralateral to the side of cerebral damage.

**Visual number dysgnosia.** Impairment of the ability to recognize the symbolic significance of numbers through visual perception.

## W

**Wernicke's encephalopathy.** A syndrome due to thiamine deficiency (vitamin $B_1$) together with other vitamins in the B complex that is frequently associated with alcoholism. The clinical features of this syndrome include ophthalmoplegia (weakness and incoordination of the eye muscles), ataxia, and dementia.

**White matter.** Tissue in the nervous system that is made up of nerve fibers (contrasting with gray matter which is made up of cell bodies).

**Word deafness (sensory aphasia).** Inability to interpret the meaning of sounds, especially speech, even though the sense of hearing is intact.

## X

**Xanthochromia.** Any yellowish discoloration, but particularly referring to the cerebrospinal fluid.

# References

# REFERENCES

Ackerly, S.S. (1935). Instinctive, emotional and mental changes following prefrontal lobe extirpation. *American Journal of Psychiatry, 92,* 717-729.

Adolffsson, R., Gottfries, C.G., Oreland, L., Roos, B.E., & Windblad, B. (1977). Reduced level of catecholamines in the brain and increased activity of monamine oxidase in platelets in Alzheimer's disease: Therapeutic implications. In R. Katzman, R.D. Terry, & K.L. Bick (Eds.), *Alzheimer's disease: Senile dementia and related disorders. Aging, Vol. 7.* New York: Raven Press.

Aguilar, M.J., & Rasmussen, T. (1960). Role of encephalitis in pathogenesis of epilepsy. *AMA Archives of Neurology, 2,* 663-676.

Aita, J.A., Armitage, S.G., Reitan, R.M., & Rabinovitz, A. (1947). The use of certain psychological tests in the evaluation of brain injury. *Journal of General Psychology, 37,* 25-44.

Alavi, A., Reivich, M., Greenberg, J.H., & Wolf, A.P. (1982). Positron emission tomography of the brain. In P.J. Ell & B.L. Holman (Eds.), *Computed emission tomography.* New York: Oxford University Press.

Albert, N.L., Goodglass, H., Helm, N.A., Rubens, A.B., & Alexander, M.P. (1981). *Clinical aspects of dysphasia.* New York: Springer-Verlag.

Alderson, P.O., Gado, M.H., & Siegal, B.D. (1977). Computerized cranial tomography and radionuclide imaging in the detection of intracranial mass lesions. *Seminars in Nuclear Medicine, 7,* 161-173.

Ambrose, J., Gooding, M.R., & Richardson, A.E. (1975). Sodium iothalamate as an aid to diagnosis of intracranial lesions by computerized transverse axial scanning. *Lancet, 2,* 669-674.

Anderson, P.G. (1970). Intracranial tumors in psychiatric autopsy material. *Acta Psychiatrica Scandinavica, 46,* 213-224.

Angevine, J.B., & Cotman, C.W. (1981). *Principles of neuroanatomy.* New York: Oxford University Press.

Bailey, P. (1927). Further remarks concerning tumors of the glioma group. *Bulletin of the Johns Hopkins Hospital, 40,* 354-389.

Bailey, P., & Bucy, P.C. (1929). Oligodendrogliomas of the brain. *Journal of Pathological Bacteriology, 32,* 735-751.

Bailey, P., & Cushing, H. (1926). *A classification of the tumors of the glioma group on a histogenetic basis with a correlated study of prognosis.* Philadelphia: J.B. Lippincott Co.

Bailey, P., & Hiller, G. (1924). The interstitial tissues of the central nervous system: A review. *Journal of Nervous and Mental Disease, 59,* 337-361.

Baker, A.B. (1962). Viral encephalitis. In A.B. Baker (Ed.), *Clinical neurology (2nd ed.) Vol. 2* (pp. 811-858). New York: Hoeber, Medical Division, Harper & Row.

Baker, A.B. (Ed.). (1971). *Clinical neurology.* Hagerstown, MD: Harper.

Ball, M.J. (1976). Neurofibrillary tangles and the pathogenesis of dementia: A quantitative time study. *Neuropathology and Applied Neurobiology, 2,* 394-410.

Ball, M.J. (1977). Neuronal loss, neurofibrillary tangles and granulovacuolar degeneration in the hippocampus with aging and dementia: A quantitative study. *Acta Neuropathologica, 37,* 111-118.

Barr, M.L., & Kiernan, J.A. (1983). *The human nervous system. An anatomical viewpoint.* Fourth Edition. Philadelphia: Harper & Row.

Barrett, L., Drayer, B., & Shin, C. (1985). High-resolution computed tomography in multiple sclerosis. *Annals of Neurology, 17,* 33-38.

Bartlett, J.R. (1971). Craniopharyngiomas: An analysis of some aspects of symptomatology, radiology and histology. *Brain, 94,* 725-732.

Bear, D.M., & Fedio, P. (1977). Quantitative analysis of interictal behavior in temporal lobe epilepsy. *Archives of Neurology, 34,* 454-467.

Beck, S.J. (1937). Psychological processes in Rorschach findings. *Journal of Abnormal and Social Psychology, 31,* 482-488.

Bell, C. (1830). *The nervous system of the human body.* London.

Benson, D.F. (1979). *Aphasia, alexia, and agraphia.* New York: Churchill Livingstone.

Benton, A.L. (1964). Contributions to aphasia before Broca. *Cortex, 1,* 314-327.

Besson, J.A.O., Glen, A.I.M., Foreman, E.I., et al. (1981). Nuclear magnetic resonance observations in alcoholic cerebral disorder and the role of vasopressin. *Lancet, 2,* 923-924.

Birren, J.E., Butler, R.N., Greenhouse, S.W. et al. (1963). Interdisciplinary relationships: Interrelations of physiological, psychological and psychiatric findings in healthy elderly men. In J.E. Birren, R.N. Butler, S.W. Greenhouse, et al. (Eds.), *Human Aging. I. A Biological and Behavioral Study.* U.S. Dept. HEW, PHS Publication No. 986. Pp. 283-305. Washington, D.C., U.S. Government Printing Office.

Blessed, G., Tomlinson, B.E., & Roth, M. (1968). The association between quantitative measures of dementia and of senile change in the cerebral gray matter of elderly subjects. *British Journal of Psychiatry, 114,* 797-811.

Bloom, H.J.G. (1975). Combined modality therapy for intracranial tumors. *Cancer, 23,* 111-120.

Boll, T.J., Heaton, R.K., & Reitan, R.M. (1974). Neuropsychological and emotional correlates of Huntington's chorea. *Journal of Nervous and Mental Disease, 158,* 61-69.

Boring, E.G. (1929). *A history of experimental psychology.* New York: Century Company.

Brazis, P.W., Masdeu, J.C., & Biller, J. (1985). *Localization in clinical neurology.* Boston: Little, Brown and Company.

Brickner, R.M. (1936). *The intellectual functions of the frontal lobes.* New York: MacMillan Co.

Brickner, R.M. (1939). Bilateral frontal lobectomy: Follow-up report of a case. *Archives of Neurology and Psychiatry, 41,* 580-585.

Broca, P. (1861). Remarques sur le siege de la faculté du langage articule, suivies d'une observation d'aphemie (perte de la parole). *Bull. Soc. Anat., 36,* 330-357.

Broders, A.C. (1920). Squamous cell epithelioma of the lip: A study of five hundred and thirty-seven cases. *Journal of the American Medical Association, 74,* 656-664.

Brody, H. (1955). Organization of the cerebral cortex. III. A study of aging in the human cerebral cortex. *Journal of Comparative Neurology, 102,* 511-556.

Brody, H. (1970). Structural changes in the aging nervous system. In H.T. Blumenthal (Ed.), *Interdisciplinary topics in gerontology. Vol. 7,* pp. 9-21. New York: Karger.

Brody, H. (1977). Cell counts in cerebrum and brain stem. In R. Katzman, R.D. Terry & K.L. Bick (Eds.), *Alzheimer's disease: Senile dementia and related disorders. Aging, Vol. 7* (pp. 345-351). New York: Raven Press.

Brody, H., & Vijayashankar, N. (1977). Anatomical changes in the nervous system. In C.E. Finch & L. Hayflick (Eds.), *Handbook of the biology of aging* (pp. 241-261). New York: Van Nostrand.

Brown, J.W. (1972). *Aphasia, apraxia, and agnosia: Clinical and theoretical aspects.* Springfield, IL: Charles C. Thomas.

Brown, J.R., Beebe, G.W., Kurtzke, J.F., Loewenson, R.B., Silberberg, D.H., & Tourtellotte, W.W. (1979). The design of clinical studies to assess therapeutic efficacy in multiple sclerosis. *Neurology (NY), 29*, 3-23.

Buchbaum, M.S., Kessler, R., Bunney, W.E., Cappelletti, J., Coppolo, R., Van Kammen, D.P., Rigal, F., Waters, R., Sokoloff, L., & Ingvar, D. (1981). Simultaneous electroencephalography and cerebral glucography with positron emission tomography (PET) in normals and patients with schizophrenia. *Journal of Cerebral Blood Flow Metabolism, 1*, Suppl. 1, S457.

Busse, E.W. (1977). Duke longitudinal study I: Senescence and senility. In R. Katzman, R.D. Terry & K.L. Bick (Eds.), *Alzheimer's disease: Senile dementia and related disorders. Aging, Vol. 7* (pp. 59-68). New York: Raven Press.

Butler, A.B., Brooks, W.H., & Netsky, M.G. (1982). Classification and biology of brain tumors. In J.R. Youmans (Ed.), *Neurological surgery*. Philadilphia: W.B. Saunders Co.

Caine, E.D., Ebert, M.H., & Weingartner, H. (1977). An outline for the analysis of dementia. *Neurology, 27*, 1087-1092.

Campbell, R.L., Campbell, J.A., Heimburger, R.F., et al. (1964). Ventriculography and myelography with absorbable radioopaque medium. *Radiology, 82*, 286.

Carpenter, M.B., & Sutin, J. (1983). *Human neuroanatomy*. Eighth Edition. Baltimore: Williams & Wilkins.

Caveness, W.F. (1963). Onset and cessation of fits following craniocerebral trauma. *Journal of Neurosurgery, 20*, 570-583.

Chusid, J.G. (1979). *Correlative neuroanatomy and functional neurology*. 17th edition. Los Altos, CA: Lange Medical Publications.

CIBA Collection of Medical Illustrations. (1983) Vol. 1. *Nervous system*. Part I. Anatomy and Physiology. Prepared by Frank H. Netter. West Caldwell, New Jersey: CIBA Pharmaceutical Company.

Claveria, Sutton, & Tress. (1977). The radiological diagnosis of meningiomas: The impact of EMI scanning. *British Journal of Radiology, 50*, 15-22.

Cobb, C.A., & Youmans, J.R. (1982). Glial and neuronal tumors of the brain in adults. In J.R. Youmans (Ed.), *Neurological surgery*. Philadelphia: W.B. Saunders Co.

Cogan, D.G. (1956). *Neurology of the ocular muscles*. Springfield, IL: Charles C. Thomas.

Collins, R.D. (1982). *Illustrated manual of neurologic diagnosis*. Second Edition. Philadelphia: J.B. Lippincott.

Colon, E.J. (1972). The elderly brain: A quantitative analysis of cerebral cortex in two cases. *Psychiatry, Neurology, and Neurochir., 75*, 261-270.

Corsellis, J. (1962). *Mental illness and the aging brain*. London: Oxford University Press.

Courville, C.B. (1967). Intracranial tumors. Notes upon a series of three thousand verified cases with some current observations pertaining to their mortality. *Bulletin of the Los Angeles Neurological Society, 32*, 1-80.

Coyle, J.T., Price, D.L., & DeLong, M.R. (1983). Alzheimer's disease: A disorder of cortical cholinergic innervation. *Science, 219*, 1184-1190.

Creasey, H., & Rapoport, S.I. (1985). The aging human brain. *Annals of Neurology, 17*, 2-10.

Cricheff, I.I., Becker, M., Schneck, S.A., & Taveras, J.M. (1964). Intracranial ependymomas: Factors influencing prognosis. *Journal of Neurosurgery, 21*, 7-14.

Crockard, H.A., Brown, F.D., et al. (1977). Physiological consequences of experimental cerebral missile injury and data analysis to predict survival. *Journal of Neurosurgery, 46*, 784-794.

Cushing, H. (1917). *Tumors of the nervus acousticus and the syndrome of the cerebellopontine angle.* Philadelphia: W.B. Saunders Co.

Cushing, H., & Eisenhardt, L. (1938). *Meningiomas: Their classification, regional behavior, life history, and surgical end results.* Springfield, IL: Charles C. Thomas.

Damadian, R. (1971). Tumor detection by NMR. *Science, 171,* 1151.

Dandy, E.W. (1918). Ventriculography following the injection of air into the cerebral ventricles. *Annals of Surgery, 68,* 5-11.

Darley, F.L., Aronson, A.E., & Brown, J.R. (1975). *Motor speech disorders.* Philadelphia: Saunders.

Dastur, D.K., Lane, M.H., Hansen, D.B., et al. (1963). Effects of aging on cerebral circulation and metabolism in man. In J.E. Birren, R.N. Butler, S.W. Greenhouse, et al. (Eds.), *Human Aging: A biological and behavioral study.* USPHS Publication No. 986. Pp. 59-76. Washington, D.C.: U.S. Government Printing Office.

Davies, P. (1979). Neurotransmitter related enzymes in senile dementia of the Alzheimer type. *Brain Research, 171,* 319-327.

Davies, P., Katz, D.A., & Crystal, H.A. (1982). Choline acetyltransferase, somatostatin and substance P in selected cases of Alzheimer's disease. In S. Corkin, K.L. Davis, J.M. Growdon, et al. (Eds.), *Alzheimer's disease: A report of progress in research. Aging, Vol. 19* (pp. 9-14). New York: Raven Press.

Davis, D.O., & Kobrine, A. (1982). Computed tomography. In J.R. Youmans (Ed.), *Neurological surgery.* Philadelphia: W.B. Saunders Company.

Davis, L., Martin, J., Padberg, F., & Anderson, R.K. (1950). A study of 182 patients with verified astrocytoma, astroblastoma, and oligodendroglioma of the brain. *Journal of Neurosurgery, 7,* 299-312.

Dax, M. (1836). Lesions de la moitie gauche de l'encephale coincident avec trouble des signes de la pensie. Paper presented at Montpelier. Cited in D. F. Benson (1979). *Aphasia, alexia and agraphia.* New York: Churchill Livingstone.

DeBakey, M.E., Crawford, E.S., & Fields, W.S. (1961). Surgical treatment of patients with cerebral arterial insufficiency associated with extracranial arterial occlusive lesions. *Neurology, 11,* 145-149.

Dekaban, A.S., & Sadowsky, D. (1978). Changes in brain weight during the span of human life: Relation of brain weights to body heights and body weights. *Annals of Neurology, 4,* 345-356.

DeMyer, W. (1980). *Technique of the neurologic examination.* Third Edition. New York: McGraw-Hill.

Dikman, S., & Reitan, R.M. (1976). Psychological deficits and recovery of functions after head injury. *Transactions of the American Neurological Association, 101,* 72-77.

Dodrill, C. (1981). Neuropsychology of epilepsy. In S.B. Filskov & T.J. Boll (Eds.), *Handbook of clinical neuropsychology.* New York: John Wiley & Sons.

Duara, R., Margolin, R.A., Robertson-Tchabo, E.A., et al. (1983). Cerebral glucose utilization as measured with positron emission tomography in 21 resting healthy men between the ages of 21 and 83 years. *Brain, 106,* 761-775.

Dublin, A.B., French, B.N., & Rennick, J.M. (1977). Computer tomography in head trauma. *Radiology, 122,* 365-369.

Dublin, A.B., & Merten, D.F. (1977). Computer tomography in evaluation of herpes simplex encephalitis. *Radiology, 125,* 133-134.

Dyck, P. (1982). Echoencephalography. In J.R. Youmans (Ed.), *Neurological surgery.* Philadelphia: W.B. Saunders Company.

Eadie, M.J., & Sutherland, J.M. (1964). Arteriosclerosis in Parkinsonism. *Journal of Neurology, Neurosurgery, and Psychiatry, 27,* 237-240.

Eastcott, H.H.G., Pickering, G.W., & Rob, C.G. (1954). Reconstruction of internal carotid artery in a patient with intermittent attacks of hemiplegia. *Lancet, 2,* 994-996.

Ellis, R.S. (1920). Norms for some structural changes in the human cerebellum from birth to old age. *Journal of Comparative Neurology, 32,* 1-34.

Ellis, W.G., Youmans, J.R., & Dreyfus, P.M. (1982). Diagnostic biopsy for neurological disease. In J.R. Youmans (Ed.), *Neurological surgery*. Philadelphia: W.B. Saunders Company.

Evans, R.G., & Jost, R.G. (1977). The clinical efficacy and cost analysis of cranial computed tomography and the radionuclide brain scan. *Seminars in Nuclear Medicine, 7,* 129-136.

Fan, K.-J., Kovi, J., & Earle, K.M. (1977). The ethnic distribution of primary central nervous system tumors: Armed Forces Institute of Pathology, 1958-1970. *Journal of Neuropathology and Experimental Neurology, 36,* 41-49.

Farrell, D.F., & Starr, A. (1968). Delayed neurological sequelae of electrical injuries. *Neurology, 18,* 601-606.

Ferrier, D. (1886). *The functions of the brain*. London: Smith Elder & Company.

Fields, W.S., & Blattner, R.J. (1958). *Viral encephalitis*. Springfield, IL: Charles C. Thomas.

Fields, W.S., Crawford, E.S., & DeBakey, M.E. (1958). Surgical considerations in cerebral arterial insufficiency. *Neurology, 8,* 801-808.

Finch, C.E. (1977a). Neurochemical and neuroendocrine changes during aging in rodent models. In R. Katzman, R.D. Terry, & K.L. Bick (Eds.), *Alzheimer's disease: Senile dementia and related disorders. Aging, Vol. 7* (pp. 461-468). New York: Raven Press.

Finch, C.E. (1977b). Neuroendocrine and autonomic functions during aging. In C.E. Finch & L. Hayflick (Eds.), *Handbook of the biology of aging* (pp. 262-280). New York: Van Nostrand.

Fisher, A.G.T. (1913). A case of complete absence of both internal carotid arteries. *Journal of Anatomy and Physiology, 48,* 37-46.

Fisher, M. (1954). Occlusion of carotid arteries. *Archives of Neurology and Psychiatry, 72,* 187-204.

Flourens, P. (1843). *Examen de la phrenologie*. Paris: Paulin.

Fogelholm, R., & Allo, K. (1973). Ischemic cerebral vascular disease in young adults. *Acta Neurologica Scandinavica, 49,* 415-433.

Ford, R., & McRae, D.L. (1966). Echoencephalography: A standardized technic for the measurement of the width of the third and lateral ventricles. In C.C. Grossman, J. Holmes, C. Joyner, & E.W. Purnell (Eds.), *Diagnostic ultrasound*. New York: Plenum Press.

Fordham, E.W. (1977). The complementary role of computerized axial transmission tomography and radionuclide imaging of the brain. *Seminars in Nuclear Medicine, 7,* 129-136.

Foster, N.L., Chase, T.N., Mansi, L., Brooke, R., Fedio, P., Patronas, N.J., & DiChiro, G. (1984). Cortical abnormalities in Alzheimer's disease. *Annals of Neurology, 16,* 649-654.

Fowler, E.P. (1936). Methods for early detection of otosclerosis: Study of sounds well above the threshold. *Archives of Otolaryngology, 24,* 731-741.

Frackowiak, R.S.J., Lenzi, G.L., Jones, T., & Heather, J.D. (1980). Quantitative measurement of regional cerebral blood flow and oxygen metabolism in man using 15-O and positron emission tomography: Theory, procedure and normal values. *Journal of Computed Assisted Tomography, 4,* 727-736.

Franz, S.I. (1907). *On the functions of the cerebrum: The frontal lobes.* Archives of Psychology, Monograph #2. New York: Science Press.

Franz, S.I., & Gordon, K. (1933). *Psychology.* New York: McGraw-Hill Book Company.

French, L.A., Wild, J.J., & Neal, D. (1950). Detection of cerebral tumors by ultrasonic pulses: Pilot studies on postmortem material. *Cancer, 3,* 705-708.

French, L.A., Wild, J.J., & Neal, D. (1951). The experimental application of ultrasonics to localization of brain tumors: Preliminary report. *Journal of Neurosurgery, 8,* 198-203.

Fritsch, G., & Hitzig, E. (1870). Ueber die electrische Erregbarkeit des Grosshirn. *Arch. f. Anat. u. Physiol., 37,* 300-332.

Gall, M.V., Becker, H., & Hacker, H. (1977). Computer tomography (CT scan) in the diagnosis of epilepsy. *Nervenarzt, 48,* 72-76.

Gelb, A., & Goldstein, K. Ueber Farbennamenamnesie. *Psychol. Forsch., 6,* 127-186.

Gerstmann, J. (1924). Fingeragnosie. Eine umschriebene storung der orientierung am eigenen korper. *Wien. Klin. Wschr., 37,* 1010-1012.

Gerstmann, J. (1927). Fingeragnosie und isolierte agraphie, ein neues syndrom. *Ztschr. Neurol. Psych., 108,* 152-177.

Geschwind, N. (1977). Behavioral change in temporal lobe epilepsy. *Archives of Neurology, 34,* 453.

Gillian, L.A. (1964). The correlation of the blood supply to the human brain stem with clinical brain stem lesions. *Journal of Neuropathology and Experimental Neurology, 23,* 78-108.

Gilman, S., & Winans, S.S. (1982). *Manter & Gatz's Essentials of clinical neuroanatomy and neurophysiology.* Philadelphia: F.A. Davis Company.

Gilroy, J., & Meyer, J.S. (1962). Auscultation of the neck in occlusive cerebral vascular disease. *Circulation, 25,* 300-310.

Gilroy, J., & Meyer, J.S. (1979). *Medical neurology.* New York: Macmillan Publishing Company.

Gissane, W. (1963). The nature and causation of road injuries. *Lancet, 2,* 695-698.

Glynn, L.E. (1940). Medial defects in the circle of Willis and their relation to aneurysm formation. *Journal of Pathological Bacteriology, 51,* 213-232.

Gol, A. (1961). The relatively benign astrocytomas of the cerebrum: A clinical study of 194 verified cases. *Journal of Neurosurgery, 18,* 501-506.

Goldberg, G., Mayer, N.H., & Taglia, J.U. (1981). Medial frontal cortex infarction and the alien hand sign. *Archives of Neurology, 38,* 683.

Goldstein, G., & Shelly, C. (1974). Neuropsychology diagnosis of multiple sclerosis in a neuropsychiatric setting. *Journal of Nervous and Mental Disease, 158,* 280-290.

Goldstein, K. (1936). The significance of the frontal lobes for mental performances. *Journal of Neurology and Psychopathology, 17,* 27-40.

Goldstein, K. (1939). Clinical and theoretic aspects of lesions of the frontal lobes. *Archives of Neurology and Psychiatry, 41,* 865-867.

Goldstein, K. (1944). The mental changes due to frontal lobe damage. *Journal of Psychology, 17,* 187-208.

Goltz, F.L. (1881). Uber die Verrichtungen des Grosshirns. Bonn: Gesammette Abhandlungen.

Gonzales, D., & Elvidge, A.R. (1962). On the occurrence of epilepsy caused by astrocytoma of the cerebral hemispheres. *Journal of Neurosurgery, 19,* 470-482.

Green, M.A., Stevenson, L.D., Fonseca, J.E., Wortis, S.B. (1952). Cerebral biopsy in patients with presenile dementia. *Diseases of the Nervous System, 13*, 303-307.

Greenberg, J.H., Reivich, M., Hand, P., Rosenquist, A., Rintelmann, W., Stein, A., Tusa, R., Dann, R., Christman, D., Fowler, G., MacGregor, B., & Wolf, A. (1981). Metabolic mapping of functional activity in human subjects with the (18F) fluorodeoxy-glucose technique. *Science (NY), 212*, 678-680.

Grunert, V., Jellinger, K., Sunder-Plassmann, M., & Wober, G. (1973). Glioblastoma multiforme: A preliminary follow-up study. *Modern Aspects of Neurosurgery, 3*, 108-115.

Guidetti, B., & Gagliardi, F.M. (1977). Epidermoid and dermoid cysts: Clinical evaluation and late surgical results. *Journal of Neurosurgery, 47*, 12-18.

Hachinski, V.C., Iliff, L.D., Zhilka, E., du Boulay, G.H.D., McAllister, V.C., Marshall, J. Russell, R.W.R. & Symon, L. (1975). Cerebral blood flow in dementia. *Archives of Neurology, 32*, 632-637.

Hachinski, B.C., Lassen, N.A., & Marshall, J. (1974). Multi-infarct dementia: A cause of mental deterioration in the elderly. *Lancet, 2*, 207-210.

Hachinski, V. (1984). Clinical physiology of the cerebral circulation. In J.R. Toole (Ed.), *Cerebral vascular disorders*. New York: Raven Press.

Halstead, W.C. (1939). Behavioral effects of lesions of the frontal lobe in man. *Archives of Neurology and Psychiatry, 42*, 780-783.

Halstead, W.C. (1940). Preliminary analysis of grouping behavior in patients with cerebral injury by the method of equivalent and non-equivalent stimuli. *American Journal of Psychiatry, 96*, 1263-1294.

Halstead, W.C. (1945). Localization of neuropsychological functions in the pre-frontal lobes. *Federation Proceedings, 4*, 13-14.

Halstead, W.C. (1947). *Brain and intelligence*. Chicago: University of Chicago Press.

Halstead, W.C., Carmichael, H.T., & Bucy, P.C. (1946). Pre-frontal lobotomy: A preliminary appraisal of the behavioral results. *American Journal of Psychiatry, 103*, 217-228.

Halstead, W.C., & Settlage, P.H. (1943). Grouping behavior of normal persons and of persons with lesions of the brain. *Archives of Neurology and Psychiatry, 49*, 489-506.

Hauge, T. (1954). Catheter vertebral angiography. *Acta Radiologica Supplement, 109*

Heaton, R.K., Nelson, L.M., Thompson, D.S., Burks, J.S., & Franklin, G.M. (1985). Neuropsychological findings in relapsing-remitting and chronic-progressive multiple sclerosis. *Journal of Consulting and Clinical Psychology, 53*, 103-110.

Hebb, D.O. (1939a). Intelligence in man after large removals of cerebral tissue: Report of four left frontal lobe cases. *Journal of General Psychology, 21*, 73-87.

Hebb, D.O. (1939b). Intelligence in man after large removals of cerebral tissue: Defects following right temporal lobectomy. *Journal of General Psychology, 21*, 437-446.

Hebb, D.O. (1941). Human intelligence after removal of cerebral tissue from the right frontal lobe. *Journal of General Psychology, 25*, 257-265.

Hebb, D.O., & Pennfield, W. (1940). Human behavior after extensive bilateral removal from the frontal lobes. *Archives of Neurology and Psychiatry, 44*, 421-438.

Hécaen, H., & Albert, M. (1978). *Human neuropsychology*. New York: John Wiley & Sons.

Heilman, K.M., & Valenstein, E. (Eds.). (1979). *Clinical neuropsychology*. New York: Oxford University Press.

Heimburger, R.F., DeMyer, W., & Reitan, R.M. (1964). Implications of Gerstmann's syndrome. *Journal of Neurology, Neurosurgery and Psychiatry, 27*, 52-57.

Henschen, S.E. (1920-1922). *Klinische und anatomosche beitrage zur pathologie des gehirns.* Stockholm: Nordiske Bokhandeln.

Henderson, G., Tomlinson, B.E., & Gibson, P.H. (1980). Cell counts in human cerebral cortex in normal adults throughout life using an image analysing computer. *Journal of Neurological Science, 46,* 113-136.

Henderson, G., Tomlinson, B.E., & Weightman, D. (1975). Cell counts in the cerebral cortex using a traditional and automatic method. *Journal of Neurological Sciences, 25,* 129-144.

Hier, D.B., David, K.R., Richardson, E.R., & Mohr, J.P. (1977). Hypertensive putaminal hemorrhage. *Annals of Neurology, 1,* 152-159.

Hoehn, M.M., Crowley, I.J., & Rutledge, C.O. (1976). Dopamine correlates of neurological and psychological status in untreated Parkinsonism. *Journal of Neurology, Neurosurgery, and Psychiatry, 39,* 941-951.

Hoffman, H.J., Hendrick, E.B., Humphreys, R.P., Buncic, J.R., Armstrong, D.L., & Jenkin, D.T. (1977). Management of craniopharyngioma in children. *Journal of Neurosurgery, 47,* 218-227.

Hunt, T. (1940). Psychological testing of psychiatric patients undergoing prefrontal lobotomy. *Psychological Bulletin, 37,* 566.

Hutchinson, E.C., & Yates, P.O. (1956). The cervical portion of the vertebral artery: A clinical-pathological study. *Brain, 79,* 319-331.

Hutchinson, E.C., & Yates, P.O. (1957). Caroticovertebral stenosis. *Lancet, 1,* 2-8.

Ivnik, R. (1978). Neuropsychological stability in multiple sclerosis. *Journal of Consulting and Clinical Psychology, 46,* 913-923.

Jacobsen, C.F. (1936). Studies of cerebral function in primates. I. The function of the frontal association areas in monkeys. *Comparative Psychology Monographs, 13,* 1-60.

Jacobsen, C.F., & Elder, J.H. (1936). Studies of cerebral function in primates. II. The effect of temporal lobe lesions on delayed response in monkeys. *Comparative Psychology Monographs, 13,* 61-65.

Jacobsen, C.F., & Nissen, H.W. (1937). Studies in the cerebral function in primates. IV. The effects of frontal lobe lesions on the delayed alternation habit in monkeys. *Journal of Comparative Psychology, 23,* 101-112.

Jacobsen, C.F., Wolfe, J.B., & Jackson, T.A. (1935). An experimental analysis of the functions of the frontal association areas in primates. *Journal of Nervous and Mental Disease, 82,* 1-14.

Jambor, K.L. (1969). Cognitive functioning in multiple sclerosis. *British Journal of Psychiatry, 115,* 765-775.

Jasper, H.H. (1970). Physiopathological mechansims of post-traumatic epilepsy. *Epilepsia, 11,* 73-80.

Jefferson, G. (1937a). Left frontal lobectomy. *Proceedings of the Royal Society of Medicine, 30,* 851-853.

Jefferson, G. (1937b). Removal of right or left frontal lobes in man. *British Medical Journal, 2,* 199-206.

Jellinger, K. (1975). Histological subtypes and prognostic problems in meningiomas. *Journal of Neurology, 208,* 279-298.

Jelsma, R., & Bucy, P.C. (1967). The treatment of glioblastoma multiforme of the brain. *Journal of Neurosurgery, 27,* 388-400.

Jennett, W.B. (1965). Predicting epilepsy after blunt head injury. *British Medical Journal, 1,* 1215-1216.

Jennett, W.B. (1969). Early traumatic epilepsy: Definition and identity. *Lancet, 1,* 1023-1025.

Jennett, W.B. (1969). Epilepsy after blunt (non-missile) head injuries. In A.E. Walker, W.F. Caveness, & M. Critchley (Eds.), *The late effects of head injury.* Springfield: Charles C. Thomas.

Jennett, W.B. (1974). Early traumatic epilepsy: Incidence and significance after nonmissile injuries. *Archives of Neurology, 30,* 384-398.

Jennett, W.B., Johnson, R., & Reid, R. (1963). Positive contrast ventriculography of pineal region tumors. *Acta Radiologica, 1,* 857-871.

Jerger, J.F. (1961). Recruitment: An allied phenomenon in differential diagnosis. *Journal of Auditory Research, 2,* 145.

Kahn, E.A., Gosch, H.H., Seeger, J.F., & Hicks, S.P. (1973). Forty-five years experience with the craniopharyngiomas. *Surgical Neurology, 1,* 5-12.

Katzman, R. (1976). The prevalence and malignancy of Alzheimer's disease. *Archives of Neurology, 33,* 217-218.

Katzman, R., & Karasu, T.B. (1975). Differential diagnosis of dementia. In W.S. Fields (ed.), *Neurological and sensory disorders in the elderly* (pp. 102-134). Miami: Symposia Specialists.

Kaufman, L., Crooks, L.E., & Margulis, A.R. (Eds.). (1981). *Nuclear magnetic resonance imaging in medicine.* New York: Igaku-Shoin.

Kernohan, J.W. (1971). Tumors of congenital origin. In J. Minckler (Ed.), *Pathology of the nervous system.* New York: McGraw-Hill Book Company.

Kernohan, J.W., & Sayers, G.P. (1952). Tumors of the central nervous system. *Atlas of Tumor Pathology,* Section V, Fascicles 35 & 37. Washington, D.C.: Armed Forces Institute of Pathology.

Kernohan, J.W., Mabon, R.F., Svien, H.J., & Adson, A.W. (1949). A simplified classification of gliomas. *Proceedings of the Staff Meetings of the Mayo Clinic, 24,* 71-75.

Kety, S.S. (1956). Human cerebral blood flow and oxygen consumption as related to aging. *Research Publications Association for Research in Nervous and Mental Disease, 35,* 31-45.

Kety, S.S., & Schmidt, C.F. (1948). The determination of cerebral blood flow in man by the use of nitrous oxide in low concentrations. *American Journal of Physiology, 143,* 53-66.

Kinkel, W.R., & Jacobs, L. (1976). Computerized axial transfers tomography in cerebral vascular disease. *Neurology, 26,* 924-930.

Kleist, K. (1934). *Gerhirnpathologie.* Leipzig: J.A. Barth.

Klopfer, B., & Kelley, D.M. (1942). *The Rorschach technique.* Yonkers-on-Hudson: World Book Company.

Knehr, C.A. (1962). Differential impairment in multiple sclerosis. *Journal of Psychology, 54,* 443-451.

Knight, S.C. (1977). Cellular immunity in multiple sclerosis. *British Medical Bulletin, 33,* 45-49.

Kooi, K.A. (1971). *Fundamentals of electroencephalography.* New York: Harper and Row.

Kuhl, D.E., & Edwards, R.Q. (1963). Image separation radioisotope scanning. *Radiology, 80,* 653-662.

Kuhl, D.E., Engel, J., Phelps, M.E., & Selin, C. (1980). Epileptic patterns of local cerebral metabolism and perfusion in humans determined by emission computed tomography of $^{18}$FDG and $^{13}$NH$_3$. *Annals of Neurology, 3,* 348-360.

Kuhl, D.E., Metter, E.J., Riege, W.H., & Phelps, M.E. (1982). Effects of human aging on patterns of local cerebral glucose utilization determined by the [$^{18}$F] fluorodeoxyglucose method. *Journal of Cerebral Blood Flow Metabolism, 2,* 163-171.

Kuhl, D.E., Phelps, M.E., Kowell, A.P., Metter, E.J., Selin, C., & Winter, J. (1980). Effects of stroke on local cerebral metabolism and perfusion: Mapping by emission computed tomography of $^{18}$FDG and $^{13}$NH$_3$. *Annals of Neurology, 8,* 47-60.

Kurland, L.T., Myrianthopoulos, N.C., & Leksell, S. (1962). Epidemiologic and genetic considerations of intracranial neoplasms. In *The biology and treatment of intracranial tumors*. Springfield, IL: Charles C. Thomas.

Kurtzke, J.F. (1955). A new scale for evaluating disability in multiple sclerosis. *Neurology (Minneap.), 5*, 580-583.

Kurtzke, J.F. (1961). On the evaluation of disability in multiple sclerosis. *Neurology (Minneap.), 11*, 686-694.

Kurtzke, J.F. (1965). Further notes on disability evaluation in multiple sclerosis, with scale modifications. *Neurology (Minneap.), 15*, 654-661.

Kurtzke, J.F. (1970). Neurologic impairment in multiple sclerosis and the Disability Status Scale. *Acta Neurologica Scandinavica, 46*, 493-512.

Kurtzke, J.F. (1983). Rating neurologic impairment in multiple sclerosis: An expanded disability status scale (EDSS). *Neurology (Cleveland), 33*, 1444-1452.

Lamb, J.F., Ingram, C.G., Johnston, I.A., & Pitman, R.M. (1982). *Essentials of Physiology*. Boston: Blackwell Scientific Publications.

Lashley, K.S. (1929). *Brain mechanisms and intelligence*. Chicago: University of Chicago Press.

Lassen, N.A., & Ingvar, D.H. (1961). The blood flow of the cerebral cortex determined by radioactive krypton. *Experientia, 17*, 42-43.

Lauterbur, P.C. (1973). Image formation by induced local interactions: Examples employing NMR. *Nature, 242*, 190-191.

Leech, R.W., & Shuman, R.M. (1982). *Neuropathology. A summary for students*. Philadelphia: Harper & Row.

Leksell, L. (1956). Echoencephalography. I. Detection of intracranial complications following head injury. *Acta Chirurgica Scandinavica, 110*, 301-315.

Leksell, L. (1958). Echoencephalography. II. Midline echo from the pineal body as an index of pineal displacement. *Acta Chirurgica Scandinavica, 115*, 255-259.

Loeb, J. (1902). *Comparative physiology of the brain and comparative psychology*. New York: G.P. Putnam and Sons.

Luckett, W.H. (1913). Air in the ventricles in the brain following a fracture of the skull. *Journal of Nervous and Mental Disease, 40*, 326-328.

MacCabe, J.J. (1975). Glioblastoma. In P.J. Vinken & G.W. Bruyn (Eds.), *Handbook of clinical neurology*. Vol. 18. Amsterdam: North Holland Publishing Company.

MacCarty, C.S., & Taylor, W.F. (1979). Intracranial meningiomas: Experiences at the Mayo Clinic. *Neurol. Med. Chir. (Tokyo), 19*, 569-574.

Malmamud, N. (1967). Psychiatric disorder with intracranial tumors of the limbic system. *Archives of Neurology, 17*, 113-123.

Marshall, J. (1964). The natural history of transient ischemic cerebral vascular attacks. *Quarterly Journal of Medicine, 33*, 309-324.

Martin, J.B. (1969). Thalamic syndrome. In P.J. Vinken & G.W. Bruyn (Eds.), *Handbook of clinical neurology*. Vol. 2. New York: American Elsivier.

Martin, F., & Lemmen, L.J. (1952). Calcification in intracranial neoplasms. *American Journal of Pathology, 28*, 1107-1131.

Martin, J.B., Reichlin, S., & Brown, G.M. (1977). *Clinical neuroendocrinology*. Philadelphia: F.A. Davis.

Marttila, R.J., & Rinne, U.K. (1976). Dementia in Parkinson's disease. *Acta Neurologica Scandinavica, 54*, 431-441.

Matsuma, H., & Nakamura, S. (1977). Senile changes in the brain in the Japanese: Incidence of Alzheimer neurofibrillary and senile plaques. In R. Katzman, R.D. Terry, & K.L. Bick (Eds.), *Alzheimer's disease: Senile dementia and related disorders. Aging, Vol. 7* (pp. 287-297). New York: Raven Press.

Matthews, C.G., Cleeland, C.S., & Hopper, C.L. (1970). Neuropsychological patterns in multiple sclerosis. *Diseases of the Nervous System, 31*, 161-170.

McAllen, P.M., & Marshall, J. (1977). Cerebral vascular incidence after myocardial infarction. *Journal of Neurology, Neurosurgery, and Psychiatry, 40*, 951-955.

McGeer, P.L., & McGeer, E.G. (1981). Neurotransmitters in the aging brain. In A.M. Davison & R.H.S. Thompson (Eds.), *The molecular basis of neuropathology*. Pp. 631-648. London: Edward Arnold.

McLaurin, R.L., & Titchener, J.L. (1982). Posttraumatic syndrome. In J.R. Youmans (Ed.), *Neurological surgery*. Philadelphia: W.B. Saunders Company.

McNaught, A.B., & Callander, R. (1983). *Illustrated physiology*. Fourth Edition. New York: Churchill Livingstone.

Michaels, L.G., Bentson, J.R., & Winter, J. (1977). Computer tomography of cerebral venous angiomas. *Journal of Computer Assisted Tomography, 1*, 149-154.

Mickey, M.R., Ellison, G.W., & Meyers, L.W. (1984). An illness severity score for multiple sclerosis. *Neurology, 34*, 1343-1347.

Miller, A.K.H., Alston, R.L., & Corsellis, J.A.N. (1980). Variation with age in the volumes of grey and white matter in the cerebral hemispheres of man: Measurements with an image analyser. *Neuropathology and Applied Neurobiology, 6*, 119-132.

Mitchell, D.E., & Hume-Adams, J. (1973). Primary focal impact damage to the brain stem in blunt head injuries. Does it exist? *Lancet, 1*, 215-218.

Moniz, E. (1927). L'encephalographie arterielle, son importance dans la localization des tumeurs cerebralles. *Revieu Neurologie, 34*, 72-90.

Moniz, E. (1936). The first attempt at operative treatment of certain psychosis. *Ancephale, 31*, 1-29.

Moniz, E. (1937). Prefrontal leukotomy in treatment of mental disorders. *American Journal of Psychiatry, 93*, 1379-1385.

Moore, G.E. (1947). Fluorescin as an agent in the differentiation of normal and malignant tissues. *Science (NY), 106*, 130-131.

Moore, G.E. (1948). Use of radioactive Dye I diodofluorescein in the diagnosis and localization of brain tumors. *Science, 107*, 569-571.

Moreno, J.B., & Deland, F.H. (1971). Brain scanning in the diagnosis of astrocytomas of the brain. *Journal of Nuclear Medicine, 12*, 107-111.

Morris, L. (1960). Arteriographic demonstration of the vertebral artery with special reference to the percutaneous subclavian puncture. *British Journal of Radiology, 32*, 673-679.

Moruzzi, G., & Magoun, H.W. (1949). Brainstem reticular formation and activation of the EEG. *Electroencephalography and Clinical Neurophysiology, 1*, 455.

Mountjoy, C.Q., Roth, M., Evans, N.J.R., & Evans, H.M. (1983). Cortical neuronal counts in normal elderly controls and demented patients. *Neurobiology of Aging, 4*, 1-11.

Muller, W., Afra, D., & Schroder, R. (1977). Supratentorial recurrences of gliomas: Morphological studies in relation to time intervals with astrocytomas. *Acta Neurochirurgica, 37*, 75-91.

Munk, H. (1890). On the visual area of the cerebral cortex, and its relation to eye movements. Translated by F.W. Mott. *Brain, 13*, 45-67.

Naritomi, H., Meyer, J.S., Sakai, F., Yamaguchi, F., & Shaw, T. (1979). Effects of advancing age on regional cerebral blood flow. *Archives of Neurology, 36*, 410-416.

Netsky, M.G. (1960). Diseases of the nervous system in the aged patient arranged by common presenting symptoms. In W. Johnson (Ed.), *The older patient.* New York: Hoeber.

Nielsen, J.M. (1946). *Agnosia, apraxia, aphasia: Their value in cerebral localization.* New York: Hoeber.

O'Brien, M.D., & Mallett, B.L. (1970). Cerebral cortex perfusion rates in dementia. *Journal of Neurology, Neurosurgery and Psychiatry, 33*, 497-500.

Obrist, W.D. (1976). Problems of aging. In G.E. Chatrian & G.C. Lairy (Eds.), *Handbook of electro-encephalography and clinical neurophysiology. Vol. 6, Part A* (pp. 274-292). Amsterdam: Elsevier.

Obrist, W.D. (1977). Electroencephalography in aging and dementia. In R. Katzman, R.D. Terry, & K.L. Bick (Eds.), *Alzheimer's disease: Senile dementia and related disorders. Aging, Vol. 7* (pp. 227-232). New York: Raven Press.

Obrist, W.D., Thompson, H.K., Wang, H.S., & Wilkinson, W.E. (1975). Regional cerebral blood flow estimated by xenon inhalation. *Stroke, 6*, 245-256.

Ojemann, G.A., & Ward, A.A. (1982). Abnormal movement disorders. In J.R. Youmans (Ed.), *Neurological surgery* (pp. 3821-3857). Philadelphia: W.B. Saunders Company.

Ommaya, A.K. (1972). Head injury in the adult. In H.F. Conn (Ed.), *Current therapy.* Philadelphia: W.B. Saunders Company.

Ommaya, A.K., Fass, F., & Yarnell, P. (1968). Whiplash injury and brain damage. *Journal of the American Medical Association, 204*, 285-289.

Ommaya, A.K., Grubb, R.L., & Naumann, R.A. (1970). Coup and contrecoup cerebral contusions. An experimental analysis. *Neurology, 20*, 388-389.

Onoyama, Y., Abe, M., Sakamoto, T., Nishidai, T., & Suyama, S. (1976). Radiation therapy in treatment of glioblastoma. *American Journal of Roentgenology, 126*, 481-492.

Oppenheimer, D.R. (1968). Microscopic lesions in the brain following head injury. *Journal of Neurology, Neurosurgery, and Psychiatry, 31*, 299-306.

Overton, M.C., Haynie, T.P., Otte, W.K., & Coe, J.E. (1965). The vertex view in brain scanning. *Journal of Nuclear Medicine, 6*, 705-710.

Pampiglione, G. (1964). Prodromal phase of measles. Some neurophysiological studies. *British Journal of Medicine, 2*, 1296-1300.

Pansky, B., & Allen, D.J. (1980). *Review of neuroscience.* New York: Macmillan Publishing Co., Inc.

Parsons, O.A., Stewart, K.D., & Arenberg, D. (1957). Impairment of abstracting ability in multiple sclerosis. *Journal of Nervous and Mental Disease, 125*, 221-225.

Penfield, W., & Roberts, L. (1959). *Speech and brain mechanisms.* Princeton, N.J.: Princeton University Press.

Peress, N.S., Kane, W.C., & Aronson, S.M. (1973). Central nervous system findings in a tenth decade autopsy population. *Progress in Brain Research, 40*, 473-483.

Perry, E.K., Blessed, G., Tomlinson, B.E. et al. (1981). Neurochemical activities in human temporal lobe related to aging and Alzheimer-type changes. *Neurobiology of Aging, 2*, 251-256.

Peyser, J.M., Edwards, K.R., Poser, D.M., & Filskov, S.D. (1980). Cognitive functions in patients with multiple sclerosis. *Archives of Neurology, 37*, 577-579.

Phelps, M.E., Hoffman, R., Mullani, G.S., & Ter-Pogossian, M.M. (1975). Application of annihilation coincidence detection to transaxial reconstruction tomography. *Journal of Nuclear Medicine, 16*, 210-224.

Phelps, M.E., Mazziotta, J.C., Engel, J., & Kuhl, D.E. (1981). Metabolic response of the brain to visual and auditory stimulation and deprivation. *Journal of Cerebral Blood Flow Metabolism, 1*, Supplement 1, S467.

Plum, F., & Van Uitert, R. (1978). Nonendocrine diseases and disorders of the hypothalamus. In S. Reichlin, R.J. Baldessarini, & J.B. Martin. *The hypothalamus*. New York: Raven Press.

Pollock, M., & Hornabrook, R.W. (1966). The prevalence, natural history and dementia of Parkinson's disease. *Brain, 89*, 429-448.

Poser, C.M., Paty, D.W., Scheinberg, L., McDonald, W.I., Davis, F.A., Ebers, G.C., Johnson, K.P., Sibley, W.A., Silberberg, D.H., & Tourtellotte, W.W. (1983). New diagnostic criteria for multiple sclerosis: Guidelines for research protocols. *Annals of Neurology, 13*, 227-231.

Poser, C.M., Paty, D.W., Scheinberg, L., McDonald, W.I., & Ebers, G.C. (Eds.), *The diagnosis of multiple sclerosis*. New York: Thieme-Stratton (in press).

Raine, C.S., & Stone, S.H. (1977). Animal model for multiple sclerosis. Chronic experimental allergic encephalomyelitis in inbred guinea pigs. *New York State Journal of Medicine, 77*, 1693-1696.

Rand, R.W., Dirks, D.D., Morgan, D.E., & Bentson, J.R. (1982). Acoustic neuromas. In J.R. Youmans (Ed.), *Neurological surgery*. Philadelphia: W.B. Saunders Co.

Rasmussen, T. (1969). Surgical therapy of post-traumatic epilepsy. In A.E. Walker, W.F. Caveness, & M. Critchley (Eds.), *The late effects of head injury*. Springfield: Charles C. Thomas.

Rasmussen, T. (1975). Surgery of epilepsy associated with brain tumors. *Advances in Neurology, 8*, 227-239.

Reed, H.B.C., & Reitan, R.M. (1963). changes in psychological test performances associated with the normal aging process. *Journal of Gerontology, 18*, 271-274.

Reilly, P.L., Graham, D.I., Hume-Adams, J., & Jennett, B. (1975). Patients with head injury who talk and die. *Lancet, 2*, 375-381.

Reitan, R.M. (1953). Intellectual functions in myxedema. *AMA Archives of Neurology and Psychiatry, 69*, 436-449.

Reitan, R.M. (1960). The significance of dysphasia for intelligence and adaptive abilities. *Journal of Psychology, 50*, 355-376.

Reitan, R.M. (1964). Psychological deficits resulting from cerebral lesions in man. In J.M. Warren and K.A. Akert (Eds.), *The frontal granular cortex and behavior*. New York: McGraw-Hill.

Reitan, R.M. (1967). Psychological changes associated with cerebral damage. *Mayo Clinic Proceedings, 42*, 653-673.

Reitan, R.M. (1976). Psychological testing of epileptic patients. In P.J. Vinken & G.W. Bruyn (Eds.), *Handbook of clinical neurology: The epilepsies*. Vols. IX and X. Amsterdam: North Holland Publishing Company.

Reitan, R.M. (1984). *Aphasia and sensory-perceptual deficits in adults*. Tucson, Arizona: Neuropsychology Press.

Reitan, R.M., & Boll, T.J. (1971). Intellectual and cognitive functions in Parkinson's disease. *Journal of Consulting and Clinical Psychology, 37*, 364-369.

Reitan, R.M., Reed, J.C., & Dyken, M.L. (1971). Cognitive, psychomotor, and motor correlates of multiple sclerosis. *Journal of Nervous and Mental Disease, 153*, 218-224.

Reitan, R.M., & Shipley, R.E. (1963). The relationship of serum cholesterol changes to psychological abilities. *Journal of Gerontology, 18*, 350-356.

Reitan, R.M., & Wolfson, D. (1985). *The Halstead-Reitan neuropsychological test battery: Theory and clinical interpretation.* Tucson, Arizona: Neuropsychology Press.

Reitan, R.M., & Wolfson, D. (in press). The Halstead-Reitan Neuropsychological Test Battery and Aging. *The Clinical Gerontologist.*

Remond, A. (Ed.), (1974). *Handbook of electroencephalography and clinical neurophysiology.* Amsterdam: Elsevier Scientific Publishing Company.

Riese, W. (1959). *A history of neurology.* New York: MD Publications.

Rob, C.G., & Wheeler, E.B. (1957). Thrombosis of internal carotid artery treated by arterial surgery. *British Medical Journal, 2*, 264-266.

Rose, F.C. (1984). Progress in aphasiology. In *Advances in Neurology*, Volume 42. New York: Raven Press.

Ross, A.T., & Reitan, R.M. (1955). Intellectual and affective functions in multiple sclerosis. *Archives of Neurology and Psychiatry, 73*, 663-677.

Rossor, M.N., Garrett, N.J., Johnson, A.L., et al. (1982). A post-mortem study of the cholinergic and GABA systems in senile dementia. *Brain, 105*, 313-330.

Russell, D.S., & Rubenstein, L.J. (1977). *Pathology of tumours of the nervous system.* 4th Edition. Baltimore: Williams & Wilkins Co.

Russell, W.R., & Whitty, C.W.M. (1952). Studies in traumatic epilepsy: Factors influencing the incidence of epilepsy after brain wounds. *Journal of Neurology, Neurosurgery, and Psychiatry, 15*, 93-98.

Rylander, G. (1947). Discussion of W.C. Halstead's paper: Specialization of behavioral functions and the frontal lobes. *Association for Research in Nervous and Mental Diseases, 27*, 64.

Sang, U.H., & Wilson, C.B. (1975). Surgical treatment of intracranial vascular malformations. *Western Journal of Medicine, 123*, 175-183.

Sarno, N.T. (Ed.). (1981). *Acquired aphasia.* New York: Academic Press.

Schaie, K.W. (1977). Quasi-experimental research designs in the psychology of aging. In J.E. Birren & K.W. Schaie (Eds.), *Handbook of the psychology of aging* (pp. 39-58). New York: Van Nostrand.

Schechter, M.M. (1982a). Cerebral angiography. In J.R. Youmans (Ed.), *Neurological surgery.* Philadelphia: W.B. Saunders Company.

Schechter, M.M. (1982b). Radiology of the skull. In J.R. Youmans (Ed.), *Neurological surgery.* Philadelphia: W.B. Saunders Company.

Scheibel, A.B. (1977). Structural aspects of the aging brain: Spine systems and the dendritic arbor. In R. Katzman, R.D. Terry, & K.L. Bick (Eds.), *Alzheimer's disease: Senile dementia and related disorders. Aging, Vol. 7* (pp. 353-373). New York: Raven Press.

Schobinger, R.A., & Ruzika, F.F. (Eds.). (1964). *Vascular roentgenology.* New York: MacMillian.

Schumacher, G.A., Beebe, G.W., Kibler, R.F., Kurland, L.T., Kurtzke, J.F., McDowell, F., Nagler, B., Sibley, W.A., Tourtellotte, W.W., & Willmon, T.L. (1965). Problems of experimental trials of therapy in multiple sclerosis. *Annals of NY Academy of Science, 122*, 552-568.

Schwab, R.S., & England, A.C. (1968-1969). Parkinson's syndromes due to various specific causes. In P.J. Vinken & G.W. Bruyn (Eds.), *Handbook of clinical neurology.* Volume 6. Diseases of the basal ganglia (pp. 227-247). Amsterdam: North Holland Publishing Company.

Schwartz, N., Creasy, H., Grady, C.L., et al. (1985). CT analysis of brain morphometrics in 30 healthy men, age 21-81 years. Annals of Neurology, in press. Cited in H. Creasy & S.I. Rapoport (1985). The aging human brain. *Annals of Neurology, 17*, 2-10.

Selby, G. (1968-1969). Parkinson's disease. In P.J. Vinken & G.W. Bruyn (Eds.), *Handbook of clinical neurology*. Volume 6. Diseases of the basal ganglia. Amsterdam: North Holland Publishing Company.

Selters, W.A, & Brackmann, D. (1977). Acoustic tumor detection with brainstem electric response and audiometry. *Archives of Otolaryngology, 103*, 181-187.

Sharbrough, F.W., & Sundt, Jr., T.M. (1982). Electroencephalography. In J.R. Youmans (Ed.), *Neurological surgery*. Pp. 195-230. Philadelphia: W.B. Saunders Company.

Shefer, V.F. (1973). Absolute number of neurons and thickness of cerebral cortex during aging, senile and vascular dementia and Pick's and Alzheimer's disease. *Neurosci. Behav. Physiol., 6*, 319-324.

Silverstein, A., Lehrer, G.M., & Mones, R. (1960). Relation of certain diagnostic features of carotid occlusion to collateral circulation. *Neurology, 10*, 409-417.

Sim, M., & Sussman, I. (1962). Alzheimer's disease: Its natural history and differential diagnosis. *Journal of Nervous and Mental Disease, 135*, 489-499.

Simpson, D. (1957). The recurrence of intracranial meningiomas after surgical treatment. *Journal of Neurology, Neurosurgery, and Psychiatry, 20*, 22-39.

Singer, J.R. (1959). Blood flow rates by NMR measurements. *Science, 130*, 1652-1653.

Smith, W.T., Turner, E., & Sim, M.R. (1966). Cerebral biopsy in the investigation of presenile dementia. II. Pathological aspects. *British Journal of Psychiatry, 112*, 127-133.

Sourander, P., & Walinder, J. (1977). Hereditary multi-infarct dementia. Morphological and clinical studies of a new disease. *Acta Neuropathologica (Berlin), 39*, 247-254.

Staples, D., & Lincoln, N.B. (1979). Intellectual impairment in multiple sclerosis and its relation to functional abilities. *Rheumatology and Rehabilitation, 18*, 153-160.

Stein, B.M. (1982). Tumors of the pineal region. In J.R. Youmans (Ed.), *Neurological surgery*. Philadelphia: W.B. Saunders Co.

Steinhoff, H., Lanksch, W., Kazner, E., Grumme, T., Meese, W., Lange, S., Aulich, A., Schinder, E., & Winde, S. (1977). Computed tomography in the diagnosis and differential diagnosis of glioblastomas. *Neuroradiology, 14*, 193-200.

Stubens, W.E. (1954). Intracranial arterial aneurysms. *Australian Annals of Medicine, 3*, 214-218.

Stopford, J.S.B. (1916). The arteries of the pons and medulla oblongata. *Journal of Anatomy, 50*, 131-164.

Strich, S.J. (1970). Lesions in the cerebral hemispheres after blunt head injury. *Journal of Clinical Pathology, 23*, (Supplement 4), 154-165.

Sutton, D. (1950). Anomalous carotid basilar anastomosis. *British Journal of Radiology, 23*, 617-619.

Sutton, D. (1962). *Arteriography*. London: E.S. Livingston, Ltd.

Talbert, O.R. (1982). General methods of clinical examination. In J.R. Youmans (Ed.), *Neurological surgery*. Philadelphia: W.B. Saunders Co.

Taveras, J.M., & Wood, E.H. (1964). *Diagnostic neuroradiology*. Baltimore, MD: Williams and Wilkins Company.

Terry, R. (1977). In M. Roth (Ed.), *Workshop conference on Alzheimer's disease, senile dementia and related disorders*. Bethesda, MD: National Institutes of Mental Health.

Tomlinson, B.E. (1970). Brain stem lesions after head injury. *Journal of Clinical Pathology, 23,* (Supplement 4), 154-165.

Tomlinson, B.E., Blessed, G., & Roth, M. (1968). Observations on the brains of non-demented old people. *Journal of Neurological Science, 7,* 331-356.

Tomlinson, B.E., Blessed, G., & Roth, M. (1970). Observations of brains of demented old people. *Journal of Neurological Sciences, 11,* 205-243.

Tomlinson, B.E., & Henderson, G. (1976). Some quantitative cerebral findings in normal and demented old people. In R. Terry & S. Gershon (Eds.), *Neurobiology of aging.* New York: Raven Press.

Toole, J.F. (1984). *Cerebral vascular disorders.* New York: Raven Press.

Toole, J.F., Yuson, C.P., Janeway, R., Johnston, F., Davis, C., Cordell, A.R., & Howard, G. (1978). Transient ischemic attacks: A prospective study of 225 patients. *Neurology, 28,* 746-753.

Tooth, H.H. (1912). Some observations on the growth and survival of intracranial tumors. *Brain, 35,* 61-108.

Tourtellotte, W.W. (1970). Multiple sclerosis and cerebral spinal fluid. In P.J. Vinken & G.W. Bruyn (Eds.), *Handbook of clinical neurology.* Vol. 9. Amsterdam: Elsevier-North Holland Publishing Company.

Tourtellotte, W.W., & Shorr, R.J. (1982). Cerebral spinal fluid. In J.R. Youmans (Ed.), *Neurological surgery.* Philadelphia: W.B. Saunders Company.

Trelles, J.O. (1978). Parasitic diseases in tropical neurology. In P.J. Vinken & G.W. Bruyn (Eds.), *Handbook of clinical neurology. Part III, Vol. 35.* Amsterdam: Elsevier-North Holland Publishing Company.

Twining, E.W. (1939). Radiology of the third and fourth ventricles. *British Journal of Radiology, 12,* 385-418.

U.S. Department of Health, Education, and Welfare: Facts of life and death. (1974). Publication Number (HRS) 74-1222, *National Center for Health Statistics,* Rockville, MD.

Veterans Administration Cooperative Study Group on Antihypertensive Agents (1970). Effects of treatment on morbidity of hypertension: Results in patients with diastolic blood pressure averaging 90-115 mm Hg. *Journal of the American Medical Association, 213,* 1143-1152.

Victor, M., Adams, R.D., & Collins, G.H. (1971). *The Wernicke-Korsakoff syndrome: A clinical and pathological study of 245 patients, 82 with postmortem examinations.* Philadelphia: Davis.

Victor, M., & Banker, B.Q. (1977). Alcohol and dementia. In R. Katzman, R.D. Terry, & K.L. Bick (Eds.), *Alzheimer's disease: Senile dementia and related disorders. Aging, Vol. 7* (pp. 149-170). New York: Raven Press.

Virchow, R. (1863-1865). *Die Krankhaften Geschwuelste.* Berlin: Hirschwald.

von Monakow, C. (1905). *Gehirnpathologie.* Vienna: A. Holder.

Vonofakos, D., Marcu, H., & Hacker, H. (1979). Oligodendrogliomas: CT patterns with emphasis on features indicating malignancy. *Journal of Computer-Assisted Tomography, 3,* 783-788.

Wagner, H.N. (1968). *Principles of nuclear medicine.* Philadelphia: W.B. Saunders Company.

Wang, H.S., & Busse, E.W. (1975). Correlates of regional cerebral blood flow in elderly community residents. In A.M. Harper, W.B. Jennett, J.D. Miller, & J.O. Rowan (Eds.), *Blood flow and metabolism in the brain.* London: Churchill-Livingstone.

Webber, M.M. (1965). Normal brain scanning. *American Journal of Roentgenology, 94,* 815-818.

Wechsler, D. (1955). *Manual for the Wechsler Adult Intelligence Scale.* New York: The Psychological Corporation.

Weigl, E. (1968). On the problem of cortical syndromes. In M.L. Simmel (Ed.), *In the search of mind: Essays in memory of Kurt Goldstein*. New York: Springer.

Westrum, L.E., White, L.E., & Ward, A.A. (1964). Morphology of the experimental epileptic focus. *Journal of Neurosurgery, 21*, 1033-1046.

White, J.C., Liu, C.T., & Mixter, W.J. (1948). Focal epilepsy: A statistical study of its causes and the results of surgical treatment. I: Epilepsy secondary to intracranial tumors. *New England Journal of Medicine, 238*, 891-899.

Wilkinson, R.H., & Goodrich, J.K. (1982). Radionuclide imaging studies. In J.R. Youmans (Ed.), *Neurological surgery*. Philadelphia: W.B. Saunders Company.

Wood, E.H. (1964). Angiographic identification of the ruptured lesion in patients with multiple cerebral aneurysms. *Journal of Neurosurgery, 21*, 182-198.

Wrenn, F.R., Good, M.L., & Handler, P. (1951). The use of positron emiting radioisotopes for the localization of brain tumors. *Science (NY), 113*, 525-527.

Yenermen, M.H., Bowerman, C.L., Haymaker, W. (1958). Colloid cysts of the third ventricle: A clinical study of 54 cases in the light of previous publications. *Acta Neuroveg., 17*, 211-277.

Young, I.R., Hall, A.S., Pallis, C.A., et al. (1981). NMR imaging of the brain in multiple sclerosis. *Lancet, 2*, 1063-1066.

Ziegler, D.K., & Hassanein, R.S. (1973). Prognosis in patients with transient ischemic attacks. *Stroke, 4*, 666-673.

Zingesser, L.H., & Schechter, M.M. (1982). Encephalography. In J.R. Youmans (Ed.), *Neurological surgery*. Philadelphia: W.B. Saunders Company.

Zuelch, K.H. (1965). *Brain tumors: Their biology and pathology*. 2nd Ed. New York: Springer.

Zuelch, K.H., & Mennel, H.D. (1975). The question of malignancy in meningiomas. *Acta Neurochirurgica, 31*, 275-276.

# Subject Index

# SUBJECT INDEX

CKKD